Infectious Disease Emergencies

Editors

STEPHEN Y. LIANG
RACHEL L. CHIN

EMERGENCY MEDICINE CLINICS OF NORTH AMERICA

www.emed.theclinics.com

Consulting Editor
AMAL MATTU

November 2018 • Volume 36 • Number 4

ELSEVIER

1600 John F. Kennedy Boulevard • Suite 1800 • Philadelphia, Pennsylvania, 19103-2899

http://www.theclinics.com

EMERGENCY MEDICINE CLINICS OF NORTH AMERICA Volume 36, Number 4
November 2018 ISSN 0733-8627, ISBN-13: 978-0-323-64322-1

Editor: Colleen Dietzler
Developmental Editor: Casey Potter

Emergency Medicine Clinics of North America (ISSN 0733-8627) is published quarterly by Elsevier Inc., 360 Park Avenue South, New York, NY, 10010-1710. Months of issue are February, May, August, and November. Business and Editorial Offices: 1600 John F. Kennedy Boulevard, Suite 1800, Philadelphia, PA 19103-2899. Customer Service Office: 6277 Sea Harbor Drive, Orlando, FL 32887-4800. Periodicals postage paid at New York, NY, and additional mailing offices. Subscription prices are $100.00 per year (US students), $336.00 per year (US individuals), $644.00 per year (US institutions), $220.00 per year (international students), $455.00 per year (international individuals), $791.00 per year (international institutions), $220.00 per year (Canadian students), $405.00 per year (Canadian individuals), and $791.00 per year (Canadian institutions). International air speed delivery is included in all *Clinics'* subscription prices. All prices are subject to change without notice. **POSTMASTER:** Send address changes to *Emergency Medicine Clinics of North America*, Elsevier Periodicals Customer Service, 11830 Westline Industrial Drive, St. Louis, MO 63146. Customer Service (orders, claims, online, change of address): Elsevier Periodicals **Customer Service, 11830 Westline Industrial Drive, St. Louis, MO 63146. Tel: 1-800-654-2452 (U.S. and Canada); 314-453-7041 (outside U.S. and Canada). Fax: 314-453-5170. E-mail: journalscustomerservice-usa@elsevier.com (for print support);** journalsonlinesupport-usa@elsevier.com (for online support).

Reprints. For copies of 100 or more of articles in this publication, please contact the Commercial Reprints Department, Elsevier Inc., 360 Park Avenue South, New York, NY 10010-1710. Tel.: 212-633-3874; Fax: 212-633-3820; E-mail: reprints@elsevier.com.

Emergency Medicine Clinics of North America is covered in *MEDLINE/PubMed (Index Medicus), Current Contents/Clinical Medicine, EMBASE/Excerpta Medica, BIOSIS, SciSearch, CINAHL, ISI/BIOMED,* and *Research Alert.*

Contributors

CONSULTING EDITOR

AMAL MATTU, MD
Professor and Vice Chair of Education, Department of Emergency Medicine, University of Maryland School of Medicine, Baltimore, Maryland

EDITORS

STEPHEN Y. LIANG, MD, MPHS
Assistant Professor of Medicine, Divisions of Emergency Medicine and Infectious Diseases, Washington University School of Medicine in St. Louis, St. Louis, Missouri

RACHEL L. CHIN, MD
Professor, Department of Emergency Medicine, Zuckerberg San Francisco General Hospital, University of California, San Francisco School of Medicine, San Francisco, California

AUTHORS

AMESH A. ADALJA, MD, FACEP, FACP, FIDSA
Senior Scholar, Johns Hopkins Center for Health Security, Baltimore, Maryland

AMELIA BREYRE, MD
Department of Emergency Medicine, Highland Hospital, Oakland, California

LAUREN CANTWELL, MD
Emergency Medicine Residency, Virginia Tech Carilion School of Medicine, Roanoke, Virginia

WAN-TSU W. CHANG, MD
Assistant Professor, Department of Emergency Medicine, University of Maryland School of Medicine, Baltimore, Maryland

JOSEPHINE FOX, MPH, RN, CIC
Infection Prevention, Barnes-Jewish Hospital, St Louis, Missouri

BRADLEY W. FRAZEE, MD
Attending Physician, Department of Emergency Medicine, Alameda Health System, Highland Hospital, Oakland, California

SUELIN M. HILBERT, MD
Assistant Professor, Department of Emergency Medicine, Washington University in St. Louis, St Louis, Missouri

RUPAL JAIN, MD
Resident, Department of Emergency Medicine, University of Maryland Medical Center, Baltimore, Maryland

DANIEL C. KOLINSKY, MD
Staff Physician, Department of Emergency Medicine, Southeast Louisiana Veterans
Health Care System, New Orleans, Louisiana

ALEX KOYFMAN, MD
Department of Emergency Medicine, The University of Texas Southwestern Medical
Center, Dallas, Texas

STEPHEN Y. LIANG, MD, MPHS
Assistant Professor of Medicine, Divisions of Emergency Medicine and Infectious
Diseases, Washington University School of Medicine in St. Louis, St Louis, Missouri

BRIT LONG, MD
Department of Emergency Medicine, San Antonio Military Medical Center, Fort Sam
Houston, Texas

LARISSA MAY, MD, MSPH
Professor, Director of Emergency Department Antibiotic Stewardship, University of
California, Davis, Sacramento, California

NICOLE MESSENGER, MD
Resident Physician, Division of Emergency Medicine, Washington University School of
Medicine in St. Louis, St Louis, Missouri

SIAMAK MOAYEDI, MD
Assistant Professor, Department of Emergency Medicine, University of Maryland School
of Medicine, Baltimore, Maryland

JACK PERKINS, MD
Associate Professor, Department of Emergency Medicine, Virginia Tech Carilion School
of Medicine, Roanoke, Virginia

MICHAEL PULIA, MD, MS
Assistant Professor, Director of Emergency Department Antibiotic Stewardship,
BerbeeWalsh Department of Emergency Medicine, University of Wisconsin-Madison
School of Medicine and Public Health, Madison, Wisconsin

ROBERT REDWOOD, MD, MPH
Clinical Adjunct Assistant Professor, Department of Family Medicine, University of
Wisconsin-Madison School of Medicine and Public Health, Madison, Wisconsin

HILARY E.L. RENO, MD, PhD
Assistant Professor, Division of Infectious Disease, Washington University in St. Louis,
St Louis, Missouri

ASHLEY C. RIDER, MD
Attending Physician, Department of Emergency Physician, Alameda Health
System–Highland Hospital, Oakland, California; Clinical Professor of Emergency
Medicine, University of California, San Francisco, San Francisco, California

MADISON RIETHMAN, MPH, CPH
Communicable Disease, Clark County Public Health, Center for Community Health,
Vancouver, Washington

MERCEDES TORRES, MD
Clinical Assistant Professor, Department of Emergency Medicine, University of Maryland
School of Medicine, Baltimore, Maryland

ELAINE YANG, MD
Resident Physician, Alameda Health System, Highland Hospital, Oakland, California

DIANA ZHONG, MD
Academic Hospitalist Fellow, Department of Medicine, University of Washington, Seattle, Washington

Contents

Infective endocarditis (IE) is an uncommon infection of cardiac valves associated with bacteremia. IE increasingly affects elderly patients with chronic disease and artificial cardiac devices. The presentation, however, remains subtle and varied, with nonspecific symptoms ranging from those resembling a mild viral infection to septic shock and multi-organ failure. IE carries potential to cause significant morbidity and mortality through its impact on cardiac function and from embolic complications. Blood cultures before administration of antibiotics and obtaining prompt echocardiography are key diagnostic steps, followed by proper selection of empiric antibiotics. Early collaboration with infectious disease, cardiology, and cardiothoracic surgery specialists may be needed.

Community-acquired pneumonia is one of the most common infections seen in emergency department patients. There is a wide spectrum of disease severity, and viral pathogens are common. After a careful history and physical examination, chest radiographs may be the only diagnostic test required. The first step in management is risk stratification, using a validated clinical decision rule and serum lactate, followed by early antibiotics and fluid resuscitation when indicated. Antibiotics should be selected with attention to risk factors for multidrug-resistant respiratory pathogens. Broad use of pneumococcal vaccine in adults and children can prevent severe community-acquired pneumonia.

Urinary tract infection (UTI) is a common infection seen in the emergency department. The spectrum of UTI includes simple versus complicated infection and lower versus upper UTI. No one history or examination finding is definitive for diagnosis. Testing often includes urinalysis and/or urine dipstick, and several pitfalls may occur in interpretation. Urine cultures should be obtained in complicated or upper UTIs but not simple and lower tract UTIs, unless a patient is pregnant. Imaging often is not required. Most patients with simple cystitis and pyelonephritis are treated as outpatients. A variety of potentially dangerous conditions may mimic UTI and pyelonephritis.

Central nervous system (CNS) infections require early recognition and aggressive management to improve patient survival and prevent long-term neurologic sequelae. Although early detection and treatment are important in many infectious syndromes, CNS infections pose unique diagnostic and therapeutic challenges. The nonspecific signs and symptoms at presentation, lack of characteristic infectious changes in laboratory and imaging diagnostics, and closed anatomic and immunologically sequestered space each present challenges to the emergency physician. This article proposes an approach to the clinical evaluation of patients with suspected CNS infection and highlights methods of diagnosis, treatment, and complications associated with CNS infections.

This article covers the diagnosis and treatment of skin and soft tissue infections commonly encountered in the emergency department: impetigo, cutaneous abscesses, purulent cellulitis, nonpurulent cellulitis, and necrotizing skin and soft tissue infections. Most purulent infections in the United States are caused by methicillin-resistant *Staphylococcus aureus*. For abscesses, the authors emphasize the importance of incision and drainage. Nonpurulent infections are usually caused by streptococcal species, and initial empiric antibiotics need not cover methicillin-resistant *Staphylococcus aureus*. For uncommon but potentially lethal necrotizing skin and soft tissue infections, the challenge is rapid diagnosis in the emergency department and prompt surgical exploration and debridement.

Bone and joint infections are potentially limb-threatening or even life-threatening diseases. Emergency physicians must consider infection when evaluating musculoskeletal complaints, as misdiagnosis can have significant consequences. Patients with bone and joint infections can have heterogeneous presentations with nonspecific signs and symptoms. *Staphylococcus aureus* is the most commonly implicated microorganism. Although diagnosis may be suggested by physical examination, laboratory testing, and imaging, tissue sampling for Gram stain and microbiologic culture is preferable, as pathogen identification and susceptibility testing help optimize long-term antibiotic therapy. A combination of medical and surgical interventions is often necessary to effectively manage these challenging infections.

Sexually transmitted infections (STIs) are very common infections in the United States. Most patients with STIs are evaluated and treated in primary care settings; however, many also present to the emergency department (ED) for initial care. Management of STIs in the ED includes appropriate testing and treatment per the **Centers for Disease Control and Prevention Sexually Transmitted Diseases Treatment Guidelines.** Although most patients with STIs are asymptomatic or may only exhibit mild symptoms, serious complications from untreated infection are possible. Pregnant women with STIs are particularly vulnerable to serious complications; therefore, empiric ED treatment combined with close follow-up care and referral to obstetrics are paramount.

Over the past 30 years, significant advances have transformed the landscape of human immunodeficiency virus (HIV) care in the emergency department. Diagnosis and management of HIV has improved, resulting in a decline in the incidence of AIDS-defining infections. Advances in pharmacology have led to fewer serious medication toxicities and more tolerable regimens. Emergency providers have played an increasingly important role in HIV screening and diagnosis of acute infection. Provision of postexposure prophylaxis is expanding from a focus on occupational exposure to include all high-risk cases.

Oncology patients are a unique patient population in the emergency department (ED). Malignancy and associated surgical, chemotherapeutic, or radiation therapies put them at an increased risk for infection. The most ominous development is neutropenic fever, which happens often and may not present with signs or symptoms other than fever. A broad differential diagnosis is essential when considering infectious disease pathology in both neutropenic and nonneutropenic oncology patients in the ED.

The emergency department (ED) is an increasingly important site of care for patients who have undergone solid organ transplantation or hematopoietic cell transplantation. It is paramount for emergency physicians to recognize infections early on, obtain appropriate diagnostic testing, initiate empirical antimicrobial therapy, and consider specialty consultation and inpatient admission when caring for these patients. This article provides emergency physicians with an approach to the assessment of transplant patients' underlying risk for infection, formulation of a broad differential diagnosis, and initial management of transplant infectious disease emergencies in the ED.

This article discusses the challenges faced by the emergency physician with recognizing and treating category. Biothreat agents and emerging infectious disease are summarized and reviewed.

EMERGENCY MEDICINE
CLINICS OF NORTH AMERICA

THE CLINICS ARE NOW AVAILABLE ONLINE!
Access your subscription at:
www.theclinics.com

PROGRAM OBJECTIVE

The goal of *Emergency Medicine Clinics of North America* is to keep practicing emergency medicine physicians and emergency medicine residents up to date with current clinical practice in emergency medicine by providing timely articles reviewing the state of the art in patient care.

LEARNING OBJECTIVES

Upon completion of this activity, participants will be able to:

1. Review clinical evaluation of patients with suspected central nervous system infection; methods of diagnosis, treatment, and complications associated with CNS infections.
2. Recognize strategies and key priorities in emergency department infection prevention.
3. Discuss emergency department management of patients with sexually transmitted Infections.

ACCREDITATION

The Elsevier Office of Continuing Medical Education (EOCME) is accredited by the Accreditation Council for Continuing Medical Education (ACCME) to provide continuing medical education for physicians.

The EOCME designates this enduring material for a maximum of 15 *AMA PRA Category 1 Credit*(s)™. Physicians should claim only the credit commensurate with the extent of their participation in the activity.

All other healthcare professionals requesting continuing education credit for this enduring material will be issued a certificate of participation.

DISCLOSURE OF CONFLICTS OF INTEREST

The EOCME assesses conflict of interest with its instructors, faculty, planners, and other individuals who are in a position to control the content of CME activities. All relevant conflicts of interest that are identified are thoroughly vetted by EOCME for fair balance, scientific objectivity, and patient care recommendations. EOCME is committed to providing its learners with CME activities that promote improvements or quality in healthcare and not a specific proprietary business or a commercial interest.

The planning committee, staff, authors and editors listed below have identified no financial relationships or relationships to products or devices they or their spouse/life partner have with commercial interest related to the content of this CME activity:

Amesh A. Adalja, MD, FACEP, FACP, FIDSA; Amelia Breyre, MD; Lauren Cantwell, MD; Wan-Tsu W. Chang, MD; Rachel Chin, MD; Josephine Fox, MPH, RN; Bradley Frazee, MD; SueLin M. Hilbert, MD; Rupal Jain, MD; Alison Kemp; Daniel C. Kolinsky, MD; Alex Koyfman, MD; Stephen Y. Liang, MD, MPHS; Brit Long, MD; Amal Mattu, MD; Amal Mattu; Nicole Messenger, MD; Siamak Moayedi, MD; Jack Perkins, MD; Katie Pfaff; Robert Redwood, MD, MPH; Hilary E. L. Reno, MD, PhD; Ashley Rider, MD; Madison Riethman, MPH, CPH; Mercedes Torres, MD; Vignesh Viswanathan; Elaine Yang, MD; Diana Zhong, MD.

The planning committee, staff, authors and editors listed below have identified financial relationships or relationships to products or devices they or their spouse/life partner have with commercial interest related to the content of this CME activity:

Larissa May, MD, MSPH: is a consultant/advisor for and receives research support from Cepheid and F. Hoffmann-La Roche Ltd; is a consultant/advisor for BioFire Diagnostics

Michael Pulia, MD, MS: is a consultant/advisor for Melinta Therapeutics, Inc. and Thermo Fisher Scientific; receives research support from F. Hoffmann-La Roche Ltd; is a consultant/advisor and receives research support from Cepheid.

UNAPPROVED/OFF-LABEL USE DISCLOSURE

The EOCME requires CME faculty to disclose to the participants:

1. When products or procedures being discussed are off-label, unlabelled, experimental, and/or investigational (not US Food and Drug Administration [FDA] approved); and
2. Any limitations on the information presented, such as data that are preliminary or that represent ongoing research, interim analyses, and/or unsupported opinions. Faculty may discuss information about pharmaceutical agents that is outside of FDA-approved labelling. This information is intended solely for CME and is not intended to promote off-label use of these medications. If you have any questions, contact the medical affairs department of the manufacturer for the most recent prescribing information.

TO ENROLL

To enroll in the *Emergency Medicine Clinics* Continuing Medical Education program, call customer service at 1-800-654-2452 or sign up online at http://www.theclinics.com/home/cme. The CME program is available to subscribers for an additional annual fee of $235 USD.

METHOD OF PARTICIPATION

In order to claim credit, participants must complete the following:

1. Complete enrolment as indicated above.
2. Read the activity.
3. Complete the CME Test and Evaluation. Participants must achieve a score of 70% on the test. All CME Tests and Evaluations must be completed online.

CME INQUIRIES/SPECIAL NEEDS

For all CME inquiries or special needs, please contact elsevierCME@elsevier.com.

Foreword
Infectious Disease Emergencies

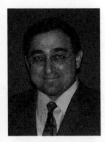

Amal Mattu, MD
Consulting Editor

For thousands of years, physicians have been battling infections. Infectious disease is likely responsible for more human deaths in history than any other cause, medical or nonmedical. In fact, it is said that mosquito-borne infections alone are responsible for more deaths than all of the wars in human history *combined*. For thousands of years, plagues and epidemics caused by infections have affected national leaders, armies, cultures, societies, and even world history. Some of the greatest physicians of recent centuries, including Lister, Jenner, Pasteur, Koch, Reed, and Ehrlich, made their mark via their discoveries that helped fight infections. It is easily argued that the very profession of medicine was born from the fight against infectious disease.[1]

In more recent decades with advances in the fight against infections, the most common cause of death worldwide has transitioned to ischemic heart disease and stroke. Yet, the World Health Organization still lists three of the top 10 causes of death worldwide as infections (lower respiratory tract disease, diarrhea, and tuberculosis).[2] Despite the advances in medical therapies and biomedical technology, the modern medical profession is still in many ways at the mercy of infections. Infections are here to stay...and kill. Therefore, it is incumbent on us as frontline medical providers in acute care to be as knowledgeable about infectious disease as possible.

In this issue of *Emergency Medicine Clinics of North America*, we have the privilege of having two emergency physician experts in infectious disease, Drs Stephen Liang and Rachel Chin, guide us through a must-know curriculum in infectious disease emergencies. These two Guest Editors have assembled an outstanding group of authors to address many of the most important topics pertaining to emergency medicine (EM) practice. Common "everyday" infections, such as urinary tract infections, skin and soft tissue infection, sexually transmitted infections, and respiratory infections are addressed. They also address the less common but highly lethal infections, such as endocarditis, central nervous system infections, and necrotizing fasciitis.

Emerg Med Clin N Am 36 (2018) xv–xvi
https://doi.org/10.1016/j.emc.2018.08.002
0733-8627/18/© 2018 Published by Elsevier Inc.

emed.theclinics.com

Separate articles are provided that address special populations, including patients with human immunodeficiency virus, cancer, transplanted organs, and victims of trauma. Important updates are also provided on emerging infections, and a critically important article is provided to discuss antimicrobial stewardship in the emergency department (ED). They conclude with a provocative article discussing the controversial topic of infection prevention in the ED.

This issue of *Emergency Medicine Clinics of North America* is a vitally important and valuable contribution to the EM literature, and it represents must-learning for all of us who practice on the frontline of medicine. Our thanks go to Drs Liang and Chin and their colleagues for their valuable work.

Amal Mattu, MD
Department of Emergency Medicine
University of Maryland School of Medicine
110 South Paca Street
6th Floor, Suite 200
Baltimore, MD 21201, USA

E-mail address:
amalmattu@comcast.net

REFERENCES

1. Mattu A. Infectious disease and emergency medicine. Emerg Med Clin N Am 2008;26(2). xv–xvi.
2. World Health Organization. Available at: http://www.who.int/en/news-room/fact-sheets/detail/the-top-10-causes-of-death.

Preface

Here to Stay: Infectious Diseases in Emergency Medicine

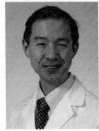
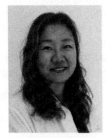

Stephen Y. Liang, MD, MPHS   Rachel L. Chin, MD
Editors

Infectious diseases are some of the most common reasons patients seek care in the emergency department (ED). While infection-related mortality in the United States has declined significantly over the past four decades, infectious diseases remain among the most frequently reported diagnoses for ED visits.[1,2] Infectious diseases account for 13.5% of all ED visits among adults aged 65 years and older.[3] The spectrum of infectious disease encountered in the practice of emergency medicine is dynamic and staggering, ranging from the commonplace (eg, community-acquired pneumonia) to the rare (eg, inhalation anthrax). The diagnosis and treatment of infectious disease is a key component of emergency medicine, stretching from the incision and drainage of a simple abscess to resuscitation and stabilization of the severely immunocompromised patient with septic shock. As sentinel health care professionals and gatekeepers to finite inpatient resources, emergency practitioners must rapidly synthesize history and examination findings with laboratory studies, imaging results, and prevailing infectious disease epidemiology to make decisions about antimicrobial therapy, patient isolation, and hospital admission.

Our aim is to provide a focused survey of the diagnosis and management of infectious diseases for and through the eyes of the busy emergency practitioner. First, our authors present contemporary updates on infectious diseases frequently encountered in the ED, including infective endocarditis, pneumonia and other respiratory infections, urinary tract infections, central nervous system infections, skin and soft tissue infections, musculoskeletal infections, and sexually transmitted infections. Next, our authors address the approach to complex ED patient populations at heightened risk for infectious complications, including those with human immunodeficiency virus infection, malignancy, and solid organ or hematopoietic cell transplantation. In keeping with the unique role of emergency medicine in public health, humanitarian, and disaster response, our authors tackle the recognition of biothreat agents and

Emerg Med Clin N Am 36 (2018) xvii–xviii
https://doi.org/10.1016/j.emc.2018.08.001
0733-8627/18/© 2018 Published by Elsevier Inc.

emerging infectious diseases in the ED and infectious diseases after hydrologic events, including hurricanes and floods. Finally, our authors close with a timely and prescient exploration of ED antimicrobial stewardship and infection prevention in the face of mounting antimicrobial resistance in an increasingly interconnected world.

We thank the dedicated and well-respected clinicians, educators, and researchers who have contributed to this issue of *Emergency Medicine Clinics of North America*. We are grateful for the opportunity to have worked with such an accomplished team of authors as well as the outstanding editorial staff at Elsevier, including Casey Potter. We are indebted to Amal Mattu, MD, for his mentorship and support of this endeavor. We hope that this work will prove an invaluable reference for emergency physicians, primary care physicians and specialists, physician assistants, nurse practitioners, residents, and medical students, who tirelessly provide acute care for patients with infectious diseases on the frontlines of emergency medicine.

Stephen Y. Liang, MD, MPHS
Divisions of Emergency Medicine and
Infectious Diseases
Washington University School of Medicine
4523 Clayton Avenue
Campus Box 8051
St. Louis, MO 63110, USA

Rachel L. Chin, MD
Department of Emergency Medicine
Zuckerberg San Francisco General Hospital
University of California
San Francisco School of Medicine
1001 Potrero Avenue, Suite 6A
San Francisco, CA 94110-1377, USA

E-mail addresses:
syliang@wustl.edu (S.Y. Liang)
rachel.chin@ucsf.edu (R.L. Chin)

REFERENCES

1. El Bcheraoui C, Mokdad AH, Dwyer-Lindgren L, et al. Trends and patterns of differences in infectious disease mortality among US counties, 1980-2014. JAMA 2018;319:1248–60.
2. Moore BJ, Scott C, Owens PL. Trends in emergency department visits, 2006-2014. HCUP statistical brief #227. Rockville (MD): Agency for Healthcare Research and Quality; 2017.
3. Goto T, Yoshida K, Tsugawa Y, et al. Infectious disease-related emergency department visits of elderly adults in the United States, 2011-2012. J Am Geriatr Soc 2016;64:31–6.

Infective Endocarditis

Elaine Yang, MD, Bradley W. Frazee, MD*

KEYWORDS

- Endocarditis • Fever • Murmur • Injection drug use (IDU) • Bloodstream infections
- Healthcare associated infections • Staphylococcal bacteremia

KEY POINTS

- Endocarditis should be considered in any patient with fever and risk factors, including significant valve damage, injection drug use, or an indwelling catheter.
- Blood cultures and echocardiography are the mainstays of diagnosis.
- Culture-negative endocarditis may result from certain fastidious or fungal organisms.
- Complications of endocarditis include heart failure, embolic stroke and metastatic infection, which may require cardiac surgery to control.

INTRODUCTION

Infective endocarditis (IE) is defined as an infection of a native or prosthetic cardiac valve, endocardial surface, or indwelling cardiac device.[1,2] Its incidence and mortality have not decreased in the past 30 years,[3] and it remains a challenging diagnosis to make and a difficult infection to treat despite new diagnostic and therapeutic strategies.[4]

The landscape of IE has changed in recent decades due to a shift in both the predominant pathogens and the most common predisposing conditions.[5] More virulent and resistant *Staphylococcus* species are becoming more common than penicillin-sensitive *Streptococcus*.[6] IE is occurring in an older, chronically ill population with more health care–associated and cardiac device–associated infections.[5] IE is no longer classified as acute versus subacute. Contemporary classification schemes vary but are all based on the distinction between native versus prosthetic valve endocarditis and community-acquired versus health care–associated infection; injection drug use (IDU)-related IE is generally considered separately.[7]

IE remains a disease with a highly variable and nonspecific presentation. Early diagnosis, particularly in the emergency department (ED) setting, depends on maintaining a high index of suspicion. IE should be suspected in any patient with a fever and unclear source of infection, new regurgitant heart murmur, and/or embolic events of unknown origin.[1] When IE is suspected, blood cultures and early formal

Disclosure Statement: The authors have no financial or nonfinancial conflicts of interest to disclose.
Alameda Health System, 1411 East 31st Street, Highland Hospital, Oakland, CA 94602, USA
* Corresponding author.
E-mail address: bradf_98@yahoo.com

Emerg Med Clin N Am 36 (2018) 645–663
https://doi.org/10.1016/j.emc.2018.06.002
emed.theclinics.com

echocardiography, the cornerstones for diagnosis, should be obtained immediately, usually while a patient is still in the ED.[8]

New consensus guidelines in the past decade have modified the approach to antibiotic therapy and prophylaxis.[8] Therapy recommendations, however, are still derived largely from expert opinion and observational cohort studies, due to the relatively low incidence of disease, lack of randomized controlled trials, and limited number of meta-analyses.[1,2] Although intravenous (IV) antibiotics are the mainstay of treatment, almost half of patients with IE eventually require surgery,[4] with common indications heart failure, perivalvular abscess formation, uncontrolled infection, and large or mobile vegetations.[8] Early consultation with cardiology and infectious disease specialists leads to improved diagnosis and management.[1]

EPIDEMIOLOGY

The annual incidence of IE is low, occurring in 3 to 10 per 100,000 people, with infection patterns varying according to geographic location. This incidence has remained stable over the past 2 decades. Globally, in 2010, IE caused the loss of 1.58 million disability-adjusted life-years (years of healthy life lost) as a result of death and illness or impairment.[4] In low-income countries, rheumatic heart disease is still the leading risk factor, underlying up to two-thirds of cases.[2,9,10] In the developed world, there has been an overall decrease in the proportion of cases related to rheumatic heart disease.[2] There is now a greater proportion of patients with other predisposing risk factors, including IDU, degenerative valve disease, congenital heart disease (CHD), prosthetic valves, and other cardiac devices.[11]

Overall, the mean patient age has increased, from approximately 45 years in the early 1980s to older than 70 in 2001 to 2006.[5] More IE patients now have comorbidities, such as chronic obstructive pulmonary disease, diabetes, cancer, and liver disease.[2] IE patients are more likely to be male. Although the overall incidence of IE has remained stable, the proportion caused by S aureus has steadily increased, now accounting for approximately 25% of cases in industrialized nations (**Table 1**). All of these shifts, in turn, highlight the growing importance of health care exposure as a risk factor for infection.[2]

A retrospective epidemiologic study examining 75,829 patients with first episodes of IE in California and New York State between 1998 and 2013 found that health care–associated IE accounted for more than half of all cases of native valve endocarditis (although in a contemporary French study the proportion of health care–associated disease was just 26.7%).[6,12] Health care–associated IE carried a 50% mortality at 1 year.[12] The proportion of patients who were dialysis dependent increased by 38.3% over the study period, accounting for 35% of health care–associated IE cases by 2010 to 2013.[12] Nosocomial (hospital-acquired) endocarditis cases actually declined over the study period, coinciding with large-scale efforts to reduce hospital-acquired infections, whereas non-nosocomial health care–associated endocarditis increased. These infections are acquired during outpatient health care encounters, for example, at dialysis and infusion centers, and often present first to the ED.

An increase in the proportion of patients with a history of valve surgery or implanted pacemakers or defibrillators has resulted in an increase in the incidence of prosthetic valve and cardiac device–related endocarditis, to 13% to 17% and 3% to 5%, respectively. Nonetheless, native valve IE still accounts for 71% to 78% of cases; 5% to 13% of cases are IDU related[1,7,12] (see **Table 1**).

Endocarditis remains rare in children, although improved survival in CHD has resulted in an increasing incidence of IE in this age group.[13] Pediatric IE is often a

Table 1
Microbiology of infective endocarditis (percentage of cases)

	Native Valve Infective Endocarditis (72%–78%)			PM/ICD-Related Infective Endocarditis (5%)	Prosthetic Valve Infective Endocarditis (13%–17%)	
	Community-Acquired (47%–55%)	Health Care–Associated[a] (18%–53%)	Injection Drug Use (5%–13%)		Early, <12 mo (4%)	Late, >12 mo (13%)
S aureus	20%–28%	25%–47%	68%–81%	23%	7%–36%	25%
Coagulase-negative staphylococcus	4%–6%	12%–25%	0%–3%	54%	0%–27%	9%
VGS	26%–28%	0%–11%	4%–10%	0	0%–7%	11%
Other streptococci	8%–18%	3%–8%	0%–4%	4%	0%–2%	12%
Enterococcus species	9%–11%	6%–42%	4%–5%	0	7%–20%	20%
Other culture negative[b]	5%–11%	0%–14%	0%–5%	24	13%–33%	20%

Percentage sum of cases may not be 100% because some patients have polymicrobial IE.

Abbreviation: PM/ICD, pacemaker/implantable cardiac defibrillator.

[a] Health care–associated includes nosocomial and non-nosocomial IE.

[b] Other culture negative species includes HACEK organisms, fungal organisms, and microorganisms not identified.

Data from Hoen B, Duval X. Infective endocarditis. N Engl J Med 2013;369(8):785; and Toyoda N, Chikwe J, Itagaki S, et al. Trends in infective endocarditis in California and New York State, 1998-2013. JAMA 2017;317(16):1652-60.

consequence of indwelling vascular catheters and invasive heart procedures, and *Staphylococcus* species continue to be the major causative organisms.[13] IE occasionally occurs in children without any history of heart murmur or heart disease.[14]

MICROBIOLOGY

Gram-positive cocci account for a majority of cases of IE (see **Table 1**).[1] *Staphylococcus* species are most frequently isolated, with *S aureus* the most common organism, causing 20% to 68% of cases in both native and prosthetic valve infections.[7] Methicillin-resistant *S aureus* (MRSA) is becoming an increasing problem, especially among high-risk groups, such as injection drug users, chronic hemodialysis patients, and patients with health care contact.[15] Compared with other pathogens, *S aureus* IE carries an increased rate of complications, including embolic disease, abscess formation, and higher in-hospital and 30-day mortality risk.[10] Coagulase-negative staphylococci (including *S epidermidis*, *S lugdunensis*, and *S capitis*) are ubiquitous skin commensals, with lower virulence potential than *S aureus* but with the ability to adhere to prosthetic material. *S epidermidis* is associated with biofilm production.[16] These species cause 17% of early prosthetic valve endocarditis and frequently infect indwelling catheters and devices.[2]

The other gram-positive cocci that are common causes of IE are the viridans streptococci species and *Enterococcus* species. Viridans group streptococcal (VGS) infection remains common in community-acquired native valve endocarditis and accounts for a higher proportion of disease in developing countries.[17] This group, which includes *Strep mutans*, *Strep salivarius*, *Strep anginosus*, *Strep mitis*, and *Strep sanguinis*, are commensals of the oral, gastrointestinal, and urogenital tract.[2] These pathogens are typically less virulent than *S aureus* and are associated with subacute/indolent disease. There is a significant incidence of VGS infection in the IDU population, likely due to the practice of using saliva to clean needles and dissolve heroin, thus introducing oral bacteria into the bloodstream.[15] Group D streptococci (*Strep bovis* and *Strep equinus* complex) cause IE associated with underlying colon cancer and advanced liver disease.[2] Enterococcal IE tends to be indolent and is associated with underlying valve disease, older age, and chronic illness. *Enterococcus* isolates are increasingly resistant to vancomycin, aminoglycosides, and ampicillin.[2]

The remaining common IE pathogens include a mixture of fastidious, zoonotic, and intracellular bacteria and fungi that often result in persistently negative blood cultures (culture-negative endocarditis). The HACEK group are fastidious gram-negative bacteria that include *Haemophilus*, *Aggregatibacter*, *Cardiobacterium*, *Eikenella corrodens*, and *Kingella kingae*. They are slow-growing commensals of the oropharynx, associated with periodontal disease and, although rarely isolated, have long been recognized as potential causes of both native and prosthetic valve endocarditis.[18] Zoonotic bacteria that cause IE are mostly intracellular pathogens and include *Coxiella burnetii* from livestock, *Bartonella henselae* from cats, and *Chlamydia psittaci* from parrots and pigeons.[1] *Tropheryma whippelii*, *Legionella* species, *Mycoplasma* species, and *Pseudomonas aeruginosa* are other rare causes of IE. Fungal causes of IE include *Candida* and *Aspergillus*; although rare overall, these are a significant cause of IE in immunocompromised patients and those with prosthetic valves.[19]

PATHOPHYSIOLOGY

Normal endothelium resists infection and thrombus formation. The development of IE results from the culmination of several factors: structural abnormalities that predispose to bacterial adherence; adhesion of circulating pathogens to a damaged valve surface; and survival of adherent organisms as they propagate as vegetation.[1] Abnormal turbulent flow and damaged endothelium expose underlying extracellular matrix proteins, leading to fibrin and platelet deposition, creating a nidus for seeding during bacteremia. With frequent bacteremia, such as in the setting of IDU or dental infection, IE may occur even without an identifiable pathologic valvular lesion.[1] In such cases, it is hypothesized that repetitive bombardment with particulate matter, such as talc present in injected material, or ischemia from drug-induced vasospasm can cause direct endothelial damage.[10]

As an infected thrombus forms, it incites an inflammatory response involving adjacent endothelium, further disrupting blood flow. Inflamed endothelial cells release cytokines, integrins, and tissue factor, which in turn attract fibronectin, monocytes, and platelets, ultimately forming an infected vegetation. Bacteria attached to the surface further activate the inflammatory cascade, becoming embedded and concealed from host defenses.[2] Production of a bacterial biofilm aids in bacterial persistence and contributes to antibiotic resistance.[16]

Valve leaflet distortion and destruction leads to regurgitant flow, impaired cardiac function, and frequently heart failure, which is the leading cause of death in patients with IE.[20] Congestive heart failure occurs in 50% to 60% of patients with IE. Aortic valve vegetations present the highest risk of heart failure due to acute aortic insufficiency.[1] Mitral valve infection can lead to rupture of chordae tendineae or papillary muscles.[1] Bacterial invasion of myocardium can also lead to abscess formation and conduction blocks.

As left-sided vegetations grow, friable material can embolize to essentially any artery, causing infarction or metastatic abscesses.[20] Infected microthrombi can incite an immunologic response, leading to vasculitic complications with immune complex deposition, such as in glomerulonephritis. Without appropriate treatment, infection may seed larger vessels, particularly of the cerebral circulation. An Intracerebral mycotic aneurysm, or a focal dilation of an arterial wall that has been weakened by infection, may cause neurologic deficits or may rupture, leading to hemorrhage.[21] Right-sided vegetations produce septic pulmonary emboli.

CLINICAL FEATURES

More than a century after IE was first described, the disease remains notorious for its diverse and nonspecific presentation, frequently leading to missed or delayed diagnosis.[1] The disease course is influenced by host factors, location of the vegetation, and microbial virulence resulting in a wide range of presentations: from indolent infection with nonspecific symptoms in a well-appearing patient to acute, severe infection presenting as septic shock and multiorgan failure.[2] Patients may complain of malaise, weight loss, dyspnea, backache, or focal neurologic symptoms—symptoms that may easily lead to misdiagnosis as a viral illness or to investigation for another infection, malignancy, rheumatologic disease, or cardiovascular or neurologic illness[1,7] **(Table 2)**.

The most common presenting symptom is fever, affecting more than 90% of patients with IE. Fever may be absent, however, in the elderly, the immunosuppressed, and those with recent antibiotic or antipyretic use.[1] A heart murmur is noted in 50% to 85% of patients with IE; however, the high prevalence of baseline murmurs in older adults makes this finding nonspecific unless the murmur is clearly new.[2] Murmurs are less often heard in right-sided IE. In 30% of cases, patients' initial presenting symptom is related to heart failure, paravalvular abscess formation, embolic stroke, or other metastatic infection, including vertebral osteomyelitis or peripheral abscesses.[20]

Table 2 Clinical features of infective endocarditis	
Symptoms	**Signs**

• Fever (90%)
 • Chills
 • Malaise
 • Dyspnea
   ○ Poor appetite
   ○ Weight loss
   ○ Weakness, focal or generalized
   ○ Back pain
	• Heart murmur (68%)
	 • Congestive heart failure
	 • New cardiac conduction disturbance
	 • Cerebral complications (stroke and meningitis)
	 • Peripheral emboli and abscesses (renal, splenic, vertebral, or peripheral arterial)
	 • Septic pulmonary emboli
	 • Fever or sepsis of unclear origin
	 • Splinter hemorrhages
	 • Roth spots
	 • Glomerulonephritis

Congestive heart failure is the most common cause of death in patients with IE and eventually occurs in up to 70% of patients.[20] Rare cases have been reported of perforation of cardiac chambers or embolization of vegetation fragments into coronary arteries, causing acute myocardial infarction.[20] Patients with left-sided IE may be relatively stable early in the course of their infection but then develop abrupt onset of pulmonary edema. Another cardiac complication of IE is paravalvular abscess formation, which can involve adjacent cardiac conduction tissue. These occur more commonly in patients with prosthetic valve endocarditis.[20] Extension into the conduction system can cause heart blocks and arrhythmias.[20]

Left-sided IE frequently results in embolic complications, which may sometimes be the presenting sign of infection. The most common embolic complication is stroke, which occurs in 10% to 20% of patients with IE and is the presenting symptom in half of these.[20] Septic cerebral emboli are much more likely to undergo hemorrhagic transformation than bland emboli, and S aureus IE is associated with the highest risk of hemorrhagic stroke.[20] Hemorrhage may develop from a ruptured mycotic aneurysm, most commonly of the middle cerebral artery.[20] Cerebral involvement may also present as nonfocal altered mental status or as frank meningitis.

Other embolic complications well described in the literature include splenic abscess (often requiring splenectomy), renal infarction, prosthetic joint infections, vertebral osteomyelitis, and spinal epidural abscess and limb ischemia.[20] Subungual or splinter hemorrhages (**Fig. 1**) and petechiae of the palate or conjunctiva are other manifestations of

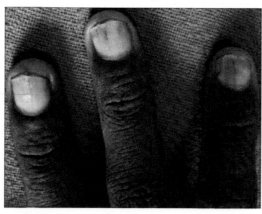

Fig. 1. Splinter hemorrhages.

small vessel metastatic infection, although these findings are nonspecific and can be seen in other disease states that result in bacteremia or vasculitis.[10]

Patients with right-sided endocarditis, involving the tricuspid or pulmonic valves, are at risk of developing septic pulmonary emboli. The initial presentation in right-sided infection may raise concern for pneumonia or pulmonary embolism. Mechanical failure of the pulmonic or tricuspid valve tends to be less consequential than that of left-sided valves but can cause signs and symptoms of right heart failure.[20] Additionally, the persistence of a patent foramen ovale with right-sided endocarditis can lead to the same systemic embolic events, as expected from a left-sided lesion.[22]

The classic textbook stigmata of IE are surprisingly uncommon, especially in high-acuity cases, which may develop other complications too quickly to manifest immunologic vascular phenomena.[4] Subacute IE, with its indolent course, allows more time for these immune-mediated findings to develop. Glomerulonephritis is a vasculitic phenomenon in which immune complexes deposit in renal microvasculature, observed in 2.3% of cases in 1 case series.[6] Janeway lesions (**Fig. 2**) are painless erythematous lesions located on the palms and soles, seen in 1.6% of cases. Osler nodes (**Fig. 3**) are painful violet lesions located on fingers and toes, seen in 2.7% of cases. Roth spots, also known as hemorrhagic cotton wool spots, are retinal hemorrhages with central white or pale centers, visualized in 0.7% of cases.[6,10]

DIAGNOSIS

Diagnosis of IE requires maintaining a high index of suspicion. It takes an astute clinician to consider the possibility of IE when faced with a constellation of suggestive findings rather than a single definitive test result.[23] IE should be considered in patients

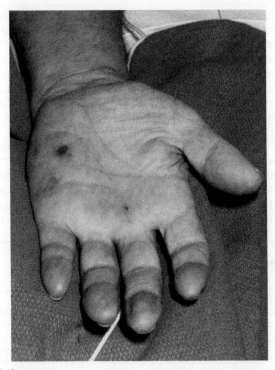

Fig. 2. Janeway lesions.

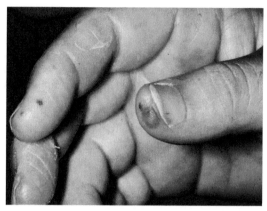

Fig. 3. Osler nodes.

who have a fever and underlying IE risk factors (**Table 3**), sepsis of unclear origin, or a new cardiac murmur. A thorough evaluation of patient risk factors includes consideration of IDU, history of significant valve abnormality, repaired CHD, indwelling vascular catheters, a prosthetic valve, or other intracardiac devices. Once suspicion of IE arises, careful auscultation in a quiet room should be performed. The diastolic murmur of aortic regurgitation can be subtle. Likewise, a thorough skin examination should be performed, looking for petechiae and other IE stigmata.

Echocardiography

In addition to data from the clinical examination and laboratory testing, formal echocardiography should be obtained as soon as possible whenever evaluating for possible IE. Results often are available while a patient is still in the ED and can assist with immediate management and disposition. **Fig. 4** highlights the fundamental role of echocardiography in making the diagnosis. Echocardiography plays a fundamental role in diagnosing endocarditis by providing direct visualization of a cardiac vegetation, abscess, or dehiscence of a prosthetic valve, as depicted in **Fig. 4**. Transthoracic echocardiography (TTE) is generally performed first when IE is suspected, often followed at some point by transesophageal echocardiography (TEE).[4] While TTE is less sensitive than TEE for detecting small vegetations, its availability and noninvasive nature make it the initial study of choice in the ED.[23] The sensitivity of TTE for detecting a new cardiac abnormality ranges from 40% to 63% compared with 90% to 100% for TEE.[24] TEE is preferred for patients with a prosthetic valve and is also more sensitive in identifying clinically important complications, such as paravalvular abscess, valve prolapse, valve leaflet perforation, pseudoaneurysm, torn chordae tendineae, and

Table 3		
Risk factors for development of infective endocarditis		
Cardiac		**Noncardiac**
Previous history of IE		IDU
Prosthetic valve or intracardiac device (pacemaker, defibrillator, or surgical baffle)		Immunosuppression (HIV, diabetes mellitus, or chronic steroid use)
Valvular or CHD		Indwelling catheter
		Chronic hemodialysis

Abbreviation: CHD, Valvular and congential heart disease.

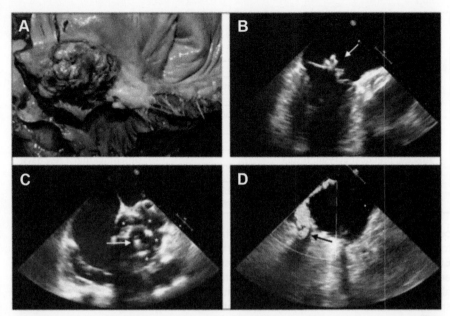

Fig. 4. Diagnosis of IE. (*A*) Vegetation in endocarditis. (*B*) TEE showing a mitral valve vegetation (*arrow*). (*C*) TEE showing the aortic valve surrounded by multiple abscesses (*asterisks*) and central vegetation (*arrow*). (*D*) Jet of mitral regurgitation (*arrow*) at the site of new prosthetic mitral valve dehiscence.

vegetations on pacemaker wires.[25] Sensitivity of TTE is higher in IDU-related cases, because frequently the vegetations are larger and right-sided and because body habitus is often favorable in this younger population. If initial TEE is negative but there remains a high suspicion for IE, repeat TTE or TEE is recommended in 5–7 days.[10]

Increasing vegetation size and mobility are associated with a higher risk of embolic complications.[26] Cardiac surgery may be indicated for a vegetation diameter greater than 10 mm as well as for other echocardiographic findings, such as severe valvular insufficiency, intracardiac abscess, pseudoaneurysm, valvular perforation or dehiscence, and decompensated heart failure (**Table 4**).[1,4]

In the ED, bedside point-of-care echocardiography can be used to detect critical IE complications, including pericardial effusion, cardiac tamponade, and valve rupture. Although not definitive, ED point-of-care ultrasound has been used to rapidly identify vegetations in both right-sided IE and left-sided IE.[14]

Blood Cultures

When IE is suspected, it is the responsibility of the emergency physician to ensure blood cultures are obtained in the ED prior to initiating antibiotics.[10] It has been shown that antibiotics significantly decrease the yield of blood cultures.[27] Three sets of blood cultures are generally recommended, drawn over at least 1 hour from different venipuncture sites.[4] Obtaining at least 10 mL per bottle greatly improves yield. Some investigators have argued that 2 sets are adequate in most situations.[28] Three sets are mandatory, however, in suspected prosthetic valve IE, because 1 of the most common pathogens, coagulase-negative staphylococcus, is also the most common blood culture contaminant. Use of a dedicated phlebotomist improves yield and reduces

Table 4
Emergency department indications for possible surgical treatment in infective endocarditis

Indication	Timing
Heart failure	
Severe aortic or mitral valve regurgitation with refractory pulmonary edema or cardiogenic shock	Emergent (within 24 h)
Fistula into cardiac chamber or pericardium with pulmonary edema or shock	Emergent
Locally uncontrolled infection	
Abscess, pseudoaneurysm, fistula	Urgent (within a few days)
Prevention of embolism	
Aortic or mitral vegetation >10 mm with embolic episode or accompanied by abscess or signs of heart failure	Urgent

contamination. Even in patients who are unstable or in septic shock, guidelines allow up to 45 minutes to obtain appropriate cultures before administering antibiotics.[29] In some ED cases, antibiotics will have been administered before the diagnosis of IE is considered. In such cases, blood cultures should still be drawn, because they retain a reasonable sensitivity for bacteremia even after antibiotics have been administered.[30] Use of special antibiotic resin bottles in patients who are already taking antibiotics is an option.[30] For patients who may be at risk of developing fungal or other rare infective organisms, the laboratory should be notified to prepare specialized cultures and additional testing, such as polymerase chain reaction or antibody titers.[10]

Newer molecular methods are being investigated and refined, including polymerase chain reaction and DNA microarray assays, which may detect bacteremia and identify the pathogen in a matter of hours, rather than relying on blood cultures, which may take days. More extensive clinical trials are required, but these methods hold great promise for rapidly detecting bacteremia and determining antibiotic resistance patterns.[31–33]

Duke Criteria

The modified Duke criteria are a widely accepted set of guidelines to aid in diagnosis of IE (**Table 5**). The criteria were originally developed for epidemiologic and clinical research rather than as a clinical decision tool.[23] Their main utility in the emergency setting is to provide a checklist of key historical and examination features to consider and a reminder of the importance of blood cultures.

Other Diagnostic Testing

Serum lactate and other tests of impaired organ perfusion should be routinely obtained along with blood cultures. Given the typical presentation of IE, a broad diagnostic workup is often ordered initially and there are several laboratory abnormalities that, although nonspecific, may suggest the correct diagnosis. These include[1]

- Anemia
- Leukocytosis
- Positive rheumatoid factor
- Elevated inflammatory markers (erythrocyte sedimentation rate, C-reactive protein, and procalcitonin)
- Urinalysis may show microscopic hematuria and occasionally red blood cell casts.

Table 5
Modified Duke criteria for the diagnosis of infective endocarditis

Major criteria	1. Blood cultures positive with typical microorganisms from 2 separate blood cultures (viridans streptococci, *Strep bovis*, HACEK group, *S aureus*, or community-acquired *Enterococci*)
	2. Persistently positive blood cultures with microorganisms consistent with IE defined as at least 2 positive cultures of blood samples >12 h apart, or at least 3 positive cultures with first and last samples drawn at least 1 h apart
	3. Single positive blood culture for *Coxiella burnetii* or anti–phase I IgG titer >1:800
	4. Evidence of endocardial involvement (echocardiographic evidence of vegetation, abscess or new partial dehiscence of prosthetic valve)
Minor criteria	1. Predisposition: predisposing heart condition or IDU
	2. Fever: temperature >38°C
	3. Vascular phenomena: major arterial emboli, septic pulmonary infarcts, mycotic aneurysm, intracranial hemorrhages, conjunctival hemorrhages, Janeway lesions
	4. Immunologic phenomena: glomerulonephritis, Osler nodes, Roth spots, rheumatoid factor
	5. Microbiological evidence: positive blood cultures not meeting major criterion or serologic evidence of active infection with organism consistent with IE
	6. Not formally included but considered: erythrocyte sedimentation rate/ C-reactive protein elevation, new clubbing, splinter hemorrhages, splenomegaly, microscopic hematuria, abnormal but nondiagnostic echocardiograph

Diagnosis of IE is definite in the presence of 2 major criteria, or 1 major and 3 minor criteria, 5 minor criteria or diagnosis of IE is possible in the presence of 1 major and 1 minor criteria, or 3 minor criteria.
  Adapted from Li JS, Sexton DJ, Mick N, et al. Proposed modifications to the Duke criteria for the diagnosis of infective endocarditis. Clin Infect Dis 2000;30(4):633–8; with permission.

An ECG may show new conduction disorders, such as first-degree atrioventricular block, bundle branch block, or complete heart block, indicating extension of infection into the His-Purkinje system. The ECG may demonstrate cardiac ischemia in the rare case of coronary artery emboli.[20] The chest radiograph is frequently abnormal in right-sided IE. Septic pulmonary emboli classically appear as peripheral, poorly marginated nodules (cotton balls), predominantly occurring in the lower lobes, and may be mistaken for multifocal pneumonia.[34] In severe left-sided infection, the chest radiographs reveal congestive heart failure.

Newer imaging modalities are being used for further evaluation of IE and its complications. Brain MR imaging has a role in identifying cerebral emboli and mycotic aneurysms. 3-D TEE allows visualization of the affected valve in multiple planes to diagnose leaflet perforation and guide surgical planning.[2] Cardiac CT or coronary CT angiography may improve the evaluation of paravalvular complications, such as abscess, prior to surgery.[4] Cardiac MR imaging can distinguish vegetation from tumor. Radionuclide studies, including PET-CT, have been used to detect peripheral embolization events, because infectious foci are metabolically active and readily take up radionuclide glucose tracer.[4]

TREATMENT AND MANAGEMENT

Treatment of IE in the ED begins with stabilization. Goal-directed therapy for sepsis, hemodynamic support, and positive pressure ventilation may be needed in the sickest subset of patients. Patients with suspected IE generally should be admitted to the hospital for further evaluation and management. Discharge to home after blood cultures is an option in well-appearing patients with nondiagnostic echocardiography who are completely reliable to follow-up. Admission is mandatory for patients with possible prosthetic valve IE, because of the high morbidity and mortality associated with prosthetic valve infections.[10] Patients with evidence of heart failure should undergo urgent consultation by a cardiothoracic surgeon, and emergency physicians should be aware of all the indications for urgent surgical intervention in IE (see **Table 4**).[4] For patients with a diagnostic echocardiogram or high likelihood of IE, early consultation with an infectious disease specialist is recommended.[1]

IDUs with fever and no definite alternative source of infection generally should be admitted to the hospital until bacteremia has been excluded with negative blood cultures at 48 hours. This approach—predicated on the notion that this patient population is unreliable to follow-up if blood cultures return positive—remains the standard of practice at urban teaching hospitals that serve large IDU populations. The problem of proper disposition of febrile but well-appearing IDUs with no apparent source of fever has been examined in numerous studies[35]; 6% to 13% of such patients are eventually diagnosed with IE. Unfortunately, these studies show it is difficult to predict which patients actually have endocarditis. A clinical decision rule to exclude IE in IDUs with a fever was recently developed, which showed that without tachycardia or a murmur, the post-test probability of IE was 5% to 7% and just 3% if an acute skin infection was present.[36] Unfortunately, only 12% of patients met all 3 low-risk criteria. The potential role of immediate formal echocardiography to risk stratify this population remains unclear.

Antibiotics

Initial antibiotic treatment of IE in the ED is almost always empiric.[1] Occasionally, patients present to the ED because previously drawn blood cultures have returned positive; in such cases, isolate or susceptibility directed antibiotics should be selected in consultation with an infectious disease specialist. With few exceptions, blood cultures should be drawn prior to administering the first dose of antibiotics (discussed previously). In cases of indolent infection, it is reasonable to withhold antibiotics entirely until culture and susceptibility results are available. Because of the inherent characteristics of vegetations and bacterial growth in IE, prolonged parenteral antibiotic therapy is required to eliminate infection, the standard course being 4 weeks to 6 weeks.[37]

Antibiotic selection for IE is a complex topic, full of esoteric issues. Consensus guidelines on IE treatment tend to focus on pathogen-specific therapy, with limited empiric treatment recommendations.[1,4] Selection of an empiric regimen should be based on key patient characteristics, in particular whether or not there is a prosthetic valve or history of IDU; some investigators also recommend tailoring the regimen to disease severity and health care exposure/risk for resistant gram-negative bacteria.[1] Hospital-specific empiric treatment recommendations, which account for local susceptibility patterns and are selected by infectious disease specialists and updated regularly, tend to trump published guidelines, which are updated infrequently (**Table 6** for a summary of published recommendations).

Recommended empiric regimens all target the most common organisms: S aureus, Streptococcus species, and Enterococci. Most regimens also provide coverage for the β-lactamase–producing HACEK organisms. Recommendations vary as to when to cover MRSA in native valve disease. Some US experts recommend empirically covering MRSA in all cases, regardless of risk factors.[38] Whether Pseudomonas and highly resistant Enterobacteriaceae strains should be covered immediately in certain patients is also controversial. Aminoglycosides are recommended in many regimens

Table 6
Empiric antibiotic therapy for suspected bacterial infective endocarditis

Infective Endocarditis Category	Recommended, Simplified Emergency Department Empiric Therapy[38,39]	European Guidelines[1]	American Heart Association and Infectious Diseases Society of America Guidelines[4]
Native valve	Vancomycin[b] 15 mg/kg q 8 h Plus Ceftriaxone[c] 2 g q 24 h	Ampicillin-sulbactam 3 g q 6 h Plus Gentamicin	No specific recommendation for empiric therapy
Prosthetic valve <12 mo	Vancomycin[b] Plus Gentamicin 1 mg/kg q 8 h	Vancomicin Plus Gentamicin Plus Rifampin 600 mg q 12 h PO	
Prosthetic valve >12 mo	Same as prosthetic valve <12 mo	Same as native valve	

Vancomycin and gentamicin dosing require regular monitoring of serum concentrations, and dosing may be adjusted according to renal function.

[a] All authors recommend withholding antibiotic therapy pending culture results in well-appearing patients with no high-risk echocardiographic signs, and obtaining infectious disease consultation as soon as possible.

[b] Substitute daptomycin 6 mg/kg q 24 hr if patient cannot tolerate vancomycin.

[c] Substitute gentamicin or meropenem 2 g q 8 hr for penicillin allergy.

because they have a synergistic effect with β-lactams and vancomycin, providing enhanced bactericidal activity, particularly against enterococcus; however, nephrotoxicity concerns and dosing difficulties arise beyond the first dose.[1] Likewise, rifampin appears in empiric regimens for suspected prosthetic valve IE, because it may be beneficial against MRSA and coagulase-negative staphylococci in this setting, but its use is fraught with rapid development of resistance and toxicity and drug interaction problems.

The authors recommend that vancomycin (15–20 mg/kg every 12 hours) be given in the ED as initial empiric therapy. Vancomycin alone for 1 dose or 2 doses is a reasonable approach in native valve and prosthetic valve disease and in IDUs. Addition of ceftriaxone can be considered to cover HACEK organisms, which are responsible for 2% of infections.[10] Adding gentamicin immediately to vancomycin is reasonable in suspected prosthetic valve infection. In patients who cannot tolerate vancomycin, daptomycin is a good alternative, with recent studies concluding that it is noninferior against S aureus, including MRSA, and Streptococcus species.[40]

Ultimately, the antibiotic regimen is tailored to isolate susceptibility, as determined by an infectious diseases specialist. Therapy is usually continued for 4 weeks to 6 weeks, with the first day counted as the first day on which blood cultures are negative.[4]

Surgery

Approximately 20% to 50% of patients with IE develop complications that can only be controlled with valve replacement surgery.[41] The main indications for valve surgery are decompensated heart failure, locally uncontrolled infection (eg, myocardial abscess), removal of large vegetations to prevent embolism, and persistent sepsis despite anti-biotic treatment.[41] Emergency physicians should consult a cardiothoracic surgeon as soon as any of these indications is identified (see **Table 4**). Virtually all cases of prosthetic valve endocarditis caused by S aureus require surgery.[42] Although valve replacement is the standard, mitral and tricuspid valve débridement or repair is sometimes possible.[20]

Early surgery for heart failure has been found to reduce the risk of death and systemic embolism.[43] The risk of embolization decreases with initiation of antibiotics; however, embolization despite treatment is likely when vegetations are large (>10 mm in diameter), highly mobile, and located on the mitral valve.[1] The presence of new left bundle branch block on preoperative electrocardiogram and presence of reduced left ventricular systolic function (ejection fraction <50%) portends a higher likelihood of need for permanent pacemaker implantation, and the presence of reduced left ventricular systolic function alone predicts in-hospital mortality.[41]

Other Management Considerations

Stroke is associated with increased mortality in patients with IE.[1] When cerebral embolic complications are suspected, immediate neurologic consultation should be obtained, along with CT or MR imaging scanning with angiography, to determine the exact location and extent of neurologic damage.[21] Patients who develop stroke syndromes from septic emboli should not receive anticoagulation because it does not reduce the risk of further embolization and the risk of hemorrhagic conversion is high, especially with S aureus infection.[1] Patients with a prosthetic valve in whom anticoagulation is deemed essential should be transitioned to IV heparin while embolic risk is high and surgical decisions are being made.[42] Patients with prosthetic valve IE who experience a cerebral embolic event should have all anticoagulation discontinued for at least 2 weeks.[4]

Successful treatment of IE ultimately requires a coordinated approach from a multidisciplinary team of providers, including emergency physicians, laboratory microbiologists, radiologists, infectious diseases specialists, cardiologists, and cardiothoracic surgeons. Development of a protocol to standardize and simplify the management of this complex disease has been shown to decrease mortality.[44]

PROGNOSIS

In addition to its up-front diagnostic utility, echocardiography is used during hospitalization to evaluate response to treatment and monitor for any signs of disease progression. Initial echocardiography serves as a baseline for comparison of vegetation size, valvular insufficiency, or changes in hemodynamic function. Repeat TEE is performed if the patient develops unexplained progression of heart failure symptoms, a new conduction block or arrhythmia, or any worsening in clinical features despite antibiotic therapy.[4]

All patients who have experienced an episode of IE are at increased risk of recurrence throughout the rest of their lifetime, at a rate of 1% to 3% per patient-year.[2] On completion of treatment, echocardiography should be performed again to establish and document a patient's new baseline valvular morphology and assess for valvular insufficiency.[4] The European Society of Cardiology recommends that patients have TTE and serum testing for inflammatory markers at 1 month, 3 months, 6 months, and 12 months after completion of treatment.[1] Patients should be monitored indefinitely for symptoms of heart failure and educated on the importance of regular dental hygiene.[4]

PREVENTION

Prevention of IE begins with minimizing bacteremia. Good oral hygiene and dental care reduces the risk of developing IE by reducing bacteremia from tooth brushing and the need for tooth extraction due to periodontal disease.[45] In-hospital and health care–associated settings, strict adherence to sterile technique, and appropriate care of central venous catheters, including early line removal, should be maintained.[2]

Historically, antibiotic prophylaxis was recommended to all patients at risk of IE, prior to undergoing procedures that could cause bacteremia. In 2008, the UK National Institute for Health and Care Excellence released new recommendations to discontinue this practice entirely, citing the low level of evidence and the potential harms of indiscriminate antibiotic use[46]; however, this guideline has been met with controversy.[47] Currently, the American Heart Association and European Society of Cardiology recommend continuing the practice, although for a more restricted set of highest-risk conditions and procedures involving infected tissue (**Box 1**).[48] Since the introduction of these recommendations limiting antibiotic prophylaxis, there has been no increased incidence of oral streptococcal endocarditis.[49]

Dental procedures that manipulate gingival tissue, involve the periapical region of teeth, or perforate oral mucosa still require prophylaxis. Unless the procedure involves a known infection, no prophylaxis is needed for the following:

Box 1
Indications for antibiotic prophylaxis

High-risk conditions (for which prophylaxis should be considered):

- Prosthetic heart valve

- Prosthetic material used for valve repair

- History of previous IE

- Unrepaired cyanotic CHD
  - Repaired congenital heart defect with prosthetic material or device or with residual shunt
  - Cardiac transplant recipients with valve regurgitation due to structurally abnormal valve

Procedures for which prophylaxis is indicated (if high-risk condition present):

- Dental procedures that manipulate gingival or periapical region of teeth, or perforation of oral mucosa

- Invasive procedures in infected tissue should receive antibiotic prophylaxis targeted against suspected bacteria

Procedures for which prophylaxis is NOT indicated:

- Local anesthetic injection in noninfected tissue

- Respiratory tract procedures, including bronchoscopy, laryngoscopy, intubation

- Gastrointestinal or urogenital procedures, including colonoscopy and cystoscopy

- Skin and soft tissue procedures (eg, laceration repair)

Data from Wilson W, Taubert KA, Gewitz M, et al. Prevention of infective endocarditis: guidelines from the American Heart Association: a guideline from the American Heart Association Rheumatic Fever, Endocarditis, and Kawasaki Disease Committee, Council on Cardiovascular Disease in the Young, and the Council on Clinical Cardiology, Council on Cardiovascular Surgery and Anesthesia, and the Quality of Care and Outcomes Research Interdisciplinary Working Group. Circulation 2007;116(15):1736–54.

- Minor dental procedures or local anesthetic injection for dental blocks
- Respiratory tract procedures, including bronchoscopy
- Genitourinary procedures, such as cystoscopy
- Skin and soft tissue procedures not involving infection, such as laceration repair[1]

For dental procedures in patients with highest-risk conditions, a single dose of amoxicillin (2 g orally) or ampicillin (2 g intramuscularly [IM]/IV) 30 to 60 minutes prior to procedure is recommended. Cephalexin (2 g orally) or clindamycin (600 mg IM/IV) may be administered in patients who are unable to tolerate penicillins.[48] Specific recommendations have not been given for prophylaxis before abscess incision and drainage. This issue is not straightforward. On one hand, there is evidence that incision and drainage of uncomplicated (afebrile) abscesses rarely cause bacteremia. On other hand, these infections are frequently due to MRSA, an important potential IE pathogen.[50] A conservative approach for patients with highest-risk conditions undergoing routine incision and drainage of an uncomplicated abscess in the ED is to give clindamycin (600 mg IM/IV) or vancomycin (20 mg/kg) 30 minutes to 60 minutes prior to the procedure.

SUMMARY

IE is an uncommon condition and a challenging diagnosis to make in the ED. Symptoms are nonspecific, murmurs are difficult to auscultate, and classic examination findings are often absent. Missed or delayed diagnosis may lead to substantial morbidity and mortality. For emergency physicians, maintaining a high index of suspicion is the key to early recognition and treatment. IE should always be considered in febrile patients with a prosthetic cardiac valve, implanted cardiac device, indwelling catheter, or a history of IDU or prior IE. Once a diagnosis is suspected, it is the responsibility of the emergency physician to ensure that blood cultures are obtained prior to administering antibiotics. Three sets of blood cultures are mandatory in suspected prosthetic valve IE. Echocardiography should be obtained while the patient is still in the ED, if possible. Cardiothoracic surgery consultation should be obtained when there are signs of heart failure, myocardial abscess, or a large vegetation associated with an embolic complication. In most cases, vancomycin alone is a reasonable immediate empiric antibiotic choice in the ED setting, with ID consultation recommended as soon as possible.

REFERENCES

1. Habib G, Hoen B, Tornos P, et al. Guidelines on the prevention, diagnosis, and treatment of infective endocarditis (new version 2009): the Task Force on the Prevention, Diagnosis, and Treatment of Infective Endocarditis of the European Society of Cardiology (ESC). Endorsed by the European Society of Clinical Microbiology and Infectious Diseases (ESCMID) and the International Society of Chemotherapy (ISC) for Infection and Cancer. Eur Heart J 2009;30(19): 2369–413.
2. Cahill TJ, Prendergast BD. Infective endocarditis. Lancet 2016;387(10021): 882–93.
3. DeSimone DC, Tleyjeh IM, Correa de Sa DD, et al. Temporal trends in infective endocarditis epidemiology from 2007 to 2013 in Olmsted County, MN. Am Heart J 2015;170(4):830–6.
4. Baddour LM, Wilson WR, Bayer AS, et al. Infective endocarditis in adults: diagnosis, antimicrobial therapy, and management of complications: a scientific

statement for healthcare professionals from the American Heart Association. Circulation 2015;132(15):1435–86.

5. Correa de Sa DD, Tleyjeh IM, Anavekar NS, et al. Epidemiological trends of infective endocarditis: a population-based study in Olmsted County, Minnesota. Mayo Clin Proc 2010;85(5):422–6.

6. Selton-Suty C, Celard M, Le Moing V, et al. Preeminence of Staphylococcus aureus in infective endocarditis: a 1-year population-based survey. Clin Infect Dis 2012;54(9):1230–9.

7. Hoen B, Duval X. Infective endocarditis. N Engl J Med 2013;369(8):785.

8. Harrison JL, Prendergast BD, Habib G. The European society of cardiology 2009 guidelines on the prevention, diagnosis, and treatment of infective endocarditis: key messages for clinical practice. Pol Arch Med Wewn 2009;119(12):773–6.

9. Marijon E, Ou P, Celermajer DS, et al. Prevalence of rheumatic heart disease detected by echocardiographic screening. N Engl J Med 2007;357(5):470–6.

10. Tintinalli JE, Stapczynski JS, Ma OJ, et al. Tintinalli's emergency medicine: a comprehensive study guide. 8th edition. New York: McGraw-Hill Education; 2016.

11. Tleyjeh IM, Abdel-Latif A, Rahbi H, et al. A systematic review of population-based studies of infective endocarditis. Chest 2007;132(3):1025–35.

12. Toyoda N, Chikwe J, Itagaki S, et al. Trends in Infective Endocarditis in California and New York State, 1998-2013. JAMA 2017;317(16):1652–60.

13. Day MD, Gauvreau K, Shulman S, et al. Characteristics of children hospitalized with infective endocarditis. Circulation 2009;119(6):865–70.

14. Cheng AB, Levine DA, Tsung JW, et al. Emergency physician diagnosis of pediatric infective endocarditis by point-of-care echocardiography. Am J Emerg Med 2012;30(2):386.e1-3.

15. Mostaghim AS, Lo HYA, Khardori N. A retrospective epidemiologic study to define risk factors, microbiology, and clinical outcomes of infective endocarditis in a large tertiary-care teaching hospital. SAGE Open Med 2017;5. 2050312117741772.

16. Becker K, Heilmann C, Peters G. Coagulase-negative staphylococci. Clin Microbiol Rev 2014;27(4):870–926.

17. Yew HS, Murdoch DR. Global trends in infective endocarditis epidemiology. Curr Infect Dis Rep 2012;14(4):367–72.

18. Chambers ST, Murdoch D, Morris A, et al. HACEK infective endocarditis: characteristics and outcomes from a large, multi-national cohort. PLoS One 2013;8(5): e63181.

19. Thuny F, Fournier PE, Casalta JP, et al. Investigation of blood culture-negative early prosthetic valve endocarditis reveals high prevalence of fungi. Heart 2010;96(10):743–7.

20. Sexton DJ, Spelman D. Current best practices and guidelines. Assessment and management of complications in infective endocarditis. Infect Dis Clin North Am 2002;16(2):507–21, xii.

21. Salgado AV, Furlan AJ, Keys TF. Mycotic aneurysm, subarachnoid hemorrhage, and indications for cerebral angiography in infective endocarditis. Stroke 1987; 18(6):1057–60.

22. Seif D, Meeks A, Mailhot T, et al. Emergency department diagnosis of infective endocarditis using bedside emergency ultrasound. Crit Ultrasound J 2013; 5(1):1.

23. Li JS, Sexton DJ, Mick N, et al. Proposed modifications to the Duke criteria for the diagnosis of infective endocarditis. Clin Infect Dis 2000;30(4):633–8.

24. Fowler VG Jr, Li J, Corey GR, et al. Role of echocardiography in evaluation of patients with Staphylococcus aureus bacteremia: experience in 103 patients. J Am Coll Cardiol 1997;30(4):1072–8.
25. Reynolds HR, Jagen MA, Tunick PA, et al. Sensitivity of transthoracic versus transesophageal echocardiography for the detection of native valve vegetations in the modern era. J Am Soc Echocardiogr 2003;16(1):67–70.
26. Sanfilippo AJ, Picard MH, Newell JB, et al. Echocardiographic assessment of patients with infectious endocarditis: prediction of risk for complications. J Am Coll Cardiol 1991;18(5):1191–9.
27. McKenzie R, Reimer LG. Effect of antimicrobials on blood cultures in endocarditis. Diagn Microbiol Infect Dis 1987;8(3):165–72.
28. Aronson MD, Bor DH. Blood cultures. Ann Intern Med 1987;106(2):246–53.
29. Levy MM, Rhodes A, Phillips GS, et al. Surviving Sepsis Campaign: association between performance metrics and outcomes in a 7.5-year study. Intensive Care Med 2014;40(11):1623–33.
30. Reimer LG, Wilson ML, Weinstein MP. Update on detection of bacteremia and fungemia. Clin Microbiol Rev 1997;10(3):444–65.
31. Rothman RE, Majmudar MD, Kelen GD, et al. Detection of bacteremia in emergency department patients at risk for infective endocarditis using universal 16S rRNA primers in a decontaminated polymerase chain reaction assay. J Infect Dis 2002;186(11):1677–81.
32. Galiana A, Coy J, Gimeno A, et al. Evaluation of the Sepsis Flow Chip assay for the diagnosis of blood infections. PLoS One 2017;12(5):e0177627.
33. Samuel LP, Tibbetts RJ, Agotesku A, et al. Evaluation of a microarray-based assay for rapid identification of Gram-positive organisms and resistance markers in positive blood cultures. J Clin Microbiol 2013;51(4):1188–92.
34. Rossi SE, Goodman PC, Franquet T. Nonthrombotic pulmonary emboli. AJR Am J Roentgenol 2000;174(6):1499–508.
35. Marantz PR, Linzer M, Feiner CJ, et al. Inability to predict diagnosis in febrile intravenous drug abusers. Ann Intern Med 1987;106(6):823–8.
36. Chung-Esaki H, Rodriguez RM, Alter H, et al. Validation of a prediction rule for endocarditis in febrile injection drug users. Am J Emerg Med 2014;32(5):412–6.
37. Gould FK, Denning DW, Elliott TS, et al. Guidelines for the diagnosis and antibiotic treatment of endocarditis in adults: a report of the Working Party of the British Society for Antimicrobial Chemotherapy. J Antimicrob Chemother 2012; 67(2):269–89.
38. Gilbert DN, Chambers HF, Eliopoulos GM, et al. 47th edition. Sanford guide to antimicrobial therapy 2017, vol.. Sperryville (VA): Antimicrobial Therapy, Inc; 2017.
39. Sexton DJ. Antimicrobial therapy of native valve endocarditis. UpToDate 2018.
40. Fowler VG Jr, Boucher HW, Corey GR, et al. Daptomycin versus standard therapy for bacteremia and endocarditis caused by Staphylococcus aureus. N Engl J Med 2006;355(7):653–65.
41. Jassal DS, Neilan TG, Pradhan AD, et al. Surgical management of infective endocarditis: early predictors of short-term morbidity and mortality. Ann Thorac Surg 2006;82(2):524–9.
42. Prendergast BD, Tornos P. Surgery for infective endocarditis: who and when? Circulation 2010;121(9):1141–52.
43. Kang DH, Kim YJ, Kim SH, et al. Early surgery versus conventional treatment for infective endocarditis. N Engl J Med 2012;366(26):2466–73.

44. Botelho-Nevers E, Thuny F, Casalta JP, et al. Dramatic reduction in infective endocarditis-related mortality with a management-based approach. Arch Intern Med 2009;169(14):1290–8.
45. Lockhart PB, Brennan MT, Thornhill M, et al. Poor oral hygiene as a risk factor for infective endocarditis-related bacteremia. J Am Dent Assoc 2009;140(10): 1238–44.
46. Centre for Clinical Practice at NICE, Prophylaxis against infective endocarditis: antimicrobial prophylaxis against infective endocarditis in adults and children undergoing interventional procedures. London: National Institute for Health and Care Excellence; 2008.
47. Dayer MJ, Jones S, Prendergast B, et al. Incidence of infective endocarditis in England, 2000-13: a secular trend, interrupted time-series analysis. Lancet 2015;385(9974):1219–28.
48. Wilson W, Taubert KA, Gewitz M, et al. Prevention of infective endocarditis: guidelines from the American Heart Association: a guideline from the American Heart Association Rheumatic Fever, Endocarditis, and Kawasaki Disease Committee, Council on Cardiovascular Disease in the Young, and the Council on Clinical Cardiology, Council on Cardiovascular Surgery and Anesthesia, and the Quality of Care and Outcomes Research Interdisciplinary Working Group. Circulation 2007;116(15):1736–54.
49. Desimone DC, Tleyjeh IM, Correa de Sa DD, et al. Incidence of infective endocarditis caused by viridans group streptococci before and after publication of the 2007 American Heart Association's endocarditis prevention guidelines. Circulation 2012;126(1):60–4.
50. Bobrow BJ, Pollack CV Jr, Gamble S, et al. Incision and drainage of cutaneous abscesses is not associated with bacteremia in afebrile adults. Ann Emerg Med 1997;29(3):404–8.

Community-Acquired Pneumonia

Ashley C. Rider, MD[a,b], Bradley W. Frazee, MD[c],*

KEYWORDS

- Acute cough illness • Pneumonia • CURB-65 • Pneumonia severity index
- Multi-drug resistant respiratory pathogen

KEY POINTS

- History, physical examination, including vital signs and saturation of peripheral oxygen, and chest radiographs results provide the essential information to clinically diagnose community-acquired pneumonia.
- Careful severity assessment is a crucial step in the emergency department management of community-acquired pneumonia and should include screening for occult sepsis with a serum lactate, followed by early antibiotics and fluid resuscitation when indicated.
- Risk stratification tools such as the PSI and CURB-65 should be used routinely to determine the most appropriate disposition.
- Emergency department providers need to be aware of risk factors for multidrug-resistant pneumonia, limiting broad spectrum antibiotics to patients satisfying guideline-recommended criteria.

INTRODUCTION

Pneumonia is a commonly encountered respiratory infection in the emergency department (ED) that is responsible for significant morbidity and mortality in our patients. Community-acquired pneumonia (CAP) is defined as an acute lung infection involving the alveoli that occurs in a patient without recent health care exposure.[1] CAP encompasses a clinical spectrum from walking pneumonia in an otherwise healthy patient to necrotizing or multilobar disease with septic shock. Pneumonia is the third leading reason for hospital admission, accounting for 544,000 hospitalizations from the ED annually.[2] Despite advances in medicine, the mortality rate from CAP has remained stable over the past 4 decades.[3] In the United States, CAP is the leading cause of

Disclosure Statement: The authors have nothing to disclose.
[a] Department of Emergency Physician, Alameda Health System – Highland Hospital, 1411 East 31st Street, Oakland, CA 94602, USA; [b] UCSF, San Francisco, CA, USA; [c] Department of Emergency Medicine, Alameda Health System – Highland Hospital, 1411 East 31st Street, Oakland, CA 94602, USA
* Corresponding author.
E-mail address: bfrazee@alamedahealthsystem.org

Emerg Med Clin N Am 36 (2018) 665–683
https://doi.org/10.1016/j.emc.2018.07.001
0733-8627/18/© 2018 Elsevier Inc. All rights reserved.

sepsis and death from infection.[3] Given the prevalence of CAP and its potential to cause severe illness, emergency providers must have a thorough understanding of this multifaceted condition and be able to take a nuanced approach to management. Emergency physicians need to recognize symptoms suggestive of CAP, order appropriate diagnostic tests, select recommended empiric antibiotics, and risk stratify the patient for proper disposition. This article provides an overview of CAP in adults and touches on drug-resistant and health care-associated disease. Opportunistic lung infections, tuberculosis, and hospital-acquired pneumonia are beyond the scope of this review.

MICROBIOLOGY

The etiology and antibiotic resistance patterns of respiratory pathogens varies by geographic region and has evolved over time with the development of vaccines. In the majority of cases requiring hospitalization, no pathogen can be identified.[1] In a 2015 US population-based surveillance study of patients admitted with CAP, only 38% of patients had a pathogen identified, and most were viral.[4] A bacterial pathogen could be isolated in only 14% of patients. The most common pathogen was rhinovirus, followed by influenza virus, then *Streptococcus pneumoniae*. *Mycoplasma pneumoniae* and *Staphylococcus aureus* were the second and third most common bacterial pathogens, respectively. Other bacterial species that commonly cause CAP include *Legionella pneumophila*, *Haemophilus influenzae*, *Chlamydophila pneumoniae*, and *Moraxella catarrhalis*.[1,4]

Common viral causes include not only human rhinovirus and influenza, but also human metapneumovirus, parainfluenza virus, respiratory syncytial virus, coronavirus, adenovirus, and Middle East respiratory syndrome coronavirus.[1] During peak influenza season, influenza may be the most common cause of CAP requiring hospitalization, although it can often be complicated by secondary bacterial infection. Fungal etiologies are generally rare in immunocompetent hosts. *Coccidioidomycosis* is a relatively common cause of pneumonia and pneumonitis in the Western United States that can mimic bacterial pneumonia. Other geographic endemic mycoses include *Histoplasma capsulatum* and *Blastomyces* in the Ohio and Mississippi River valleys. Opportunistic fungal pneumonias frequently seen in patients with AIDS and solid organ transplant include *Pneumocystic jiroveci* pneumonia, *Aspergillus*, *Candida albicans*, and *Cryptococcus neoformans* (**Table 1**).

MICROBIOLOGY: DRUG-RESISTANT PATHOGENS

The categorization of pneumonia is evolving. Until recently, pneumonia was divided into 4 categories: CAP, health care-associated pneumonia (HCAP), hospital-acquired pneumonia, and ventilator-associated pneumonia. Hospital-acquired pneumonia and ventilator-associated pneumonia are outside the scope of this article. HCAP is a category that includes patients who have been in regular contact with the health care system, including nursing home residents, patients undergoing home infusion therapy or wound care, dialysis patients, and patients hospitalized for 2 days or more in the prior 90 days.[5] Such patients are thought to have a higher risk of pneumonia caused by multidrug-resistant (MDR) bacteria, warranting broad spectrum antibiotic coverage, similar to hospital-acquired pneumonia. Common MDR pathogens include *Pseudomonas aeruginosa*, methicillin-resistant *S aureus* (MRSA), and gram-negative *Enterobacteriaceae* species. This topic is currently in flux because HCAP criteria are neither sensitive nor specific for identifying patients infected with MDR organisms. Treating these patients with the same regimen as for

Table 1
List of pneumonia pathogens according to patient population

Patient Population	Pathogens
Otherwise healthy adult, bacterial	*Streptococcus pneumoniae* *Mycoplasma pneumoniae* *Staphylococcus aureus* *Legionella pneumophila* *Haemophilus influenzae* *Chlamydophila pneumoniae* *Moraxella catarrhalis*
Otherwise healthy adult, viral	Human rhinovirus Influenza Human metapneumovirus Parainfluenza virus Respiratory syncytial virus Coronavirus Adenovirus
Adults with health care exposure	*Pseudomonas aeruginosa* *S aureus* *Klebsiella pneumoniae* *Escherichia coli*
Pediatric patients – by age Birth to 20 d	*E coli* *Listeria monocytogenes* Group B streptococci
20 d to 4 mo	*Chlamydia trachomatis* *Streptococcus pneumoniae*
4 mo to 5 y	*C trachomatis* *Streptococcus pneumoniae* *M pneumoniae* Respiratory syncytial virus Influenza Parainfluenza Adenovirus Rhinovirus
School-aged children	*C pneumoniae* *M pneumoniae* *Streptococcus pneumoniae* *M catarrhalis* *H influenzae* *S aureus*
Unusual and opportunistic infectious etiologies	*Pneumocystic jiroveci* *Histoplasma capsulatum* *Blastomyces* *Coccidioidomycosis* *Aspergillus* *Candida albicans* *Mucorales* *Cryptococcus neoformans* *Coxiella burnetii* *Mycobacterium tuberculosis*

hospital-acquired pneumonia leads to overtreatment with broad spectrum antibiotics.[6] Excess mortality in HCAP may be largely attributable to patient comorbidities rather than drug-resistant pathogens.[6] The Infectious Diseases Society of America (IDSA) and American Thoracic Society are removing the HCAP category from their guidelines.[7] Forthcoming guidelines will recommend that the group formally known as HCAP be divided into 2 groups, those appropriate for limited spectrum therapy and those with 2 of 3 risk factors for MDR, who do require broad spectrum therapy.[8] **Table 2** lists risk factors for the most important MDR organisms. Although evidence on this topic remains incomplete and exact recommendations are not yet clear, it remains very important to identify ED patients who require broad spectrum empiric antibiotics.

Historically, penicillin was sufficient treatment for S pneumoniae, but over the past 3 decades the prevalence of drug resistant pneumococcus has increased.[9] Alteration in the penicillin-binding protein is the main resistance mechanism. In the United States, pneumonia owing to penicillin nonsusceptible strains increased from 18% in 1991 to 35% in 2002.[10] The clinical significance of penicillin-resistant S pneumoniae remains unclear, with mixed data on mortality impact and associated costs and durations of stay.[9,11] However, adverse outcomes are associated with high-level penicillin resistance (minimum inhibitory concentration of ≥ 4) and these infections require treatment with a cephalosporin or fluoroquinolone.

Macrolide-resistant pneumococcus is also a growing problem. The mechanism for high-level resistance involves methylation of a ribosomal binding site, whereas lower level resistance involves drug efflux via a membrane transporter. A study conducted in Japan, where macrolide-resistant strains exceed 90% in some areas, found that 83%

Table 2	
Risk factors for drug-resistant pneumonia pathogens	
Drug-Resistant Pathogen	**Risk Factors**
Drug-resistant *streptococcus*	Age >65
	Beta-lactam or macrolide therapy within 3 mo
	Immunosuppression
	Alcoholism
	Daycare centers
	Medical comorbidities
Enteric gram negative	Residence in a nursing home
	Recent hospitalization
	Recent antibiotics
	Cardiopulmonary disease
	Smoking
	Underlying malignancy
MRSA	Age >74 y
	Dialysis
	Prior MRSA infection
	Prior hospitalization
	Recent nursing home stay
	Medical comorbidities
Pseudomonas	Chronic obstructive pulmonary disease
	Immunosuppression
	Recent steroid exposure
	Hemiplegia
	Recent antibiotics against gram positive organisms
	Recent hospitalization

Abbreviation: MRSA, methicillin-resistant *Staphylococcus aureus*.

of patients still had a good clinical response to azithromycin, suggesting that the clinical significance of resistance is unclear in vivo.[12] In the United States, macrolide-resistant pneumococcus averages 27.9%, with the greatest prevalence in Louisiana and state-by-state variation as high as 33%.[13] Macrolide resistance should be considered in high-resistance regions, particularly when there has been recent antibiotic exposure and macrolide monotherapy is being considered.

Macrolide-resistant *M pneumoniae* emerged around 2000 as another concerning drug-resistant CAP pathogen.[14] Resistance is conferred from point mutations where the macrolide binds to the ribosome subunit. A study of 6 centers throughout the United States revealed an *M pneumoniae* macrolide resistance rate of 13.2%.[14]

PATHOPHYSIOLOGY

Pneumonia is an alveolar infection that occurs when the innate immune system is unable to clear a pathogen from the lower airway and alveoli.[15] Local inflammatory factors and cytokines cause additional harm to the lung parenchyma and lead to systemic inflammation, which causes secondary symptoms such as fever, chills, and fatigue.[16] At a histologic level, the inflammatory response causes congestion, which progresses to red and gray hepatization, and may resolve with minimal fibrosis.[17] In terms of lung mechanics and physiology, pus in the parenchyma leads to decreased compliance and shunt, which increases the work of breathing and worsens hypoxemia and tachypnea—the most important physical examination signs of severe pneumonia for emergency physicians to focus on at the bedside.[17]

CAP affects patients of all ages across the spectrum of health, with certain organisms having a predilection for specific patient subgroups. Any condition that causes decreased mucociliary clearance and cough, like cigarette smoking, puts patients at increased risk, as do conditions that lead to aspiration such as cerebral vascular accidents, esophageal disorders, and neuromuscular disorders.[15] Old age and dehydration affect how pneumonia manifests and can make recognition more difficult. Underlying cardiopulmonary disease or structural lung disease can also delay recognition.[18]

EPIDEMIOLOGY

Pneumonia carries the highest mortality of any infectious disease.[19] Lower respiratory tract infections are the most common infectious cause of death in the world, with 3.5 million deaths annually worldwide (World Health Organization). In the United States, influenza and pneumonia are listed together as the 9th leading cause of death.[20] The highest rates are among elderly adults aged 65 to 79 years.[4] Outcomes in patients requiring hospitalization for pneumonia are poor: the 30-day mortality is 10% to 12% and the readmission rate is 18%.[1] Interestingly, mortality after a CAP hospitalization remains increased at 1 year and 5 years. Patients with chronic obstructive pulmonary disease, diabetes mellitus, renal failure, congestive heart failure, coronary artery disease, and liver disease have an increased incidence of CAP.[21] Fortunately, the use of the pneumococcal conjugate vaccine may be responsible for up to a 35% decrease in the incidence of pneumonia.[22]

DIFFERENTIAL DIAGNOSIS

In day-to-day practice, the main differential diagnosis in an immunocompetent ambulatory patient presenting with acute cough illness is CAP versus viral bronchitis. Correctly distinguishing between the two depends in large part on elements of the history and physical examination, particularly age, upper respiratory infection symptoms, pulse oximetry, and lung sounds. In EM practice, chest radiographs also plays a central role. CAP is distinguished by the presence of an alveolar infiltrate on chest radiographs, whereas those with bronchitis will have a normal chest radiographs (with the possible exception of peribronchial thickening). Accurately distinguishing pneumonia from acute bronchitis is one of the most important ways that emergency physicians can improve antibiotic stewardship.

In the case of acute cough with a negative radiographs, possible diagnoses include viral bronchitis, asthma, gastroesophageal reflux disease, postnasal drip, sinusitis, or medication side effect, particularly an angiotensin-converting enzyme inhibitor–induced cough (**Table 3**).[23] When an infiltrate is present on radiographs, important noninfectious causes to consider include pulmonary edema, pulmonary embolism with pulmonary infarction, lung cancer, alveolar hemorrhage (arteriovenous malformation, Goodpasture's syndrome, Wegener's granulomatosis), bronchiectasis, cryptogenic organizing pneumonia, acute eosinophilic pneumonia, interstitial lung diseases, vasculitis, cocaine-induced lung injury, pulmonary contusion, drug reaction, and high altitude pulmonary edema, among others.[18]

When the chest radiograph is abnormal, in addition to the common bacterial and viral infectious etiologies, emergency physicians need to keep in mind less common infectious causes of pneumonia. Immunocompetent hosts may develop infections from endemic mycoses such as histoplasmosis, blastomycosis, or coccidiomycosis. Septic emboli should be considered in patients with multiple sites of infection or history of injection drug use. Immunocompromised hosts, particularly patients infected with the human immunodeficiency virus (HIV), are at risk for opportunistic lung infections, including from fungal pathogens, such as *P jiroveci* (*P jiroveci* pneumonia), *Aspergillus, C albicans, Mucormycosis, C neoformans*, as well as *Mycobacterium*

Table 3
Differential diagnosis of noninfectious causes of an infiltrate on chest radiographs, and differential diagnosis of cause of a normal chest radiographs in the setting of acute cough illness

Chest Radiograph Findings	Causes
Abnormal chest radiograph, infectious	Refer to micro table
Abnormal chest radiograph, noninfectious	Cardiogenic pulmonary edema Bronchiectasis Pulmonary infarction Arteriovenous malformation Interstitial lung disease Cryptogenic organizing pneumonia Acute eosinophilic pneumonia Pneumonitis Vasculitis Cocaine-induced lung injury Pulmonary contusion Drug reaction High altitude pulmonary edema Lung cancer
Normal chest radiograph	Bronchitis Asthma Gastroesophageal reflux disease Upper respiratory tract infection Medication side-effect

tuberculosis and *Mycobacterium avium complex*. Tuberculosis and *P jiroveci* pneumonia are remarkably common and easily misdiagnosed causes of pneumonia in HIV-infected patients with CD4 counts of less than 500 cells/mm^3. When evaluating pneumonia, emergency physicians should consider the possibility that the patient has HIV or is otherwise immunocompromised.

Diagnosis: History and Physical Examination

Although the diagnostic criteria for CAP seem relatively straightforward, making the correct diagnosis can be difficult. A thoughtful history and physical examination with close attention to the actual respiratory rate and core temperature, as well as careful interpretation of chest radiographs, are required. This caution is especially true in the elderly. The clinical diagnosis of CAP is made on the basis of respiratory symptoms such as cough, sputum production, dyspnea, chest pain, signs of fever, and hypoxemia, as well as an infiltrate on chest imaging.[24] Additional symptoms may include myalgia, fatigue, abdominal pain, and headache, making CAP difficult to distinguish from viral infection, particularly influenza, based on history alone.[25] Possible chest examination findings include dullness to percussion, decreased breath sounds, and inspiratory crackles.

Because patients in the ambulatory setting with symptoms suggestive of a respiratory infection have a prevalence of pneumonia of only about 5%, it is possible to rule out CAP without a chest radiograph. Nonelderly patients without any abnormal vital signs and without a focally abnormal auscultatory examination have a probability of CAP (abnormal chest radiographs) of less than 1%. Ruling out CAP without an radiographs should not be attempted, however, in elderly patients, because many will not mount typical signs and symptoms. As many as 30% of elderly patients with CAP are afebrile in the ED and preexisting oxygenation problems and lung disease can further complicate the picture.[1]

Fig. 1 outlines a simplified diagnostic approach for ambulatory patients with cough and a suspicion for CAP. Patients who are not elderly, with normal vital signs and normal auscultatory examination, can generally be given a diagnosis of bronchitis and discharged home without antibiotics. If vital signs or examination are abnormal,

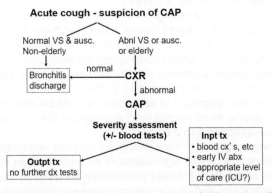

Fig. 1. Summary of the diagnostic approach to acute cough illness in ambulatory patients. This shows the central role of the chest radiographs and, in cases of community-acquired pneumonia (CAP), severity assessment (typically with a clinical decision rule). Abnl, abnormal; abx, antibiotics; ausc., auscultation; cx, culture; CXR, chest radiograph; ICU, intensive care unit; inpt, inpatient; IV, intravenous; outpt, outpatient; tx, treatment; VS, vital signs.

or the patient is elderly, a chest radiograph should be obtained. If the film is normal, the correct diagnosis is usually bronchitis. Rarely, very early in the disease course, or in severely dehydrated patients, the chest radiographs will be normal in CAP, but this is an uncommon issue in ambulatory patients less than 65 years old. If the chest radiographs confirms the diagnosis of CAP, the next step is risk stratification (see Severity Assessment and Clinical Decision Rules). In many patients who are determined to be at low risk for mortality by a clinical decision rule, no further diagnostic testing is required before discharge. The only important remaining step in such patients is proper oral antibiotic selection (see **Fig. 1**).

Diagnosis: Imaging

A chest radiograph is the crucial diagnostic test for CAP in adults. Physical examination alone is less sensitive and specific than a chest radiograph.[24] Infiltrates may be subtle, so a study that includes both the posteroanterior and lateral views is preferred. Opacities typically develop within 12 hours.[26] The most common findings include peribronchial nodules, silhouette sign, parapneumonic effusions, and ground glass opacities.[26,27] More severe pneumonia is characterized by multilobar involvement, cavitation, and bilateral pleural effusions.[28] However, the radiographic appearance does not necessarily correspond with clinical severity and infiltrates may evolve independent of clinical improvement or worsening.

Although etiology cannot be reliably predicted by chest radiograph appearance, the following classic associations between radiographic findings and etiology are described in the literature. S pneumoniae typically appears as alveolar or lobar pneumonia. The lower lobe and multilobar involvement is frequently seen.[26] Bilateral disease and interstitial infiltrates are found in 50% of cases. Mycoplasma typically produces reticulonodular opacities or patchy consolidations. Mycoplasma targets bronchial epithelium and, therefore, can cause bronchial wall thickening (peribronchial cuffing) in central bronchi like respiratory viruses. Similarly, Chlamydia pneumoniae classically shows patchy consolidations or reticular opacities. Viral pneumonitis/pneumonia can be radiographically indistinguishable from bacterial CAP, but ground glass opacities are the most common findings after a normal chest radiographs. Finally, aspiration pneumonia commonly affects the posterior and inferior segments of the lung and may cavitate if subacute or chronic.[27]

The interpretation of a chest radiographs, however, is an imperfect practice. Not only do these radiographic patterns poorly predict etiology, but radiologists may miss infiltrates in up to 15% of cases.[29] The timing of CAP presentation may also affect radiographic appearance. The chest radiographs may seems to be normal in the first few hours of S pneumoniae, in patients with HIV with early P jirovecii infection, or in the setting of severe dehydration, as is common in patients from skilled nursing facilities.[25] In such cases, a clinical diagnosis of pneumonia should be considered even if the chest radiograph seems to be normal, and it is reasonable to treat for pneumonia and repeat the radiograph in 1 to 2 days.[24]

Computed tomography (CT) is more sensitive than plain radiographs for detecting pneumonia. Although the clinical significance of an infiltrate seen on CT but not on chest radiographs is debated, a recent prospective surveillance study showed that illness severity, pathogens, and clinical outcomes were comparable between patients with CAP with an abnormal chest radiographs and those diagnosed by CT scan without an obvious infiltrate on radiographs.[30] If clinical suspicion for pneumonia remains high despite a negative chest radiograph, advanced imaging should be considered and empiric treatment initiated. CT scans may be better at visualizing certain areas of the lung, such as the upper lobes and lingula, and at elucidating interstitial infiltrates as seen with atypical pathogens.[31] CT scanning is useful to further characterize necrotizing infection, multilobar disease, empyema, and pleural involvement. It can also help to differentiate CAP from tuberculosis or lung cancer, which can be difficult to distinguish on chest radiographs alone.

Guidelines do not support the use of ultrasound examination for the diagnosis of pneumonia in adults when other imaging modalities are available. However, a metaanalysis concluded that, in the hands of experienced operators, ultrasound examination may have a sensitivity and specificity as high as 94% and 96%, respectively.[32] Ultrasound examination may offer an ideal alternative diagnostic modality in pediatric patients and critically ill patients in whom it is difficult to obtain a 2-view film (**Fig. 2**).

Diagnosis: Additional Testing

When history, physical examination, and imaging studies confirm the diagnosis of CAP, additional etiologic testing may or may not be required depending on the patient's clinical status and disposition. This area holds considerable controversy in emergency medicine. Identification of the causative organism uses resources and is costly; even when it reveals the pathogen, etiologic testing only rarely leads to a change in treatment.[18] In contrast, cases in which an organism is identified may allow for deescalation from broad to more narrow spectrum treatment during the hospitalization, thereby decreasing cost of care and preventing adverse effects.[1] Etiologic testing is also important from a public health standpoint, allowing for epidemiologic monitoring of drug susceptibility and the incidence of specific pathogens.

The IDSA recommends directing testing toward patients with the highest expected yield. For outpatients, etiologic testing, with the exception of a rapid diagnostic tests for influenza, is rarely indicated.[24] If obtained before antibiotic administration, blood cultures grow a pathogen in 5% to 14% of CAP cases, depending on disease severity. The sensitivity of blood cultures is halved if antibiotics have already been administered. The most common isolate is *S pneumoniae.* Although pneumococcal infections rarely require a change in therapy based on isolate susceptibility, these isolates do allow surveillance for penicillin and macrolide resistance. Among hospitalized patients, blood cultures should always be drawn in those with severe CAP requiring

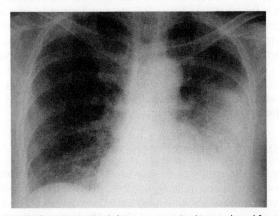

Fig. 2. Chest radiograph demonstrating lobar pneumonia. (*Reproduced from* Medscape Drugs & Diseases (https://emedicine.medscape.com/), typical bacterial pneumonia imaging. 2015. Available at: https://emedicine.medscape.com/article/360090-overview; with permission.)

admission to the intensive care unit (ICU). In patients admitted to the floor, blood cultures are optional, but should be performed in patients with alcohol abuse, liver disease, leukopenia, effusion, or asplenia.[24]

Patients with severe CAP should also have a respiratory specimen obtained for culture and Gram stain. Sputum should be obtained within 12 hours of initiation of antibiotics.[1] The yield of respiratory cultures is significantly higher from endotracheal aspirates or bronchoscopic sampling and should be sent on all intubated patients with CAP.[24] Absence of S aureus or gram-negative rods in a respiratory specimen suggests these pathogens are not the cause of illness and can allow the antibiotic regimen to be narrowed early in the hospitalization.

Although use of polymerase chain reaction has increased the detection of viral respiratory pathogens in CAP, the role of these tests, other than for influenza, remains unclear.[1] Influenza testing is recommended for admitted patients when local influenza activity is high. It is also recommended that patients with severe CAP have urinary antigen tests for S pneumoniae as well as Legionella pneumophilia if Legionella serogroup 1 is suspected. S pneumoniae urinary antigen tests remain positive for 3 days after initiating therapy.[24] Local health department notification is required if Legionella is detected because this may indicate an outbreak. In general, more etiologic testing should be done for patients with a history of alcohol abuse, liver disease, lung disease, leukopenia, cavitary infiltrates, asplenia, pleural effusion, and recent travel.[24]

Serum lactate is a widely recommended screening test for severe sepsis. When elevated in the setting of infection, the lactate level independently predicts mortality. A prospective observational study comparing CURB-65 and serum lactate in 1641 patient with CAP showed that lactate better predicted 28-day mortality, hospitalization, and ICU admission.[33] Lactate should routinely be drawn along with blood cultures as part of the workup for patients being hospitalized with severe CAP to help guide resuscitation, treatment, and disposition.

Testing for acute phase reactants has a growing role in evaluation of CAP and other infectious diseases, particularly in pediatric populations. Procalcitonin is an acute phase reactant that has a very low circulating level (<0.15 ng/mL) normally, but increases with inflammatory diseases, particularly in response to bacterial toxins. The procalcitonin level may be helpful in distinguishing bacterial from viral infections, although the data are not consistent.[3,15] Procalcitonin may also serve as a marker of disease severity; if low or decreasing, it may allow for the deescalation or termination of antibiotics in the inpatient setting. In a metaanalysis of 14 randomized trials, the use of procalcitonin was associated with a decrease in the duration of antibiotic therapy from 8 to 4 days, without a change in mortality.[34] Another metaanalysis showed lower mortality among critically ill patients who were allowed to have procalcitonin-guided cessation of antibiotics.[35] Other biomarkers currently under investigation to differentiate viral from bacterial illness include C-reactive protein and cortisol.[15] Although biomarkers may have a future role in risk-stratification of CAP in the ED setting, ED studies are limited at this time (**Fig. 3**).

SEVERITY ASSESSMENT AND CLINICAL DECISION RULES

Owing to the very wide spectrum of disease severity in CAP, it is strongly recommended that emergency physicians routinely use a structured, clinical decision rule to risk stratify patients with CAP. A number of rules have been developed and validated, all of which are used to determine the intensity of diagnostic testing and optimal safe disposition of the patient—to home, inpatient ward, or inpatient ICU. Besides helping to identify the sickest subset of patients, another important benefit of clinical decision

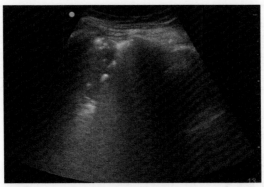

Fig. 3. Ultrasound image showing air bronchograms suggestive of pneumonia. (*Courtesy of Highland Emergency Medicine, Oakland, CA.*)

rules is that they promote safe discharge of low-risk patients who might otherwise be admitted to the hospital unnecessarily.

The IDSA divides the signs of severe CAP into major and minor criteria. Approximately 10% of patients hospitalized with CAP will require an ICU stay. It is absolutely crucial that emergency physicians recognize the signs of severe disease to ensure appropriate disposition. The minor criteria include:

- Respiratory rate of greater than 30 breaths per minute;
- Pao_2/Fio_2 of less than 250;
- Multilobar infiltrates;
- Confusion;
- Uremia;
- Leukopenia;
- Thrombocytopenia;
- Hypothermia; and
- Hypotension.

The clinically less helpful major criteria are mechanical ventilation and septic shock requiring vasopressors.[24] ICU admission is recommended with any major criteria or 3 or more minor criteria. The minor signs represent a valuable guide to identifying subtle organ system dysfunction and hypoperfusion. A careful assessment for these subtle signs of poor organ perfusion is the key to effective care of patients with CAP.[36] Critical early interventions include prompt antibiotic treatment, monitoring serial blood gases and serum lactate levels, and frequent reassessment.

The 2 most widely validated and used CAP clinical decision rules are the Pneumonia Severity Index (PSI) and CURB-65. The PSI was developed in 1997 by the Pneumonia Patient Outcomes Research Team in an effort to predict short-term CAP mortality (**Table 4**).[37] It is intended for immunocompetent adults based on data available at presentation. The higher the score, the higher the risk of death or eventual admission to the ICU. In practice, the score helps emergency providers to determine an appropriate disposition destination. PSI class IV and V patients should be hospitalized, with class V usually requiring ICU admission. Class III patients may be appropriate for 23-hour observation, 1 or 2 doses of intravenous antibiotics, and hydration.[38] Classes I and II patients can usually be safely managed as outpatients. The PSI has been externally validated in several large trials and a randomized control trial at 19 hospitals confirmed that using it safely reduces low risk admissions.[39]

Table 4
Clinical decision rules

Clinical Decision Rule	Factors	Points			Score and Stratification		
						Risk class	Mortality
Pneumonia Severity Index (PSI)	Male	Age	Point total			I	Class I: 0.1%–0.4%
	Age >50	Age + 10	If all are absent ≤70 low risk			II	Class II: 0.6%–0.7%
	Nursing home resident	30	71–90 low risk			III	Class III: 0.9%–2.8%
	Neoplastic disease	30	91–130 moderate			IV	Class IV: 8.2%–12.5%
	Congestive heart failure	10	>130 high risk			V	Class V: 27.1%–31.1%
	Cerebrovascular disease	10					
	Renal disease	10					
	Liver disease	20					
	Altered mental status	20					
	HR ≥125 beats/min	10					
	RR ≥30 breaths/min	20					
	Systolic BP <90 mm Hg	20					
	Temperature <35°C or ≥40°C	15					
	Arterial pH <7.35	30					
	BUN ≥30 mg/dL	20					
	Sodium <130 mmol/L	20					
	Glucose ≥250 mg/dL	10					
	Hematocrit <30%	10					
	Partial pressure arterial O$_2$ <60 mm Hg or O$_2$ sat <90%	10					
	Pleural effusion	10					

Suggested Disposition

I, II: outpatient
III: observation
IV, V: hospitalize

Clinical Decision Rule	Factors	Points	Score and Stratification	
			Score total	Mortality (30-d)
British Thoracic Society (BTS) modified	Confusion/orientation	1	0–5	0 factors: 0.7%
	BUN >20 mg/dL (7 mmol/L)	1		1 factors: 2.1%
	RR ≥30 breaths/min	1		2 factors: 9.2%
Or	Low BP: <90 SBP, ≤60 DBP	1		3 factors: 14.5%
CURB-65	Age ≥65 y	1		4 factors: 40%
				5 factors: 57%

Suggested Disposition

0–1: treat as outpatients
2: admit to floor
≥3: ICU

Abbreviations: BP, blood pressure; BUN, blood urea nitrogen; DBP, diastolic blood pressure; HR, heart rate; ICU, intensive care unit; RR, respiratory rate; SBP, systolic blood pressure.

The CURB-65 score combines just 5 variables to determine disease severity, placing more emphasis on physiologic parameters.[40] It is much easier to calculate than the PSI (see **Table 4**). One point each is assigned for confusion, blood urea nitrogen of 20 mg/dL or greater, respiratory rate of 30 or greater, blood pressure less than 90 mm Hg or diastolic 60 mm Hg or greater, and age greater than 65.[18] Patients with a score of 2 or higher should be admitted to the hospital. The CURB-65 is not as well-validated as the PSI and when the 2 measures are compared, the PSI with its 20 variables boasts a slightly higher discriminatory power for mortality and classifies a slightly higher percentage of patients as low risk, and in that sense has greater usefulness.[24,41]

Other pneumonia clinical decision rules that are less-widely used in the United States include SMART-COP, A-DROP, and CAP-PIRO. The Australian SMART-COP score assigns points for low systolic blood pressure, multilobar infiltrates, low albumin, tachypnea, tachycardia, confusion, hypoxemia, and acidemia. A score of 3 or more points identified 92% of patients who would later receive vasopressor or ventilator support.[42] The A-DROP scoring system, developed by the Japanese Respiratory Society, uses the variables age (males $\geq$70, females $\geq$75), dehydration (blood urea nitrogen >210 mg/mL), respiratory failure (SaO_2 $\leq$90%), confusion, and hypotension.[43] Similarities between these clinical decision rules are not surprising. The CURB-65 seems to have emerged as the preferred score in the ED because of its simplicity, although the PSI still has a role because it is better at identifying patients who seem to be "on the fence" but can actually be safely discharged.

In addition to clinical decision rules, assessment of nonmeasurable factors is important when determining disposition. Before patient discharge, emergency physicians must consider the likelihood of direct complications of the pneumonia, such as hypoxemia or pleural effusion, exacerbation of underlying disease, the patient's ability to take oral medication, and availability of a caregiver.[24] Discharge is appropriate when the respiratory rate is less than 24 breaths per minute, the saturation of peripheral oxygen is greater than 90%, mental status is normal, and the patient can tolerate oral intake.[38] Finally, psychosocial factors and patient preference must be considered. Outpatient care of CAP costs 25 times less than hospitalization and patients resume normal activity faster, so providers should encourage discharge when it is deemed clinically and socially safe.[24]

TREATMENT

Antibiotic therapy for CAP should be directed at the most common pathogens with consideration of local resistance patterns and patient disposition. Once the diagnosis is made, antibiotics should be administered as soon as possible. There is no longer a CMS quality metric regarding time to treatment, but a widely accepted target is within 6 hours of presentation.[1,44] Patients who exhibit signs of sepsis should receive antibiotics within 1 hour.

If available, local empiric antibiotic treatment guidelines that reflect the hospital antibiogram should be followed. In nonsevere cases, the goal is to reliably cover S pneumoniae and atypical bacterial pathogens. The decision to provide broader coverage is based on health care exposure risk factures, a history of structural lung disease, or other specific conditions (eg, known MRSA colonization).[18]

For outpatients without coexisting illnesses or recent antibiotic use, the IDSA recommends a macrolide (azithromycin, clarithromycin) or doxycycline.[1,24] If coexisting illness is present or the patient has recently used antibiotics, a respiratory fluoroquinolone (moxifloxacin, levofloxacin) is recommended; a beta-lactam (eg, amoxicillin) plus macrolide may also be used. Risk factors for drug-resistant *Streptococcus pneumoniae* include comorbidities such as heart disease, liver disease, renal disease, diabetes, alcoholism, immunosuppression, or antimicrobial use within the previous 3 months (see **Table 2**). For these patients, a respiratory fluoroquinolone should be prescribed or a beta-lactam plus a macrolide.[24] In 1 cohort of patients treated for CAP in the ED, approximately one-half had 1 risk factor for drug-resistant *S pneumonia*, raising concern for potential overuse of fluoroquinolones.[45] In areas such as Louisiana with a large percentage (48%) of macrolide-resistant *S pneumoniae* (defined as a minimum inhibitory concentration of ≥16), a respiratory fluoroquinolone or beta-lactam plus macrolide can be used.[24] See **Tables 5** for treatment guidelines.

For hospitalized patients, the IDSA guidelines recommends a beta-lactam plus a macrolide (eg, ceftriaxone plus azithromycin). There is increasing evidence that patients do better with a combination of antibiotics rather than fluoroquinolone monotherapy, possibly related to immunomodulation.[3] During high local influenza activity, hospitalized patients generally should also be treated with oseltamivir. Droplet and contact precautions should be used when influenza is suspected.

The risk for MDR pathogens must be considered before selecting a treatment regimen for hospitalized patients (see **Table 2**). In those with 2 or more MDR risk factors such as medical comorbidities, recent hospitalization, or recent antibiotics, immunosuppression coverage for *P aeruginosa* is recommended. *Pseudomonas*, which is invariably MDR, may cause 1% to 8% of severe CAP cases, and is associated with a case fatality rate of 50% to 100%. To cover MDR organisms, an antipseudomonal cephalosporin (eg, cefepime, ceftazidime), carbapenem (eg, meropenem, imipenem), or antipseudomonal penicillin (eg, piperacillin-tazobactam) plus an antipseudomonal fluoroquinolone is recommended.[5] MRSA coverage with vancomycin or linezolid should be added in patients with suspected recent or coinfection with influenza, chronic glucocorticoid use, or other risk factors for MRSA (see **Table 2**).[18,46]

Table 5
Treatment of adults with community-acquired pneumonia

Patient Characteristics	Regimen
Outpatient: previously healthy	Macrolide Doxycycline
Outpatient: with comorbidities (heart, lung renal disease, diabetes, alcoholism) or recent use of antibiotics concerning for drug-resistant *Streptococcus pneumoniae*	Respiratory fluoroquinolone Beta-lactam plus macrolide
Outpatient: macrolide-resistance streptococcus areas (>25% of infection)	Respiratory fluoroquinolone Beta-lactam plus macrolide
Inpatient: floor	Respiratory fluoroquinolone Beta-lactam plus macrolide
Inpatient: intensive care unit	Beta-lactam plus azithromycin or respiratory fluoroquinolone Penicillin allergic: respiratory fluoroquinolone plus aztreonam
Inpatient: Pseudomonas	Antipseudomonal beta-lactam such as piperacillin-tazobactam, cefepime, meropenem, imipenem plus ciprofloxacin or levofloxacin
Inpatient: methicillin-resistant *Staphylococcus aureus*	Vancomycin or linezolid

The recommended duration for CAP therapy is 5 to 7 days. Evidence suggests there is no difference in outcomes when treatment duration is 7 days or less compared with 8 days or more.[47] Exceptions include S aureus lobar pneumonia, which may require extended treatment for 2 weeks, and S aureus bacteremia, which generally requires 4 weeks of intravenous treatment.[48] Atypical infections are also an exception; if M pneumoniae or C pneumoniae are known to be the causative organism, 10 to 14 days is recommended. For Legionella, 14 to 21 days of therapy is recommended.[49] For hospitalized patients, an early switch from intravenous to oral antibiotics does not compromise outcome and decreases the duration of stay.[3]

In addition to antimicrobials and symptomatic care, other CAP treatment adjuncts should be considered, corticosteroids being the most important and widely debated. Steroids may attenuate the inflammatory response, reduce the frequency of acute respiratory distress syndrome, and decrease the length of illness. A systematic review and metaanalysis suggested that steroids reduce the need for mechanical ventilation and rate of acute respiratory distress syndrome by 5% (estimated number needed to treat of 20).[50] Despite this evidence in favor of steroids, there are many high-quality studies showing no benefit.[51] The case for adjunctive steroids is stronger in severe CAP.[50] Steroids should be trialed in patients with vasopressor-dependent shock and selectively in patients with severe CAP and evidence of inadequate cortisol response.[24] Early physical therapy is another important treatment adjunct in hospitalized patients. A single-center retrospective study showed an association between physical therapy for 30 minutes or more and lower 30-day readmission rate.[52]

Long-Term Host Effects

Discharged patients should be informed about the usual course of illness in CAP. In previously healthy adults with pneumococcal pneumonia, fevers typically resolve within 3 days of initiating antibiotics.[53] One week after presentation, 80% of patients will still have fatigue and 50% will have dyspnea.[54] Overall, patients improve clinically much faster than radiographs clear. Patients hospitalized for CAP have a 1-year mortality rate 2.5 times greater than controls and mortality remains elevated for 2 years, even in patients with no comorbidities.[55–57] Excess cardiovascular risk has been observed for 5 to 10 years after infection. This phenomenon is likely due to the fact that systemic inflammation destabilizes coronary plaques and produces a procoagulant effect.[58,59] Primary care providers should ensure that after a pneumonia diagnosis patients receive aspirin and statin if they are eligible.[60,61]

PREVENTION

In the primary care setting, the most important measure to reduce a patient's risk of CAP is to encourage smoking cessation, because tobacco use interferes with immune system and lung function. Children should be vaccinated against S pneumoniae and H influenza with PCV13 and HIB.[45] All healthy adults over the age of 65 should receive vaccination against S pneumoniae. The PCV13 should be given to adults 65 and older who have not previously received a dose and the PPSV23 should be given at least 1 year later.[62] This regimen is especially important for patients with chronic obstructive pulmonary disease in whom pneumococcal vaccine has been shown to reduce the likelihood of CAP (needed to treat = 21) and exacerbations of chronic obstructive pulmonary disease.[63] Influenza vaccines should be given yearly to all eligible patients. Finally, frequent hand washing should be encouraged to patients and providers alike, primarily to prevent spread of respiratory viruses.

SUMMARY

- History, physical examination, including vital signs and saturation of peripheral oxygen, and chest radiographs results provide the essential information to clinically diagnose CAP.
- CAP is caused by both bacterial and viral pathogens.
- It is essential to query the patient's past medical history for risk factors that predispose to drug-resistant pneumonia.
- The concept of HCAP is changing; ED providers need to be aware of risk factors for MDR pneumonia, limiting broad spectrum antibiotics to patients satisfying guideline-recommended criteria.
- In severe CAP, ED providers should collect blood cultures before administering antibiotics and sputum cultures when applicable, although in most cases etiologic testing does not reveal the causative pathogen.
- Careful severity assessment is a crucial step in ED CAP management and should include screening for occult sepsis with a serum lactate, followed by early antibiotics and fluid resuscitation when indicated.
- Risk stratification tools such as the PSI and CURB-65 should be used routinely to determine the most appropriate disposition for a patient.
- Emergency providers should be familiar with the latest guidelines for antimicrobial treatment for both outpatient and inpatient CAP, which will continue to change as resistance patterns in respiratory pathogens evolve.
- Vaccination must be encouraged to continue to prevent respiratory infections in children and adults.

REFERENCES

1. Musher DM, Thorner AR. Community-acquired pneumonia. N Engl J Med 2014; 371:1619–28.
2. Rui P, Kang K. National hospital ambulatory medical care survey: 2015 emergency department summary tables. Available at: http://www.cdc.gov/nchs/data/ahcd/nhamcs_emergency/2015_ed_web_tables.pdf.
3. Waterer GW, Rello J, Wunderink RG. Management of community-acquired pneumonia in adults. Am J Respir Crit Care Med 2011;183:157–64.
4. Jain S, Self WH, Wunderink RG. Community-acquired pneumonia requiring hospitalization among U.S. adults. N Engl J Med 2015;373(5):415–27.
5. American Thoracic Society, Infectious Diseases Society of America. Guidelines for the management of adults with hospital-acquired, ventilator-associated, and healthcare-associated pneumonia. Am J Respir Crit Care Med 2005;171: 388–416.
6. Chalmers JD, Rother C, Salihh W, et al. Healthcare-associated pneumonia does not accurately identify potentially resistant pathogens: a systematic review and meta-analysis. Clin Infect Dis 2014;58(3):330–9.
7. Kalil AC, Metersky ML, Klompas M, et al. Executive summary: management of adults with hospital-acquired and ventilator- associated pneumonia: 2016 clinical practice guidelines by the Infectious Diseases Society of America and the American Thoracic Society. Clin Infect Dis 2016;63(5):575–82.
8. Kollef MH, Sherman G, Ward S, et al. Inadequate antimicrobial treatment of infections: a risk factor for hospital mortality among critically ill patients. Chest 1999; 115(2):462–74.
9. File TM Jr. Clinical implications and treatment of multiresistant Streptococcus pneumoniae pneumonia. Clin Microbiol Infect 2006;12(3):31–41.

10. Doern GV, Richter SS, Miller A, et al. Antimicrobial resistance among Strepto-coccus pneumonaie in the United States: have we begun to turn the corner on resistance to certain antimicrobial classes? Clin Infect Dis 2005;41:139–48.

11. Rothermel C. Penicillin and macrolide resistance in Pneumococcal pneumonia: does in vitro resistance affect clinical outcomes? Clin Infect Dis 2004;38(4): S346–9.

12. Yanagihara K, Izumikawa K, Higa F, et al. Efficacy of azithromycin in the treatment of community-acquired pneumonia, including patients with macrolide-resistant Streptococcus pneumoniae infection. Intern Med 2009;48:527–35.

13. Farrell DJ, Jenkins SG. Distribution across the USA of macrolide resistance and macrolide resistance mechanisms among Streptococcus pneumoniae isolates collected from patients with respiratory tract infections: PROTEKT US 2001-2002. J Antimicrob Chemother 2004;54(S1):i17–22.

14. Zheng X, Lee S, Selvarangan R, et al. Macrolide-resistant mycoplasma pneumo-niae, United States. Emerg Infect Dis 2015;21(8):1470–2.

15. Brar NK, Niederman MS. Management of a community-acquired pneumonia: a review and update. Ther Adv Respir Dis 2011;5(1):61–78.

16. van der Poll T, Opal SM. Pathogenesis, treatment, and prevention of pneumo-coccal pneumonia. Lancet 2009;374:1543–56.

17. Reid PT, Innes JA. Respiratory disease. In: Colledge NR, Walker BR, Ralston SH, editors. Davidson's principle and practice of medicine. 21st edition. Edinburgh: Elsevier Publications; 2010. p. 680–2.

18. Wunderink RG, Waterer GW. Community-acquired pneumonia. N Engl J Med 2014;370:543–51.

19. Bartlett JG, Mundy LM. Community-acquired pneumonia. N Engl J Med 1995; 333(24):1618–24.

20. Murphy SL, Xu J, Kochanek KD. Deaths: preliminary data for 2010. Natl Vital Stat Rep 2012;60:1–51.

21. Lim WS, Baudouin SV, George RC, et al. BTS guidelines for the management of community acquired pneumonia in adults. Thorax 2009;64(S3):iii1–55.

22. Black S, Shinefield H, Fireman B, et al. Efficacy, safety and immunogenicity of heptavalent pneumococcal conjugate vaccine in children. Pediatr Infect Dis J 2000;19:187–95.

23. Turner RD, Bothamley GH. Chronic cough and a normal chest X-ray - a simple systematic approach to exclude common causes before referral to secondary care: a retrospective cohort study. NPJ Prim Care Respir Med 2016;26:15081.

24. Mandell LA, Wunderink RG, Anzueto A, et al. Infectious Diseases Society of America/American Thoracic Society consensus guidelines on the management of community-acquired pneumonia in adults. Clin Infect Dis 2007;44(S2):S27–72.

25. Akter S, Shamsuzzaman, Jahan F. Community acquired pneumonia. Int J Respir Pulm Med 2015;2:2.

26. Amanullah S, et al. Typical bacterial pneumonia imaging. Medscape 2018. Avail-able at: https://emedicine.medscape.com/article/360090-overview#a2.

27. Nambu A, Ozawa K, Kobayashi N, et al. Imaging of community-acquired pneu-monia: roles of imaging examinations, imaging diagnosis of specific pathogens and discrimination from noninfectious diseases. World J Radiol 2014;6(10): 779–93.

28. Hasley PB, Albaum MN, Li YH, et al. Do pulmonary radiographic findings at pre-sentation predict mortality in patients with community-acquired pneumonia? Arch Intern Med 1996;156(19):2206–12.

29. Albaum MN, Hill LC, Murphy M, et al. Interobserver reliability of the chest radiograph in community-acquired pneumonia. Chest 1996;110:343–50.

30. Upchurch CP, Grijalva CG, Wunderink RG, et al. Community-acquired pneumonia visualized on ct scans but not chest radiographs pathogens, severity, and clinical outcomes. Chest 2018;153(3):601–10.

31. Syrjälä H, Broas M, Suramo I, et al. High-resolution computed tomography for the diagnosis of community-acquired pneumonia. Clin Infect Dis 1998;27:358–63.

32. Chavez MA, Shams N, Ellington LE, et al. Lung ultrasound for the diagnosis of pneumonia in adults: a systematic review and meta-analysis. Respir Res 2014; 15:50.

33. Chen YX, Chun-Shen L. Lactate on emergency department arrival as a predictor of mortality and site-of-care in pneumonia patients: a cohort study. Thorax 2015;1–7. https://doi.org/10.1136/thoraxjnl-2014-206461.

34. Schuetz P, Müller B, Christ-Crain M, et al. Procalcitonin to initiate or discontinue antibiotics in acute respiratory tract infections. Cochrane Database Syst Rev 2012;(9):CD007498.

35. Lam SW, Bauer SR, Fowler R, et al. Systematic review and meta-analysis of procalcitonin-guidance versus usual care for antimicrobial management in critically ill patients: focus on subgroups based on antibiotic initiation, cessation, or mixed Strategies. Crit Care Med 2018. https://doi.org/10.1097/CCM.0000000000002953.

36. Lim HF, Phua J, Mukhopadhyay A, et al. IDSA/ATS minor criteria aided pre-ICU resuscitation in severe community-acquired pneumonia. Eur Respir J 2014; 43(3):852–62.

37. Fine MJ, Auble TE, Yealy DM, et al. A prediction rule to identify low-risk patients with community-acquired pneumonia. N Engl J Med 1997;336:243–50.

38. Halm EA, Teirstein AS. Management of community-acquired pneumonia. N Engl J Med 2002;347:2039–45.

39. Marrie TJ, Lau CY, Wheeler SL, et al. A controlled trial of a critical pathway for treatment of community- acquired pneumonia. JAMA 2000;283:749–55.

40. Lim WS, van der Eerden MM, Laing R, et al. Defining community acquired pneumonia severity on presentation to hospital: an international derivation and validation study. Thorax 2003;58:377–82.

41. Aujesky D, Fine MJ. The Pneumonia Severity Index: a decade after the initial derivation and validation. Clin Infect Dis 2008;47:S133–9.

42. Charles PG, Wolfe R, Whitby M, et al. SMART-COP: a tool for predicting the need for intensive respiratory or vasopressor support in community-acquired pneumonia. Clin Infect Dis 2008;47(3):375–84.

43. The Committee for the Japanese Respiratory Society Guidelines in the Management of Respiratory Infections. The Japanese Respiratory Society guidelines for the management of community-acquired pneumonia in adults. Respirology 2006; 11:S79–133.

44. Wilson KC, Schünemann HJ. An appraisal of the evidence underlying performance measures for community-acquired pneumonia. Am J Respir Crit Care Med 2011;183:1454–62.

45. Jenkins TC, Sakai J, Knepper BC, et al. Risk Factors for drug-resistant Streptococcus pneumoniae and antibiotic prescribing practices in outpatient community-acquired pneumonia. Acad Emerg Med 2012;19:703–6.

46. Sicot N, Khanafer N, Meyssonnier V, et al. Methicillin resistance is not a predictor of severity in community-acquired Staphylococcus aureus necrotizing

pneumonia: results of a prospective observational study. Clin Microbiol Infect 2013;19:E142–8.

47. Li JZ, Winston LG, Moore DH, et al. Efficacy of short-course antibiotic regimens for community-acquired pneumonia: a meta-analysis. Am J Med 2007;120: 783–90.

48. Liu C, Bayer A, Cosgrove SE, et al. Clinical practice guidelines by the Infectious Diseases Society of America for the treatment of methicillin-resistant Staphylococcus aureus infections in adults and children. Clin Infect Dis 2011;52(3): e18–55.

49. Niederman MS, Bass JB Jr, Campbell GD, et al. Guidelines for the initial management of adults with community- acquired pneumonia: diagnosis, assessment of severity, and initial antimicrobial therapy. American Thoracic Society. Medical Section of the American Lung Association. Am Rev Respir Dis 1993;148:1418–26.

50. Siemieniuk RAC, Meade MO, Alonso-Coello P, et al. Corticosteroid therapy for patients hospitalized with community-acquired pneumonia. A systematic review and meta-analysis. Ann Intern Med 2015;163:519–28.

51. Chalmers JD. Corticosteroids for community-acquired pneumonia: a critical view of the evidence. Eur Respir J 2016;48:984–6.

52. Kim SJ, Lee JH, Han B, et al. Effects of hospital-based physical therapy on hospital discharge outcomes among hospitalized older adults with community-acquired pneumonia and declining physical function. Aging Dis 2015;6:174–9.

53. Austrian R, Winston AL. The efficacy of penicillin V (phenoxymethyl- penicillin) in the treatment of mild and of moderately severe pneumococcal pneumonia. Am J Med Sci 1956;232:624–8.

54. Metlay JP, Fine MJ, Schulz R, et al. Measuring symptomatic and functional recovery in patients with community-acquired pneumonia. J Gen Intern Med 1997;12: 423–30.

55. Kaplan V, Clermont G, Griffin MF, et al. Pneumonia: still the old man's friend? Arch Intern Med 2003;163:317–23.

56. Brancati FL, Chow JW, Wagener MM, et al. Is pneumonia really the old man's friend? Two-year prognosis after community-acquired pneumonia. Lancet 1993; 342:30–3.

57. Waterer GW, Kessler LA, Wunderink RG. Medium-term survival after hospitalization with community-acquired pneumonia. Am J Respir Crit Care Med 2004;169: 910–4.

58. Koivula I, Sten M, Makela PH. Prognosis after community-acquired pneumonia in the elderly: a population-based 12-year follow-up study. Arch Intern Med 1999; 159:1550–5.

59. Stoll G, Bendszus M. Inflammation and atherosclerosis: novel insights into plaque formation and destabilization. Stroke 2006;37:1923–32.

60. Cangemi R, Calvieri C, Falcone M, et al. Relation of cardiac complications in the early phase of community-acquired pneumonia to long-term mortality and cardiovascular events. Am J Cardiol 2015;116:647–51.

61. Hadfield J, Bennett L. Determining best outcomes from community-acquired pneumonia and how to achieve them. Respirology 2018;23(2):138–47.

62. National Center for Immunization and Respiratory Diseases. Pneumococcal Vaccine Recommendations. 2017. Available at: https://www.cdc.gov/vaccines/vpd/ pneumo/hcp/recommendations.html. Accessed January 22, 2018.

63. Walters JAE, Qing TN, Poole P, et al. Vaccines for preventing pneumonia in chronic obstructive pulmonary disease. Cochrane Database Syst Rev 2017;(1):CD001390.

The Emergency Department Diagnosis and Management of Urinary Tract Infection

Brit Long, MD[a],*, Alex Koyfman, MD[b]

KEYWORDS

- Urinary tract infection • Cystitis • Pyelonephritis • Sepsis • Obstruction
- Hydronephrosis • Mimic

KEY POINTS

- The evaluation and management of urinary tract infections (UTIs) in the emergency department depend on illness severity, patient hemodynamic status, and underlying comorbidities. A variety of potentially deadly conditions may mimic cystitis or pyelonephritis.
- Dysuria, urinary frequency, and urinary urgency in the absence of vaginitis or cervicitis with vaginal discharge are supportive of UTI.
- Most patients with simple cystitis and pyelonephritis can be treated as outpatients, and the specific antibiotic used depends on the region's antibiogram and diagnosis.
- Urinary testing with urinalysis or urine dipstick is associated with several pitfalls but can be helpful when used appropriately. Urine cultures should be obtained in complicated or upper UTI. Simple and lower tract UTIs do not require urine cultures, unless the patient is pregnant. Asymptomatic bacteriuria should only be treated in specific circumstances; otherwise, it does not require antibiotics.

INTRODUCTION

Urinary tract infection (UTI) is a common condition evaluated and managed in the emergency department (ED). Emergency physicians evaluate a wide spectrum of UTIs, including uncomplicated cystitis, pyelonephritis, and even septic shock. When compared with other hospital or outpatient settings, patients in the ED are often sicker. Emergency physicians are faced with several challenges when managing patients with UTI with limited history, absence of follow-up, lack of culture results, and less ability to care for patients in a longitudinal manner. Patients in the ED may have little to no ability to follow-up.

[a] Department of Emergency Medicine, San Antonio Military Medical Center, 3841 Roger Brooke Drive, Fort Sam Houston, TX 78234, USA; [b] Department of Emergency Medicine, The University of Texas Southwestern Medical Center, 5323 Harry Hines Boulevard, Dallas, TX 75390, USA
* Corresponding author.
E-mail address: Brit.long@yahoo.com

Emerg Med Clin N Am 36 (2018) 685–710
https://doi.org/10.1016/j.emc.2018.06.003
0733-8627/18/Published by Elsevier Inc.
emed.theclinics.com

Emergency physicians are tasked with several decisions. The first is determining if an infection is complicated versus uncomplicated, second is assessing what laboratory and imaging evaluation is necessary, and third is determining the need for antibiotics and patient disposition.[1–4] Potential mimics of UTI should also be considered. This review addresses these factors through a focused evaluation of the literature.

DEFINITIONS

UTIs can be classified by location and the presence of functional or structural abnormalities. This classification is important, because evaluation and treatment depend on accurate assessment. Infection of the bladder defines acute cystitis or lower tract UTI. Pyelonephritis, which most commonly occurs when bacteria ascend to the kidney from the bladder, is the most common presentation of upper UTI.[1–5] Symptoms are typically more severe, although it usually starts as simple cystitis.[1–7] Untreated, pyelonephritis has the potential in some cases to progress to septic shock and death.[8,9]

An uncomplicated UTI, or cystitis, occurs in young, healthy premenopausal women.[1,2,5,6] These women are not pregnant and do not possess structural or functional urinary tract abnormalities.[5–7] Uncomplicated infections of the lower urinary tract are at low risk for treatment failure and are usually not associated with antibiotic-resistant organisms, although resistance rates are continually increasing.[6–8,10–14] All other patients meet criteria for complicated infection, a heterogenous definition (**Box 1**).[8,15] Complicated infections are at risk for drug-resistant organisms and may require further evaluation and more extensive treatment.[3,4]

Epidemiology

UTIs are a common disease: approximately half of women experience one infection during their lifetime.[1–3,16] Premenopausal women demonstrate an incidence of 0.5 to 0.7 cases per person-year in sexually active women.[7,16] UTI risk factors for this population include sexual intercourse, spermicidal use, and prior UTI.[1,2,6,7] Men demonstrate lower rates of UTI, with 5 to 8 UTIs per 10,000 in young and middle-aged men.[17,18] Men older than 50 years, however, demonstrate a higher risk of UTI (20%–50% prevalence) due to prostate enlargement, debilitation, and potential urinary tract instrumentation.[17–19] ED visits approached more than 3 million visits in the United States in 2010, with more than 80% of visits made by women and 50% in patients 18 years to 44 years old.[2,3,20,21] Most of these patients are diagnosed

---

Box 1
Complicated urinary tract infection

- Pyelonephritis/upper UTI
- Male
- Pregnancy
- Anatomic abnormalities (vesicoureteral reflux, stricture, and neurogenic bladder)
- Urolithiasis
- Catheter, stent, or tube present in urinary system
- Malignancy, chemotherapy, and immunosuppression
- Failure of antibiotics
- Hospital/health care–associated UTI

with simple acute cystitis, although pyelonephritis accounts for as much as 13% of UTI ED evaluations.[2,3,6] The annual incidence of pyelonephritis ranges from 459,000 to 1,138,000 patients in the United States.[8,22] Patients presenting to the ED with UTIs are typically sicker; in other settings, pyelonephritis accounts for 1 in 28 cystitis cases.[5,6] Pyelonephritis accounts for up to 4000 deaths in the United States annually.[5,8,23]

The most common pathogen for UTI is *Escherichia coli* (more than 80%), followed by *Staphylococcus saprophyticus*, with rates approaching 15%.[1–5,24] Although these two microbes cause a majority of uncomplicated and complicated UTIs, other gram-negative bacilli, such as *Klebsiella* and *Proteus mirabilis*, and gram-positive bacteria, such as enterococcus and group B streptococcus, can also result in UTI.[25,26] Complicated UTIs, including catheter-associated UTIs, can be caused by a larger range of organisms and are often polymicrobial. *Pseudomonas aeruginosa* and *Enterococcus faecium*, as well as extended-spectrum β-lactamase (ESBL)-producing bacteria, more commonly result in complicated infection.[2,3,7,25,26] Prevalence of resistance to fluoroquinolones is increasing for uncomplicated and complicated pyelonephritis, 6.3% and 19.9%, respectively; and the prevalence of ESBL bacteria is also concerning in uncomplicated and complicated pyelonephritis, 2.6% and 12.2%, respectively.[27] Infection due to *S aureus* is more likely due to bacteremic seeding of the urogenital tract from another source.[2,3] Other populations, such as young men and women with vaginal discharge, pruritus, or other pelvic complaints, may be due to sexually transmitted infection (STI) or uropathogenic *E coli*.[4–7] Elderly men with history of urinary obstruction have greater risk of polymicrobial infection and resistant organisms.[3,8,15,19]

HISTORY AND EXAMINATION IN THE EMERGENCY DEPARTMENT

When a patient with concern or suspicion for UTI presents to the ED, several key questions should be asked. First, does the patient require resuscitation due to hemodynamic instability from sepsis? Second, are the symptoms or presentation due to a UTI, or is a mimic present? If it is a UTI, is it simple or complicated and lower or upper? Is the patient pregnant, and could this be a STI? What antimicrobial should be used if it is a UTI? Finally, what is the appropriate disposition?[3]

The type of UTI and location of infection often determine patient signs and symptoms, although history and examination are not 100% reliable in every patient.[3,6,28,29] Patients with acute, uncomplicated cystitis typically experience dysuria, urinary frequency, and urinary urgency.[28,29] Although these are the classic findings in UTI, they are by no means definitive for UTI. As discussed previously, these patients are typically premenopausal nonpregnant women.[1–5,28,29] Unfortunately, these symptoms can also occur with STI, vaginitis, and chemical or allergic irritant exposure, although UTI typically is not associated with vaginal discharge.[3,6,7] No one specific history or physical examination finding can rule in or rule out UTI. Specificity is 60% for frequency, 78% to 88% for urgency, 52% to 58% for dysuria, and 69% to 91% for fever.[28] Dysuria, frequency, and hematuria, however, increase the probability of simple UTI.[2,3,28,29] The absence of symptoms of vaginitis or cervicitis (vaginal bleeding, discharge, and irritation) and presence of dysuria increase the likelihood of UTI more than 90%, with positive likelihood ratio (LR) over 24.[29] Importantly, self-diagnosis of UTI carries a positive LR of 4.[29]

Differentiating lower tract UTI and upper tract UTI is predominantly clinical, based on history and examination. Close evaluation of a patient's hemodynamic status may lead to clues of systemic toxicity and diagnosis of sepsis.[3,5,6,8] Diagnosing pyelonephritis in a patient with fever, flank pain, and other urinary symptoms is straightforward.[8,28,29] Many patients with lower tract UTI, however, may also describe vague back/flank pain or subjective fever. Patients with symptoms for more than 7 days, with history of recurrent UTI, or who have failed prior UTI therapy; men; and patients with complicating factors (diabetes, immunosuppression, elderly, and pregnancy) require consideration of pyelonephritis and longer duration of treatment.[3,8,30] If a patient fails a shorter course antibiotic therapy for simple cystitis, a diagnosis of pyelonephritis requiring further treatment is recommended. Pyelonephritis often presents with fevers, chills, nausea/vomiting, and flank pain with lower tract symptoms.[3,8,31] Patients may also describe pain in other regions, such as the abdomen, and this is more common in patients who present atypically (elderly and immunocompromised). Fever is often present in pyelonephritis at some point in the disease course.[8,31] Up to 20% of patients with pyelonephritis, however, do not have urinary symptoms, and clinical presentation and disease severity can vary significantly.[32,33] Patients lacking fever more commonly have another condition, such as pelvic inflammatory disease (PID), diverticulitis, or cholecystitis.[3] Elderly patients are more commonly afebrile, are unable to describe symptoms, may present with pain in other locations, and may demonstrate altered mental status or weakness. A genitourinary examination should be considered in women with vaginal complaints (discharge) and men with suspected UTI as well as close abdominal and back examination for potential UTI mimics.

LABORATORY EVALUATION

Definitive diagnosis of UTI includes urine culture displaying significant numbers of bacteria. However, urine cultures are not routinely performed in the ED. When urine cultures are obtained, results are not readily available. In the ED, lower UTI is a clinical diagnosis, and urinary testing may not be required if the patient meets criteria for uncomplicated cystitis.[2–4] Urine testing can be helpful in specific situations, especially in intermediate-risk patients.

Traditionally, urine is obtained for testing in the appropriate clinical setting. The bladder and urine within the bladder are normally sterile. Several options are available for urine collection: clean-catch midstream sample, suprapubic aspiration, and urethral catheterization.[2–4,34] The most common means is clean-catch midstream specimen, although this may be difficult to obtain in pediatric and elderly patients.[34–36] For midstream collection, surrounding areas are typically appropriately cleansed.[34–36] One study, however, found contamination rates were similar between those with and without cleansing.[37] Collection of midstream urine with or without cleansing produces a reasonable specimen. Catheterization may be required for ill or immobilized patients. Once urine is collected, it should be analyzed as quickly as possible, because a delay of more than 2 hours can result in unreliable results, and, if it cannot be analyzed quickly, the specimen should be refrigerated.[3,34–36]

Urine cultures are usually not available at the time of ED evaluation, and other urinary assessments can be used to assist in diagnosis, including urinary dipstick, microscopic examination, and urine flow cytometry.[2,3] The definition of UTI varies, however, limiting routine use of several methods. Pyuria is the presence of whole or lysed white blood cells (WBCs) in the urine and is one of the most reliable signs of UTI.[38–40] An abnormal result is greater than 10 WBCs/mm^3 in an unspun voided midstream urine sample, which occurs in approximately 96% of patients with UTI.[38,40] A centrifuged urinalysis demonstrating 2 WBCs/mm^3 to 5 WBCs/mm^3 or greater than or equal to 15 bacteria per high-power field (HPF) suggests UTI.[39] WBC casts are evidence of pyelonephritis, and hematuria is also helpful, because hematuria is typically absent in urethritis and vaginitis.[40]

The most prevalent means for diagnosing a UTI is by way of urine dipstick, as it is inexpensive and convenient, and this test possesses sensitivity and specificity similar to microscopic urinalysis.[41,42] Dipsticks are reagent strips that can detect leukocyte esterase (LE) and nitrite.[40] LE reflects pyuria and is released by leukocytes, typically in the setting of greater than 10 WBCs per HPF.[40,43,44] To properly evaluate for pyuria, the dipstick requires 30 seconds to 1 minute of urine contact. LE displays sensitivity of 75% to 96% and specificity of 94% to 98% for UTI diagnosis.[29,40,41,43] False-positive results occur with contaminated specimens, trichomonas infection, and drugs or food that color urine red. False-negative results occur with intercurrent or recent antibiotic therapy, glycosuria, proteinuria, high urine-specific gravity, and low bacteria counts.[40]

Nitrites are evidence of the presence of Enterobacteriaceae, which convert urine nitrates to nitrite.[40,44,45] A positive test is extremely specific but not sensitive.[45,46] More than 10,000 bacteria/mL urine are required to result in a positive nitrite test.[40,45,46] Unfortunately, the nitrite dipstick reagent strip is sensitive to air. After 1 week of exposure to air, up to one-third of strips provide a false-positive result, which increases to three-fourths at 2 weeks.[40,47] Nitrite testing possesses a sensitivity of 35% to 85% and specificity of 95% for UTI diagnosis.[44,48] Although specific, sensitivity is poor, because S saprophyticus and enterococcus do not reduce nitrate to nitrite, and certain drugs and food that result in red urine can also result in false-negative tests.[44,49] The test also requires time for urinary incubation within the bladder. The combination of LE and nitrite results in a sensitivity of 75% to 90% and specificity approaching 100%.[48] Results of this test display several limitations. A history strongly suggestive of UTI, even in the setting of negative LE and nitrite, may require treatment.[7,44] A positive LE or nitrite test without symptoms, however, does not necessarily require antibiotics.[44] Several pitfalls can exist in the interpretation of urine dipstick results (Table 1).

Urine cultures provide the definitive diagnosis of UTI, with greater than or equal to 10^5 colony-forming units (CFUs)/mL of bacteria or 10^2 CFUs/mL in the presence of symptoms considered diagnostic.[6,7,44] Urine cultures for uncomplicated cystitis are not recommended.[6,7] On a routine basis, urine cultures provide little diagnostic utility in the ED. Pretreatment urine cultures in this patient population are not cost effective, do not predict treatment outcomes, and do not affect patient management.[35,36,52,53] One prospective, double-blind, randomized placebo-controlled trial evaluated women ages 16 years to 50 years with dysuria and frequency but negative urine dipstick for LE and nitrites.[36] Women receiving antibiotics reported complete resolution of dysuria in 76% of patients compared with 26% of the placebo arm. By day 7, more than 90% of women receiving antibiotics experienced symptom resolution versus 59% in the placebo group.[54] Patients not improving with standard antimicrobial therapy, however, require urine culture. Urine cultures are recommended for patients with complicated UTI, pyelonephritis, and recent antimicrobial therapy.[3,6,7]

If urine cultures are obtained in the ED, a system should be in place for following results and ensuring that results are sent to the physician actively caring for a patient.[3,6] If a culture result suggests resistance to the prescribed antibiotic, the patient should be contacted. Patients with improved symptoms may not need a different antimicrobial. This is in part due to high urinary antibiotic concentrations, which may result in clinical cure despite in vitro resistance. If symptoms have not improved, a different treatment should be provided.

Table 1
Pitfalls in urinary tract infection diagnosis using urine dipstick

Pitfall	Explanation
Cloudy and smelly urine = UTI	Odor and degree of transparency are not reliable in diagnosis of UTI. Diet, urine crystals, hydration status, and other factors affect urine appearance and smell.[37,47–49]
Squamous cells are present = contamination	SECs are poor markers of urine culture contamination.[50,51] One study evaluated a quantitative threshold of SECs.[50] In this study, samples with fewer than 8 SECs/low-power field demonstrated greater ability to predict bacteriuria on urinalysis, but SECs did not accurately identify contaminated urine.[50]
Positive LE or pyuria = UTI	Positive LE demonstrates sensitivity 80%–90% and specificity 95%–98% for pyuria. WBC counts 6–10 cells/mL occur with dehydration, oliguria, or anuria. Contamination, interstitial nephritis, nephrolithiasis, tumor, interstitial cystitis, intraabdominal pathology, and atypical organisms cause pyuria.[38,41,46]
Positive nitrites in UA = UTI	The test does have high specificity (95%) for gram-negative bacteriuria, but it cannot be used alone and may be negative with insufficient urine dwell time in the bladder or in infection with organisms unable to convert nitrate to nitrite.[37,41,45,49]

Abbreviations: LPF, low power field; UA, urinalysis; SEC, squamous epithelial cell.

Blood cultures are advised for only certain situations. They are not recommended for uncomplicated cystitis.[3,6,7] In pyelonephritis, blood cultures do not usually change management, although bacteremia can be present in up to 40% of patients with pyelonephritis.[55–60] Blood and urine cultures are concordant in up to 97% of nonpregnant adult women with simple pyelonephritis.[58] In 1 study evaluating nonpregnant patients with simple and complicated cases of pyelonephritis, 23% of patients had positive blood cultures; of these, only 2 were discordant with urine culture results and did not affect management.[61] Several other studies suggest that blood culture results do not affect management in patients with pyelonephritis.[55,62] Blood cultures are most commonly positive in patients with severe illness, immunocompromised state, those with urinary tract obstruction, and patients greater than 65 years old.[8,58,63] In severe sepsis or septic shock, blood cultures may be positive in up to 42% of patients, with an odds ratio of 4.76 (95% CI, 1.43–15.84).[60]

IMAGING

Most patients with uncomplicated and complicated UTIs do not require imaging in an ED, although no formal guidelines for imaging are present. Imaging may assist in patients where diagnostic uncertainty exists, those with toxic appearance and hemodynamic instability, those with suspected urolithiasis with UTI, and those who have failed therapy or have recurrent infection.[3,8] In the setting of septic shock, imaging to further determine the source of infection may be needed, because source control is a key element in sepsis management.[3,8,64] One recent study evaluated a clinical prediction rule for use of radiologic imaging consisting of urine pH greater than 7.0, history of urolithiasis, and/or renal insufficiency in patients with febrile UTI, which led to a reduction in imaging tests by 40%.[64] Imaging modalities include abdominal radiograph, ultrasound (US), and CT.[64] Plain film radiography demonstrates lower sensitivity for complication and is typically not used.[3,6,65–68] A standard kidneys, ureter, and bladder view has a sensitivity of 45% to 59% and specificity approaching 77% for detection of renal pathology.[65–69] US is a valuable examination in unstable patients who may not tolerate CT. It is rapidly available, is not associated with radiation, and is cost-effective.[68–72] It can demonstrate hydronephrosis, abscess, and hydroureter,[71,73] with sensitivity approaching 80% and specificity 73% for hydronephrosis.[68–73] Evidence of hydronephrosis on US in the setting of UTI requires further evaluation for obstruction.[70–72] The most sensitive test for renal pathology is CT, however, which provides information on the presence of anatomic complications (calculi), hydroureter, gas, and abscess. If air is present on CT, emphysematous pyelonephritis should be considered, which is lethal.[3,65,69] Renal artery or vein occlusion due to embolus or thrombus requires IV contrast. Any concern for severe renal pathology or UTI mimic warrants imaging, often with CT.[65,69,72–76]

URINARY TRACT INFECTION MANAGEMENT

Treatment depends on patient comorbidities, diagnosis, and hemodynamic status. Although up to 42% of infections may resolve on their own, antibiotics are typically recommended.[3,4,6,7] Antibiotic therapy must be individualized and selected based on patient diagnosis, medication allergies, compliance history, cost, availability, and local antibiograms (E coli and Klebsiella continue to demonstrate increasing resistance to beta lactam antibiotics and fluoroquinolones) (**Table 2**).[3,4,6,7,25,27] One of the most important considerations is the institutional/regional antibiogram. If treating pyelonephritis, fosfomycin and nitrofurantoin are not recommended, because they concentrate in the bladder and not the kidneys.[3,4,6,7] Fluoroquinolone resistance is increasing,[25,27,77,78] and in regions with greater than 10% resistance to fluoroquinolones, a long-acting parenteral cephalosporin is recommended in the ED.[6,7] Resistance to trimethoprim/sulfamethoxazole is also increasing.[77,78] In areas of the United States with high prevalence of ESBLs and severe sepsis or septic shock with UTI, empiric treatment with a carbapenem is recommended.[25,27,77,78] Ceftazidime/avibactam and ceftolozane/tazobactam are two recently approved agents for use in anticipated resistant Pseudomonas infection or carbapenem resistance.[2] Patients with hemodynamic instability and concern for sepsis from UTI require intravenous (IV) fluids and potentially vasopressors if the patient is unresponsive to IV fluids.[8,9,79] Evaluation for urinary obstruction in a patient with septic shock is necessary, because close to 10% of patients with septic shock due to urinary source have an associated obstruction, necessitating emergent urologic intervention.[8,9,79]

Source control is also vital in patients with sepsis from a urinary source. Hydronephrosis and obstruction due to a urinary source require percutaneous or endourologic drainage.[3] Renal abscess may warrant drainage if a patient is unstable or if an abscess is large enough. Emphysematous pyelonephritis, although rare, requires immediate surgery for partial or total nephrectomy.[3,4,80,81]

CLINICAL MIMICS AND EMERGENCY DEPARTMENT APPROACH

Given the multitude of signs and symptoms associated with upper and lower UTIs, maintaining a broad differential diagnosis is necessary. There are a significant number of potentially dangerous mimics for lower UTIs and upper UTIs (**Table 3**). Nonemergent diagnoses include bladder carcinoma, varicella zoster, bladder calculi, overactive bladder, endometriosis, interstitial cystitis, pelvic congestion syndrome,

Table 2			
Antibiotic therapy for urinary tract infection			
Diagnosis	**Antibiotic**	**Dosing/Delivery Route**	**Therapy Duration**
Acute uncomplicated cystitis	Nitrofurantoin	100 mg PO twice daily	5 d
	TMP/SMX[a]	1 DS tablet (160/800 mg) PO twice daily	3 d
	Fosfomycin trometamol	3 g PO	Once
	Cefpodoxime	100 mg PO twice daily	3–7 d
	Cephalexin	500 mg PO twice daily	3–7 d
	Cefuroxime	250 mg PO twice daily	3–7 d
Acute complicated cystitis	Ciprofloxacin[a]	500 mg PO twice daily or 1000 mg XR once daily	7 d
	Levofloxacin[a]	750 mg IV/PO once daily	Once
	TMP/SMX	1 DS tablet (160/800 mg) PO twice daily	5 d
	Cefepime	2 g IV twice daily	3 d
	Ampicillin and centamicin	Ampicillin, 1 g IV 4× daily, and gentamicin, 5–7 mg/kg/d IV	Transition to PO medication once able
	Imipenem/cilastatin	500 mg IV 4× daily (reserve for suspected ESBL)	Transition to PO medication once able
Pyelonephritis—outpatient	TMP/SMX[a]	1 DS tablet (160/800 mg) PO twice daily	14 d
	Ciprofloxacin[a]	500 mg PO twice daily or 1000 mg XR once daily	7 d
	Levofloxacin[a]	750 mg PO once daily	5 d
	Cephalexin	500 mg PO 3× daily	10–14 d
	Amoxicillin-clavulanate	875 mg/125 mg PO 3× daily	10–14 d
	Cefixime	400 mg PO once daily	10–14 d
	Cefpodoxime	200 mg PO twice daily	10–14 d
Pyelonephritis—inpatient	*Not suspecting enterococcus:*		Switch to PO therapy when able
	Ceftriaxone	1 g IV once daily	
	Ciprofloxacin[a]	400 mg IV twice daily	
	Levofloxacin[a]	750 mg IV once daily	
	Cefepime	1 g IV 3× daily	
	Imipenem	500 mg IV 4× daily	
	Aztreonam	2 g IV 3× daily	
	Suspecting enterococcus:		
	Ampicillin and gentamicin	Ampicillin, 2 g IV 4× daily, and gentamicin, 1 mg/kg IV 3× daily	
	Piperacillin/tazobactam	4.5 g IV 3× daily	
	Ampicillin/sulbactam	3 g IV 4× daily	

Abbreviations: DS, double-strength; TMP/SMX, trimethoprim/sulfamethoxazole; XR, extended release.

[a] If local resistance to a fluoroquinolone is greater than 10%, then an initial IV dose of a long-acting parenteral antimicrobial agent should be administered (1 g ceftriaxone or a 24-h consolidated dose of an aminoglycoside). TMP/SMX should be avoided if local resistance greater than 20% or prescribed for UTI in the previous 3 mo. TMP/-SMX DS tablets may be utilized twice daily for 14 d, however not in cases of enterococcal or pseudomonal infection.

Data from Refs.[2–7]

Table 3
Urinary tract infection mimics requiring emergency department intervention

Diagnosis	Presentation/Evaluation	Management
Abdominal aortic aneurysm[82]	• Often asymptomatic until time of rupture. • Insidious presentation, including weeks of progressive back pain (slow leak) vs sudden severe abdominal, flank, or back pain with or without hypotension or syncope. • Rare presentations: massive GI bleeding (aortoenteric fistula), hemorrhagic shock (rupture into the peritoneum), high-output heart failure (aortocaval fistula), or femoral neuropathy (secondary to aneurysmal rupture and enlarging hematoma). • Risk factors: hypertension, smoking, male gender, white ethnicity, age >60, and disease occurring in a primary relative. • Symptomatic or clinically unstable patient: bedside US (95%–100% sensitive, 100% specific), type and cross. • Stable patient: CT	• Symptomatic or unstable patient: consult vascular surgery and transfuse blood products. • Emergent surgery for rupture: mortality 34%–85%. • Stable patient: abdominal aorta >3 cm requires referral and surveillance by US or CT every 6–12 mo. Consult vascular surgery for aneurysms ≥5 cm; annual risk of rupture 25%–40%.

Cholecystitis[83,84]	• Patients often experience right upper quadrant or midepigastric pain and nausea; may report fever and pain radiating to the flanks.
	• Diagnosis is clinical: history, physical examination, and US findings.
	  ○ Risk factors: oral contraceptives or estrogen replacement therapy, diseases of the terminal ileum, cirrhosis, hemolytic diseases, pregnancy, obesity, and TPN.
	• Physical examination findings: Murphy sign (positive LR: 2.8; 95% CI, 0.8–8.62).
	• US (sensitivity 95%, specificity 98%): sonographic Murphy sign, pericholecystic fluid, gallstones/biliary sludge, gallbladder wall thickening >3 mm.
	• Laboratory evaluation: CBC often demonstrates leukocytosis, and LFTs may be elevated.
		• Initiate antibiotic therapy:
		  ○ Mildly ill: ciprofloxacin, 400 mg IV, and metronidazole, 500 mg IV.
		  ○ Critically ill: vancomycin, 20 mg/kg (up to 2 g) IV, and piperacillin/tazobactam, 4.5 g IV, or carbapenem.
		• Consult general surgery.
		• Diabetes is a risk factor for emphysematous cholecystitis. If diagnosed, initiate antibiotic therapy directed against gram-negative rods and anaerobes, and consult surgery.

(continued on next page)

Table 3
(continued)

Diagnosis	Presentation/Evaluation	Management
Spinal epidural abscess[85]	• Spinal epidural abscess may present with back pain in addition to fever, myalgias, and focal neurologic deficit. • Hematogenous spread of infection is most common (*S aureus* indicated in 60%–90% of cases). • Frequently localized to the thoracic spine in adults (50%–80% of cases). • Risk factors: spinal surgeries, lumbar punctures, trauma, advanced age, pregnancy, sickle cell disease, IV drug abuse, diabetes, and immunosuppression. • Laboratory studies: CBC (nonspecific, leukocytosis may be absent), ESR (commonly elevated; may be falsely low in the setting of hyperglycemia, systemic corticosteroid therapy, and high-dose aspirin therapy), CRP (frequently elevated), and blood cultures. • Imaging: MR imaging of the whole spine with and without contrast.	• Initiate broad-spectrum antibiotic therapy. • Consult neurosurgery for further treatment.
Urolithiasis[86,87]	• Patients may report severe, waxing, and waning pain localized to the flanks or back with radiation to the abdomen, inguinal area, or groin. • Risk factors: inflammatory bowel disease, bariatric surgery, hyperparathyroidism, renal tubular acidosis, gout, and diabetes. • History should include an inquiry regarding the aforementioned risk factors and medications related to stone formation. • Physical examination: assess for signs of sepsis, which may indicate concomitant infection. • Laboratory analysis: β-hCG for women, urinalysis, CBC (WBCs may be elevated), renal function (assess for renal injury). • Imaging: noncontrast helical CT is the gold standard (95%–100% sensitivity, 94%–96% specificity). Consider US in pregnant women (19% sensitivity, limited because only observational data, eg, hydronephrosis, may be obtained).	• Calculi ≤5 mm have a 70%–90% chance of passing; those 5–10 mm <50% chance of passing. • Patients without concomitant infection, signs of obstruction, or inherent renal pathology: consult urology for follow-up. Discharge with medical expulsive therapy (tamsulosin) of stones >5 mm, pain control, and antiemetic as needed. • Patients with renal calculi >5 mm, signs consistent with obstruction, renal injury, concomitant infection, or pregnant patients with calculi: consult urology. • Initiate antibiotic therapy in the setting of infection.

| Pneumonia[88,89] | • Predominant clinical findings include cough, dyspnea, sputum production, and fever. May report flank pain (secondary to lower lobe pathology).
• Common pathogens: *S pneumoniae*, nontypeable strains of *Haemophilus influenzae*, and *Moraxella catarrhalis*; *Mycoplasma pneumoniae* frequent in adolescents and young adults.
• If recent dental procedures, seizures, alcoholism, or loss of consciousness, suspect anaerobic pathogens.
• Risk factors: congestive heart failure, diabetes, alcoholism, COPD, and HIV.
• History: inquire as to IV antibiotic utilization in the previous 90 d (risk factor for hospital acquired pneumonia).
• Physical examination: evaluate for evidence of sepsis and hemodynamic instability.
• Laboratory evaluation: blood cultures for all patients who are clinically ill and in whom a diagnosis of sepsis is suspected; serology ([*Pneumocystis jirovecii*, etc.] or urine antigens [*Legionella*]) as appropriate.
• Imaging: chest radiograph; US may assist. | • Patients may be appropriate for discharge based on hemodynamic status, functional status, and clinical scoring with antibiotics.
• Clinically ill patients: initiate early goal-directed therapy: broad-spectrum antibiotics and fluid resuscitation and admit |
| PE[90] | • Patients with PE often present with dyspnea, tachypnea, and pleuritic chest pain, which may radiate to the flanks or abdomen.
• Temperature >38°C may be found.
• Evaluation: history and examination and risk-stratification.
• Bedside echocardiography may be used for rapid triage in the unstable patient (evidence of right ventricular strain).
• ECG and chest radiography commonly nonspecific.
• Utilize D-dimer and PERC criteria as appropriate.
• Imaging: CT pulmonary angiography remains the gold standard for diagnosis. | • Anticoagulate as indicated. |

(continued on next page)

Table 3
(continued)

Diagnosis	Presentation/Evaluation	Management
Thromboembolic renovascular disease[91,92]	• Thromboembolic renovascular disease (renal artery thrombosis, renal vein thrombosis, or renal artery embolism) may present with flank pain. • Flank pain or pain radiating to the groin is present in 90% of patients with radiographically diagnosed renal artery embolism. • Renal vein thrombosis may be confused for pyelonephritis. • Risk factors for renal artery embolism: atrial fibrillation, cardiac thrombus after infarction, atrial myxoma, endocarditis, and paradoxic emboli. • Risk factors for renal artery thrombosis: renal artery atherosclerosis, renal artery or aortic dissection, renal artery or aortic aneurysms, trauma, hypercoagulable disorders, and malignancy. • Risk factor for renal vein thrombosis: nephrotic syndrome. • Men with renal vein thrombosis may present with left-sided hydrocele. Patients with renal artery embolism or thrombosis may demonstrate hypertensive emergency. • Laboratory evaluation: renal vein thrombosis may have leukocytosis. Renal artery or vein pathology may have variable renal function. Acute kidney injury to acute renal failure. • Urinalysis: hematuria in up to 72% of cases of renal artery embolism. • Imaging: CT angiogram for renal artery thrombus, with venography for renal vein thrombus.	• Consult vascular surgery. • Renal artery embolism or thrombosis: endovascular thrombolysis vs angioplasty or stenting. • Renal vein thrombosis: systemic anticoagulation vs catheter-directed thrombolytic therapy. • 30-d mortality in patients presenting with renal artery embolism secondary to atrial fibrillation: 10%–13%.
Appendicitis[93,94]	• Lifetime risk of appendicitis is 8.6% in men and 6.7% in women. • 50%–60% of adolescent and adult patients with appendicitis report periumbilical pain migrating to the right lower quadrant. This presentation is rare in elderly patients (15%–30%). • Patients with signs/symptoms suggestive of peritonitis: immediate surgical consult. • Laboratory studies: leukocytosis and elevated acute-phase inflammatory markers common but not definitive. • Imaging: IV contrast CT considered the imaging study of choice (94% sensitivity, 95% specificity). US (86% sensitivity and 81% specificity) and MR imaging (pediatric patients, pregnant women) may be used for definitive diagnosis.	• Fluid resuscitation, IV antibiotics, and surgical consultation.

Condition	Clinical Features	Management
Diverticulitis[95,96]	• Diverticulitis and diverticular abscess may present with lower quadrant pain associated with fever, nausea, emesis, and diarrhea. • Laboratory evaluation: CBC (leukocytosis common), UA may have sterile pyuria. • Imaging: systemically ill patient with concern for complicated diverticulitis (requiring surgical evaluation and management) or those who are immunosuppressed, have numerous medical comorbidities or are elderly: CT with IV contrast approaches 100% sensitivity. • Uncomplicated diverticulitis: patients with a history of diverticular disease or diverticulitis who are not systemically ill may not require imaging.	• Uncomplicated diverticulitis: patients who are PO tolerant may be discharged home with antibiotic therapy. Failure to respond to outpatient therapy within 48–72 h: consider repeat investigation for alternative diagnoses or surgical consultation. • Complicated diverticulitis: fluid resuscitation, parenteral antibiotic therapy, and surgical consultation with consideration for interventional radiology if localized abscess.
Ectopic pregnancy[97]	• Currently accounts for 2% of pregnancies in the United States. • Suspect in women of childbearing age presenting with amenorrhea and abdominal pain, with or without vaginal bleeding. • Signs of rupture and subsequent hemorrhage: hypotension with or without syncope. • Risk factors: PID, endometriosis, infertility treatments, previous tubal procedures, previous ectopic pregnancy, and multiple sexual partners. • Physical examination: pelvic examination to assess cervical os. Bimanual examination reveals adnexal tenderness or mass in 50% of cases. • Laboratory evaluation: serum β-hCG level, perform CBC with type and screen or type and cross as appropriate. • Imaging: transvaginal US. US expected to demonstrates signs consistent with pregnancy (gestational sac and yolk sac) at serum β-hCG levels >2000 mIU/mL.	• Emergent obstetric consultation for all patients with an identified ectopic pregnancy. • Patients with US absent findings: obstetric follow-up in 1–7 d with repeat serum β-hCG and repeat US; considered an ectopic pregnancy until proved otherwise. • Rhesus factor negative patients experiencing bleeding during pregnancy require RhoGAM administration.
Epididymitis/orchitis[98,99]	• Patients frequently report pain and swelling of the scrotum. Pain frequently radiates to the groin and suprapubic area. • Epididymitis may occur secondary to bacterial infection (Pseudomonas or coliform species in men >age 35), STI, or rarely with trauma. Mumps: spread of hematogenous infection or viral infection (mumps in 20%). Pyogenic form may occur due to E coli, Klebsiella, P aeruginosa, staphylococci, or streptococci. • Physical examination: tenderness with palpation of the posterior aspect of the scrotum. Hydrocele may occur secondary to secretion of inflammatory fluid between the layers of the tunica vaginalis. Orchitis often presents with unilateral pain, though pyogenic causes associated with systemic illness. • Laboratory evaluation: UA and STI laboratory tests. • Imaging: color-flow Doppler US useful for the differential diagnosis of complicated cases.	• Epididymitis: initiate antibiotic therapy as appropriate. Complications: testicular infarction, abscess, or pyocele of the scrotum. • Orchitis: bacterial orchitis should receive antibiotic therapy. Viral orchitis resolves in 4–5 d (mild cases) to 3 wk (severe cases).

(continued on next page)

Table 3
(continued)

Diagnosis	Presentation/Evaluation	Management
Ovarian torsion[100,101]	• Women with ovarian torsion present with severe lower abdominal pain with or without nausea and emesis. • Risk factors: infertility therapy, pregnancy, and history of ovarian cysts. • Physical examination: 50%–90% of patients display a tender adnexal mass or adnexal fullness on examination. • Imaging: transvaginal US should be used for evaluation. The most consistent finding indicating torsion is a unilaterally enlarged ovary; however, up to 50% of patients may have a normal US. The presence or absence of arterial and venous Doppler flow does not exclude the diagnosis.	• Surgical emergency: consult gynecology as soon as the diagnosis is suspected.
Testicular torsion[102]	• Sudden onset of testicular pain without fever or urinary symptoms. Pain may radiate to the groin or suprapubic region. • Intravaginal torsion (malrotation of the spermatic cord within the tunica vaginalis) occurs in 90% of cases. • Physical examination may include a firm, high-riding testis with horizontal lie, and absent cremasteric reflex. • Imaging: US may demonstrate absent/decreased testicular blood flow.	• Consult urology. • Perform manual detorsion (external rotation of testis toward the thigh) without delay if clinical diagnosis apparent. • 80% testicular salvage if detorsion occurs within 6–12 h of onset.

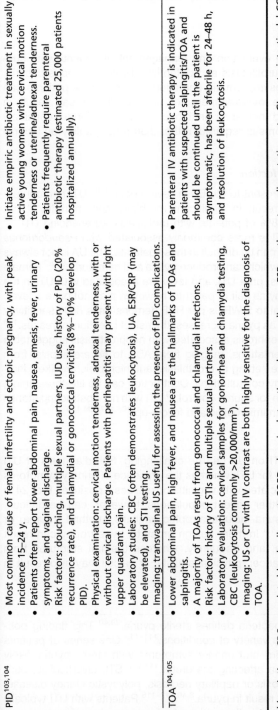

PID[103,104]	• Most common cause of female infertility and ectopic pregnancy, with peak incidence 15–24 y. • Patients often report lower abdominal pain, nausea, emesis, fever, urinary symptoms, and vaginal discharge. • Risk factors: douching, multiple sexual partners, IUD use, history of PID (20% recurrence rate), and chlamydial or gonococcal cervicitis (8%–10% develop PID). • Physical examination: cervical motion tenderness, adnexal tenderness, with or without cervical discharge. Patients with perihepatitis may present with right upper quadrant pain. • Laboratory studies: CBC (often demonstrates leukocytosis), UA, ESR/CRP (may be elevated), and STI testing. • Imaging: transvaginal US useful for assessing the presence of PID complications.	• Initiate empiric antibiotic treatment in sexually active young women with cervical motion tenderness or uterine/adnexal tenderness. • Patients frequently require parenteral antibiotic therapy (estimated 25,000 patients hospitalized annually).
TOA[104,105]	• Lower abdominal pain, high fever, and nausea are the hallmarks of TOAs and salpingitis. • A majority of TOAs result from gonococcal and chlamydial infections. • Risk factors: history of STIs and multiple sexual partners. • Laboratory evaluation: cervical samples for gonorrhea and chlamydia testing, CBC (leukocytosis commonly >20,000/mm³). • Imaging: US or CT with IV contrast are both highly sensitive for the diagnosis of TOA.	• Parenteral IV antibiotic therapy is indicated in patients with suspected salpingitis/TOA and should be continued until the patient is asymptomatic, has been afebrile for 24–48 h, and resolution of leukocytosis.

Abbreviations: CBC, complete blood cell count; COPD, chronic obstructive pulmonary disease; ESR, erythrocyte sedimentation rate; GI, gastrointestinal; hCG, human chorionic gonadotropin; LFT, liver function test; PE, pulmonary embolism; PERC, Pulmonary Embolism Rule-out Criteria; TOA, tubo-ovarian abscess; TPN, total parenteral nutrition; UA, urinalysis.

nonvenereal vulvovaginitis, prostadynia, and vulvodynia, which are not further explored in this article. These conditions may be managed in the outpatient setting.

SPECIAL POPULATIONS

Other important aspects in the evaluation and management of patients with suspected UTI include those with urolithiasis and potential UTI, noninfectious dysuria, sterile pyuria, and those with asymptomatic bacteriuria (ASB). These patients can produce a quandary, because overtreatment for suspected UTI can result in adverse medication events and increased antibiotic resistance. Careful consideration of the patient and symptoms is required, rather than relying solely on laboratory assessment.

Urolithiasis and Urinary Tract Infection

Patients with urolithiasis often present to the ED in severe pain.[86,87] UTI can complicate this condition and may result in significant morbidity and mortality if not adequately treated, with up to 8% of patients with urolithiasis experiencing UTI.[106] In the setting of urolithiasis, UTI is more commonly associated with *Pseudomonas* or *Proteus*.[3,107] Diagnosis of UTI can be difficult in these patients. The UA is not always easily interpreted in urolithiasis, which can produce pyuria and hematuria.[86,87] Female gender, dysuria, frequency, chills, prior UTI, and fever are associated with UTI in the setting of urolithiasis.[106] As many as half of patients, however, may not have a fever. Pyuria with greater than or equal to 5 WBCs per HPF demonstrates 86% sensitivity and 79% specificity for UTI and, as pyuria increases, the risk of infection increases.[106] One study of patients with pyonephrosis associated with nephrolithiasis suggested a wide spectrum of clinical presentations, ranging from ASB to severe sepsis, from UTI.[108] If UTI is suspected in the setting of urolithiasis, antimicrobials are likely indicated in conjunction with urology consultation.[3] Obstruction can be life-threatening, warranting emergent intervention for source control.[79] UTI with nonobstructing stones can be treated with outpatient antimicrobials and follow-up.[106,107,109,110]

Noninfectious Dysuria

Dysuria without evidence of UTI on UA can be challenging. Self-diagnosis of UTI demonstrates a positive LR of 4 for UTI, whereas the presence of urinary symptoms and absence of symptoms associated with vaginitis possesses a positive LR of 24 in reproductive-aged women.[29] Other patient populations, however, can be difficult. Etiologies of noninfectious dysuria include atrophic vaginitis, urethral trauma, or reaction to hygiene products.[2–4,6] In men, benign prostatic hypertrophy can result in urethral obstruction, dysuria, and frequency, whereas urethral strictures from STI, urethral instrumentation, cancer, physical activity, or calculi may also result in dysuria.[2,3]

Sterile Pyuria

Urinalysis with WBCs and no bacteria defines sterile pyuria.[29,40] This finding possesses a wide differential with a variety of conditions.[111–115] One series of patients with appendicitis found one-third had urinary symptoms with sterile pyuria, likely due to appendiceal inflammation affecting the ureter.[111,112] STI, diverticulitis, perinephric abscess, renal tuberculosis or papillary necrosis, polycystic kidney disease, nephropathy, and nephritis may result in pyuria.[3,40,113–115] Patients with UTI typically demonstrate bacteriuria with pyuria in the setting of urinary symptoms.[44]

Urinary Tract Infection and Sexually Transmitted Infection

Differentiating UTI and STI can be difficult, as these conditions are common in reproductive-aged healthy patients.[2–4] A genitourinary examination may be needed for further differentiation and specimen collection. One cross-sectional study of sexually active women found a prevalence of 17% for UTI, 33% for STI, and 4% for both.[116] Urinary symptoms in this population did not predict STI.[116] Another study, however, found an incidence of 9% for STI compared with 57% for UTI.[117] UTI and STI can overlap with symptoms, including dysuria, although UTI is typically not associated with vaginal discharge as with STI.[3,28,29] STI typically presents with more gradual onset of symptoms, vaginal discharge/bleeding, lower abdominal pain, pruritis, dyspareunia, external dysuria, new sexual partner, and no change in frequency or urgency.[118] *Chlamydia trachomatis* and *Neisseria gonorrhoeae* are the most common causes of cervicitis or PID in women and epididymitis or prostatitis in reproductive-aged men.[3,103–105] Unfortunately, point-of-care testing for identification of these organisms is not available in all EDs, although several tests demonstrate promise.[119,120] Clinicians may treat empirically for UTI or STI or treat for both concurrently.[3] If the clinician decides to treat only one, follow-up must be in place to evaluate for continued symptoms and assessment of testing completed in the ED.

Asymptomatic Bacteriuria

Bacteria in the urine without symptoms of UTI defines ASB, specifically in women with 2 consecutive clean-catch voided specimens with the same organism in greater than 10^5 CFUs/mL and in men with 1 specimen and the same organism count.[121–123] This finding does not definitively diagnose UTI, and ASB rates increase with age.[40,44,121,124,125] One study found 5% of sexually active young women demonstrate ASB.[123] Rates of ASB approach 25% to 50% of women and 15% to 49% of men without indwelling catheters.[124] These rates increase in the elderly due to altered elimination, anatomic variations of the urogenital tract, poor hygiene, hormonal changes, and neurologic impairment.[121,125] Many of these organisms are not harmful but rather commensal organisms.[44] A symptomatic UTI in the elderly patient is less common than ASB,[125] and ASB is not associated with long-term adverse outcomes, such as pyelonephritis, sepsis, or renal failure.[126] ASB has not been shown to increase the risk of hypertension, kidney disease, or death in patients with otherwise normal immune status.[127] Renal transplant patients, however, are at higher risk of pyelonephritis with ASB.[128,129] Bacteria obtained from urine culture is also not definitive for diagnosis of UTI.[7,44]

Clinical signs and symptoms of UTI are needed for treatment, but many patients are not able to provide these.[44,121] Emergency physicians regularly evaluate older patients unable to provide history and examination. A 2014 study recommended treatment if patients demonstrated bacteriuria and pyuria with two of the following: fever, worsening urinary frequency or urgency, acute dysuria, suprapubic tenderness, and costovertebral angle tenderness.[130] Other possible formulas to differentiate UTI and bacteriuria are the following: pyuria + bacteriuria + nitrites = infection; bacteriuria but no pyuria = colonization/bacteriuria; and pyuria alone but no bacteria = inflammation.[131] Patients undergoing instrumentation or surgery of the bladder may require antibiotics.[3,39] ASB in pregnancy also requires treatment with antibiotics to decrease the risk of maternal-fetal morbidity and pyelonephritis.[132,133] Treating patients without true UTI can increase antimicrobial resistance as well as expose patients to dangerous side effects and diseases, such as *Clostridium difficile* colitis.[121,134–136] Antibiotics are used inappropriately in close to half of patients with ASB.[136] Educational programs and knowledge of ASB, however, can effectively reduce inappropriate treatment.[136]

What About the Older Patient with Altered Mental Status or Recurrent Falls?

Altered mental status, "failure to thrive," or recurrent falls in an elderly patient encompass a large differential. History and examination are often unrevealing, resulting in further testing, often with urinalysis. If UTI is a contributor, systemic signs or symptoms should be present, along with evidence of UTI, such as dysuria.[44,134] In patients with clinical suspicion of UTI without a catheter, acute change in mental status is associated with bacteriuria and pyuria.[135] Several studies suggest that urinary testing in a patient with a history of falls but no signs or symptoms of UTI is unlikely to yield evidence of pyuria or bacteriuria.[44,136–140]

Patients with chronic dementia and recurrent falls or those who are altered and unable to provide a history of urinary symptoms can be challenging. Evaluation for suprapubic or CVA tenderness in conjunction with UA can be helpful.[44] UA with positive nitrites, pyuria, and bacteriuria may be suggestive of UTI.[44,141] In patients for whom history and examination are unreliable but with no other explanation for AMS, one study recommends using bacteriuria with other markers of systemic inflammation, including fever/hypothermia, elevated WBC/C-reactive protein (CRP), elevated blood glucose in absence of diabetes, and acutely altered mental status to diagnose UTI and begin treatment.[141] If urine dipstick demonstrates negative LE and nitrite, then UTI is not present.[3,44,141] Other causes of altered mental status must be excluded before diagnosing UTI as the sole cause of altered mental status. If a patient meets criteria for sepsis or has elevated markers of inflammation and the UA is consistent with UTI, then treatment is warranted.[3,4,8,44]

DISPOSITION

Patient disposition is a key component of every patient evaluation in the ED. No validated decision rule is available for patients with UTI, unlike pneumonia. The majority of patients with uncomplicated and even complicated UTIs are appropriate for discharge.[2–7] Possible reasons for admission are discussed in **Box 2**. Patients with pyelonephritis are more likely to warrant admission due to fever, vomiting, and tachycardia, but those who improve after IV fluids, antibiotics, and antiemetics can potentially be discharged with close follow-up.[3,7,8] Patients without any of the findings listed in **Box 2** are otherwise appropriate for discharge.

Box 2
Indications for admission

Inability to tolerate oral intake with severe nausea and vomiting

Hemodynamic instability

Obstruction or complication along urinary tract

Failure of outpatient therapy, including antibiotics

Poor social support, inability to obtain medications, and unable to attend follow-up

Concern for resistant organism with no option for oral antibiotic therapy

Pregnancy with pyelonephritis

For patients discharged with an oral antibiotic, follow-up is recommended to ensure the patient is improving.[2–7] If a urine culture is obtained, a follow-up process should be in place to ensure that antibiotic treatment was adequate. A patient who is not improving or is worsening after 1-2 days of antibiotics requires reevaluation with further testing. Imaging to evaluate for a UTI mimic, complicated UTI, or obstruction may be needed as well as urine culture.

SUMMARY

UTI presents along a wide spectrum, commonly evaluated and managed in the ED. No single history or examination finding is definitive for diagnosis, but dysuria, urinary frequency, and urinary urgency in the absence of vaginal discharge strongly suggest UTI. History and examination should be used in combination with urine testing for diagnosis. Imaging is often not needed, except in specific circumstances. Most patients with simple cystitis and pyelonephritis can be treated as outpatients, and prescribed antibiotic depends on the region's antibiogram and diagnosis. A variety of potentially dangerous conditions can mimic UTI and pyelonephritis.

REFERENCES

1. Stamm WE, Hooton TM, Johnson JR, et al. Urinary tract infections: from pathogenesis to treatment. J Infect Dis 1989;159:400–6.
2. Gupta K, Grigoryan L, Trautner B. Urinary tract infection. Ann Intern Med 2017; 167(7):ITC49–64.
3. Takhar SS, Moran GJ. Diagnosis and management of urinary tract infection in the emergency department and outpatient settings. Infect Dis Clin North Am 2014;28:33–48.
4. Stamm WE, Hooton TM. Management of urinary-tract infections in adults. N Engl J Med 1993;329(18):1328–34.
5. Warren JW, Abrutyn E, Hebel JR, et al. Guidelines for antimicrobial treatment of uncomplicated acute bacterial cystitis and acute pyelonephritis in women. Clin Infect Dis 1999;29(4):745–58.
6. Hooton TM. Uncomplicated urinary tract infection. N Engl J Med 2012;366(11): 1028–37.
7. Gupta K, Hooton TM, Naber KG, et al. International clinical practice guidelines for the treatment of acute uncomplicated cystitis and pyelonephritis in women: a 2010 update by the infectious diseases society of America and the European society for microbiology and infectious diseases. Clin Infect Dis 2011;52(5): E103–20.
8. Johnson JR, Russo TA. Acute pyelonephritis in adults. N Engl J Med 2018;378: 48–59.
9. Singer M, Deutschman CS, Seymour CW, et al. The third international consensus definitions for sepsis and septic shock (Sepsis-3). JAMA 2016; 315:801–10.
10. Dalhoff A. Global fluoroquinolone resistance epidemiology and implications for clinical use. Interdiscip Perspect Infect Dis 2012;2012:976273.
11. Johnson SW, Anderson DJ, May DB, et al. Utility of a clinical risk factor scoring model in predicting infection with extended-spectrum β-lactamase-producing enterobacteriaceae on hospital admission. Infect Control Hosp Epidemiol 2013;34:385–92.

12. Hayakawa K, Gattu S, Marchaim D, et al. Epidemiology and risk factors for isolation of Escherichia coli producing CTX-M-type extended-spectrum β-lactamase in a large U.S. medical center. Antimicrob Agents Chemother 2013;57:4010–8.

13. Doi Y, Park YS, Rivera JI, et al. Community-associated extended-spectrum β-lactamase-producing Escherichia coli infection in the United States. Clin Infect Dis 2013;56:641–8.

14. Peirano G, van der Bij AK, Gregson DB, et al. Molecular epidemiology over an 11-year period (2000 to 2010) of extended-spectrum β-lactamase-producing Escherichia coli causing bacteremia in a centralized Canadian region. J Clin Microbiol 2012;50:294–9.

15. Neal DE. Complicated urinary tract infections. Urol Clin North Am 2008;35(1):13–22.

16. Hooton TM, Scholes D, Hughes JP, et al. A prospective study of risk factors for symptomatic urinary tract infection in young women. N Engl J Med 1996;335:468–74.

17. Krieger JN, Ross SO, Simonsen JM. Urinary tract infections in healthy university men. J Urol 1993;149:1046.

18. Vorland LH, Carlson K, Aalen O. An epidemiological survey of urinary tract infections among outpatients in Northern Norway. Scand J Infect Dis 1985;17:277.

19. Foxman B. Epidemiology of urinary tract infections: incidence, morbidity, and economic costs. Am J Med 2002;113(Suppl 1A):5S–13S.

20. HCUPnet. Healthcare cost and utilization project (HCUP). Rockville (MD): Agency for Healthcare Research and Quality; 2010. Available at: http://hcupnet.hhrq.gov/. Accessed November 9, 2017.

21. National Center for Health Statistics. National hospital ambulatory medical care survey (NHAMCS), 2010. Hyattsville (MD). Public-use data file and documentation. Available at: ftp://ftp.cdc.gov/pub/Health_Statistics/NCHS/Datasets/NHAMCS/. Accessed November 2, 2017.

22. Czaja CA, Scholes D, Hooton TM, et al. Population-based epidemiologic analysis of acute pyelonephritis. Clin Infect Dis 2007;45:273–80.

23. Lagu T, Rothberg MB, Shieh M-S, et al. Hospitalizations, costs, and outcomes of severe sepsis in the United States 2003 to 2007. Crit Care Med 2012;40:754–61.

24. Jordan PA, Iravani A, Richard GA, et al. Urinary-tract infection caused by Staphylococcus-saprophyticus. J Infect Dis 1980;142(4):510–5.

25. Talan DA, Krishnadasan A, Abrahamian FM, et al. Prevalence and risk factor analysis of trimethoprim-sulfamethoxazole- and fluoroquinolone-resistant Escherichia coli infection among emergency department patients with pyelonephritis. Clin Infect Dis 2008;47(9):1150–8.

26. Gupta K, Sahm DF, Mayfield D, et al. Antimicrobial resistance among uropathogens that cause community-acquired urinary tract infections in women: a nationwide analysis. Clin Infect Dis 2001;33(1):89–94.

27. Talan DA, Takhar SS, Krishnadasan A, et al, EMERGEncy ID Net Study Group. Fluoroquinolone-resistant and extended-spectrum β-lactamase–producing Escherichia coli infections in patients with pyelonephritis, United States. Emerg Infect Dis 2016;22(9):1594–603.

28. Meister L, Morley EJ, Scheer D, et al. History and physical examination plus laboratory testing for the diagnosis of adult female urinary tract infection. Acad Emerg Med 2013;20(7):631–45.

29. Bent S, Nallamothu BK, Simel DL, et al. Does this woman have an acute uncomplicated urinary tract infection? JAMA 2002;287(20):2701–10.

30. Fairley KF, Carson NE, Gutch RC, et al. Site of infection in acute urinary-tract infection in general practice. Lancet 1971;2(7725):615–8.
31. Pinson AG, Philbrick JT, Lindbeck GH, et al. Fever in the clinical diagnosis of acute pyelonephritis. Am J Emerg Med 1997;15(2):148–51.
32. Piccoli GB, Consiglio V, Colla L, et al. Antibiotic treatment for acute 'uncomplicated' or 'primary' pyelonephritis: a systematic, 'semantic revision'. Int J Antimicrob Agents 2006;28(Suppl 1):S49–63.
33. Owens RC Jr, Johnson JR, Stogsdill P, et al. Community transmission in the United States of a CTX-M-15-producing sequence type ST131 Escherichia coli strain resulting in death. J Clin Microbiol 2011;49:3406–8.
34. Hooton TM, Roberts PL, Cox ME, et al. Voided midstream urine culture and acute cystitis in premenopausal women. N Engl J Med 2013;369(20):1883–91.
35. Wilson ML, Gaido L. Laboratory diagnosis of urinary tract infections in adult patients. Clin Infect Dis 2004;38(8):1150–8.
36. Walter FG, Knopp RK. Urine sampling in ambulatory women - midstream clean-catch versus catherization. Ann Emerg Med 1989;18(2):166–72.
37. Lifshitz E, Kramer L. Outpatient urine culture: does collection technique matter? Arch Intern Med 2000;160:2537–40.
38. Cunha B. Introduction: urinary tract infections. In: Cunha B, editor. Urinary tract infections: current issues in diagnosis and treatment. Antibiotics for Clinicians. 1998;2(suppl 2):3–4.
39. Orenstein R, Wong ES. Urinary tract infections in adults. Am Fam Physician 1999;59(5):1225–34. Available at: www.aafp.org/afp/990301ap/1225.html. Accessed November 12, 2017.
40. Simerville JA, Maxted WC, Pahira JJ. Urinalysis: a comprehensive review. Am Fam Physician 2005;71(6):1153–62.
41. Lammers RL, Gibson S, Kovacs D, et al. Comparison of test characteristics of urine dipstick and urinalysis at various test cutoff points. Ann Emerg Med 2001;38(5):505–12.
42. Stamm WE. Measurement of pyuria and its relation to bacteriuria. Am J Med 1983;75(1B):53–8.
43. Pappas PG. Laboratory in the diagnosis and management of urinary tract infections. Med Clin North Am 1991;75:313.
44. Schulz L, Hoffman RJ, Pothof J, et al. Top ten myths regarding the diagnosis and treatment of urinary tract infections. J Emerg Med 2016;51(1):25–30.
45. Williams GJ, Macaskill P, Chan SF, et al. Absolute and relative accuracy of rapid urine tests for urinary tract infection in children: a meta-analysis. Lancet Infect Dis 2010;10:240.
46. Pels RJ, Bor DH, Woolhandler S, et al. Dipstick urinalysis screening of asymptomatic adults for urinary tract disorders. II. Bacteriuria. JAMA 1989;262:1221–4.
47. Gallagher EJ, Schwartz E, Weinstein RS. Performance characteristics of urine dipsticks stored in open containers. Am J Emerg Med 1990;8:121–3.
48. Deville WL, Yzermans JC, van Duijn NP, et al. The urine dipstick test useful to rule out infections. A meta-analysis of the accuracy. BMC Urol 2004;4:4.
49. Leman P. Validity of urinalysis and microscopy for detecting urinary tract infection in the emergency department. Eur J Emerg Med 2002;9(2):141–7.
50. Foley A, French L. Urine clarity inaccurate to rule out urinary tract infection in women. J Am Board Fam Med 2011;24:474–5.
51. Nicolle LE. The chronic indwelling catheter and urinary infection in long-term-care facility residents. Infect Control Hosp Epidemiol 2001;22:316–21.

52. Stapleton AE. Urine culture in uncomplicated UTI: interpretation and significance. Curr Infect Dis Rep 2016;18:15.
53. Carlson KJ, Mulley AG. Management of acute dysuria - a decision-analysis model of alternative strategies. Ann Intern Med 1985;102(2):244-9.
54. Little P, Moore MV, Turner S, et al. Effectiveness of five different approaches in management of urinary tract infection: randomised controlled trial. BMJ 2010; 340:c199.
55. Thanassi M. Utility of urine and blood cultures in pyelonephritis. Acad Emerg Med 1997;4(8):797-800.
56. Otto G, Sandberg T, Marklund BI, et al. Virulence factors and pap genotype in Escherichia coli isolates from women with acute pyelonephritis, with or without bacteremia. Clin Infect Dis 1993;17(3):448-56.
57. Finkelstein R, Kassis E, Reinhertz G, et al. Community-acquired urinary tract infection in adults: a hospital viewpoint. J Hosp Infect 1998;38(3):193-202.
58. Velasco M, Martinez JA, Moreno-Martinez A, et al. Blood cultures for women with uncomplicated acute pyelonephritis: are they necessary? Clin Infect Dis 2003; 37(8):1127.
59. Chen Y, Nitzan O, Saliba W, et al. Are blood cultures necessary in the management of women with complicated pyelonephritis? J Infect 2006;53(4):235-40.
60. Hsu CY, Fang HC, Chou KJ, et al. The clinical impact of bacteremia in complicated acute pyelonephritis. Am J Med Sci 2006;332(4):175-80.
61. Smith WR, McClish DK, Poses RM, et al. Bacteremia in young urban women admitted with pyelonephritis. Am J Med Sci 1997;313:50-7.
62. McMurray BR, Wrenn KD, Wright SW. Usefulness of blood cultures in pyelonephritis. Am J Emerg Med 1997;15:137-40.
63. Kim Y, Seo MR, Kim SJ, et al. Usefulness of blood cultures and radiologic imaging studies in the management of patients with community-acquired acute pyelonephritis. Infect Chemother 2017;49:22-30.
64. van Nieuwkoop C, Hoppe BP, Bonten TN, et al. Predicting the need for radiologic imaging in adults with febrile urinary tract infection. Clin Infect Dis 2010; 51:1266-72.
65. Jindal G, Ramchandani P. Acute flank pain secondary to urolithiasis: radiologic evaluation and alternate diagnoses. Radiol Clin North Am 2007;45(3):395-410.
66. Levine JA, Neitlich J, Verga M, et al. Ureteral calculi in patients with flank pain: correlation of plain radiography with unenhanced helical CT. Radiology 1997; 204(1):27-31.
67. Catalano O, Nunziata A, Altei F, et al. Suspected ureteral colic: primary helical CT versus selective helical CT after unenhanced radiography and sonography. AJR Am J Roentgenol 2002;178(2):379-87.
68. Fowler KA, Locken JA, Duchesne JH, et al. US for detecting renal calculi with nonenhanced CT as a reference standard. Radiology 2002;222(1):109-13.
69. Sheafor DH, Hertzberg BS, Freed KS, et al. Nonenhanced helical CT and US in the emergency evaluation of patients with renal colic: prospective comparison. Radiology 2000;217(3):792-7.
70. Henderson SO, Hoffner RJ, Aragona JL, et al. Bedside emergency department ultrasonography plus radiography of the kidneys, ureters and bladder vs intravenous pyelography in the evaluation of suspected ureteral colic. Acad Emerg Med 1998;5(7):666-71.
71. Kartal M, Eray O, Erdogru T, et al. Prospective validation of a current algorithm including bedside US performed by emergency physicians for patients with acute flank pain suspected for renal colic. Emerg Med J 2006;23(5):341-4.

72. Rosen CL, Brown DF, Sagarin MJ, et al. Ultrasonography by emergency physicians in patients with suspected ureteral colic. J Emerg Med 1998;16(6):865–70.

73. Gaspari RJ, Horst K. Emergency ultrasound and urinalysis in the evaluation of flank pain. Acad Emerg Med 2005;12(12):1180–4.

74. Miller OF, Kane CJ. Unenhanced helical computed tomography in the evaluation of acute flank pain. Curr Opin Urol 2000;10(2):123–9.

75. Dalrymple NC, Verga M, Anderson KR, et al. The value of unenhanced helical computerized tomography in the management of acute flank pain. J Urol 1998;159(3):735–40.

76. Miller OF, Rineer SK, Reichard SR, et al. Prospective comparison of unenhanced spiral computed tomography and intravenous urogram in the evaluation of acute flank pain. Urology 1998;52(6):982–7.

77. Walker E, Lyman A, Gupta K, et al. Clinical management of an increasing threat: outpatient urinary tract infections due to multidrug-resistant uropathogens. Clin Infect Dis 2016;63:960–5.

78. Grigoryan L, Trautner BW, Gupta K. Diagnosis and management of urinary tract infections in the outpatient setting: a review. JAMA 2014;312:1677–84.

79. Reyner K, Heffner AC, Karvetski CH. Urinary obstruction is an important complicating factor in patients with septic shock due to urinary infection. Am J Emerg Med 2016;34(4):694–6.

80. Ubee SS, McGlynn L, Fordham M. Emphysematous pyelonephritis. BJU Int 2011;107:1474–8.

81. Rubenstein JN, Schaeffer AJ. Managing complicated urinary tract infections: the urologic view. Infect Dis Clin North Am 2003;17:333–51.

82. Aggarwal S, Qamar A, Sharma V, et al. Abdominal aortic aneurysm: a comprehensive review. Exp Clin Cardiol 2011;16(1):11–5.

83. Welch J, Chike V, Bowens N, et al. Acute cholecystitis. First consult. Philadelphia: Elsevier; 2011.

84. Trowbridge R, Rutkowski N, Shojania K. Does this patient have acute cholecystitis? JAMA 2003;289(1):80–6.

85. Alerhand S, Wood S, Long B, et al. The time-sensitive challenge of diagnosing spinal epidural abscess in the emergency department. Intern Emerg Med 2017; 12(8):1179–83.

86. Bushinsky D. Nephrolithiasis. In: Goldman L, Schafer AI, editors. Goldman-cecil medicine. 25th edition. Philadelphia: Saunders Elsevier; 2016. p. 811–6.e1.

87. Gottlieb M, Long B, Koyfman A. Urolithiasis. Am J Emerg Med 2018. https://doi.org/10.1016/j.ajem.2018.01.003.

88. Long B, Long D, Koyfman A. Emergency medicine evaluation of community-acquired pneumonia: history, examination, imaging and laboratory assessment, and risk scores. J Emerg Med 2017;53(5):642–52.

89. Mandell L, Wunderink R, Anzueto A, et al. Infectious Diseases Society of America/American Thoracic Society consensus guidelines on the management of community-acquired pneumonia in adults. Clin Infect Dis 2007;44(Suppl 2): S27–72.

90. Freeman A, Abernethy A. Pulmonary embolism. Philadelphia: First Consult. Elsevier; 2014.

91. Hazanov N, Somin M, Attali M, et al. Acute renal embolism. Forty-four cases of renal infarction in patients with atrial fibrillation. Medicine (Baltimore) 2004;83(5): 292–9.

92. Greco B, Dwyer J, Lewis J. Thromboembolic renovascular disease. In: Johnson RJ, Feehally J, Floege, editors. Comprehensive clinical nephrology, vol. 66, 5th edition. Philadelphia: Saunders Elsevier; 2015. p. 767–78.

93. Sarosi G. Appendicitis. In: Feldman M, Friedman LS, Brandt LJ, editors. Sleisenger and Fordtran's gastrointestinal and liver disease. 10th edition. Philadelphia: Saunders Elsevier; 2016. p. 2112–22.e3.

94. Terasawa T, Blackmore C, Bent S, et al. Systematic review: computer tomography and ultrasonography to detect acute appendicitis in adults and adolescents. Ann Intern Med 2004;141:537–46.

95. Sifri C, Madoff L. Diverticulitis ad typhlitis. In: Mandell G, Bennett J, Dolin R, editors. Mandell, Douglas, and Bennett's principles and practice of infectious diseases, vol. 81, 8th edition. Philadelphia: Saunders Elsevier; 2015. p. 986–9.e1.

96. Ferzoco L, Raptopoulos V, Silen W. Acute diverticulitis. N Engl J Med 1998;338: 1521–6.

97. Robertson JJ, Long B, Koyfman A. Emergency medicine myths: ectopic pregnancy evaluation, risk factors, and presentation. j. Emerg Med 2017;53(6): 819–28.

98. McGowan C, Krieger J. Prostatitis, epididymitis, and orchitis. In: Mandell G, Bennett J, Dolin R, editors. Mandell, Douglas, and Bennett's principles and practice of infectious diseases, vol. 112, 8th edition. Philadelphia: Saunders Elsevier; 2015. p. 1381–7.e2.

99. Chan P, Schlegel P. Inflammatory conditions of the male excurrent ductal system. Part I. J Androl 2002;23:453–60.

100. Robertson JJ, Long B, Koyfman A. Myths in the evaluation and management of ovarian torsion. J Emerg Med 2017;52(4):449–56.

101. Asfour V, Varma R, Menon P. Clinical risk factors for ovarian torsion. J Obstet Gynaecol 2015;35(7):721–5.

102. Ferri F. Testicular torsion. In: Ferri F, editor. Ferri's clinical advisor 2017. Philadelphia: Elsevier; 2017. p. 1251–2.e1.

103. Kim A, Pearson R, Scherger J, et al. Pelvic inflammatory disease. Philadelphia: First Consult. Elsevier; 2010.

104. Soper D. Infections in the female pelvis. In: Mandell G, Bennett J, Dolin R, editors. Mandell, Douglas, and Bennett's principles and practice of infectious diseases. 8th edition. Philadelphia: Saunders Elsevier; 2014. p. 1372–80.e2.

105. Osborne N. Tubo-ovarian abscess: pathogenesis and management. J Natl Med Assoc 1986;78(10):937–51.

106. Abrahamian FM, Krishnadasan A, Mower WR, et al. Association of pyuria and clinical characteristics with the presence of urinary tract infection among patients with acute nephrolithiasis. Ann Emerg Med 2013;62(5):526–33.

107. Dobardzic AM, Dobardzic R. Epidemiological features of complicated UTI in a district hospital of Kuwait. Eur J Epidemiol 1997;13(4):465–70.

108. Stlezin M, Hofmann R, Stoller ML. Pyonephrosis - diagnosis and treatment. Br J Urol 1992;70(4):360–3.

109. Dielubanza EJ, Mazur DJ, Schaeffer AJ. Management of non-catheter-associated complicated urinary tract infection. Infect Dis Clin North Am 2014; 28(1):121–34.

110. Mariappan P, Loong CW. Midstream urine culture and sensitivity test is a poor predictor of infected urine proximal to the obstructing ureteral stone or infected stones: a prospective clinical study. J Urol 2004;171(6 Pt 1):2142–5.

111. Tundidor Bermúdez AM, Amado Diéguez JA, Montes de Oca Mastrapa JL. Urological manifestations of acute appendicitis. Arch Esp Urol 2005;58(3):207–12 [in Spanish].

112. Dieter RS. Sterile pyuria: a differential diagnosis. Compr Ther 2000;26(3):150–2.

113. Sobel J, Kaye D. Urinary tract infections. In: Mandell G, Bennett J, Dolin R, editors. Mandell, Douglas, and Bennett's principles and practice of infectious diseases, vol. 74, 8th edition. Philadelphia: Saunders Elsevier; 2015. p. 886–913.e3.

114. Eagan JW. Urinary tract cytology. In: Hill GS, editor. Uropathology, vol. 2. Philadelphia: Churchill Livingstone; 1989. p. 873.

115. Wise GJ, Schlegel PN. Sterile pyuria. N Engl J Med 2015;372:1048.

116. Huppert JS, Biro F, Lan D, et al. Urinary symptoms in adolescent females: STI or UTI? J Adolesc Health 2007;40:418–24.

117. Prentiss KA, Newby PK, Vinci RJ. Adolescent female with urinary symptoms: a diagnostic challenge for the pediatrician. Pediatr Emerg Care 2011;27(9): 789–94.

118. Bent S, Saint S. The optimal use of diagnostic testing in women with acute uncomplicated cystitis. Am J Med 2002;113(Suppl 1A):20S–8S.

119. Natoli L, Maher L, Shephard M, et al. Point-of-care testing for chlamydia and gonorrhoea: implications for clinical practice. PLoS One 2014;9(6):e100518.

120. Herbst de Cortina S, Bristow CC, Joseph Davey D, et al. A systematic review of point of care testing for chlamydia trachomatis, neisseria gonorrhoeae, and trichomonas vaginalis. Infect Dis Obstet Gynecol 2016;2016:4386127.

121. Nicolle LE, Bradley S, Colgan R, et al. Infectious Diseases Society of America guidelines for the diagnosis and treatment of asymptomatic bacteriuria in adults. Clin Infect Dis 2005;40:643–54.

122. Mohr NM, Harland KK, Crabb V, et al. Urinary squamous epithelial cells do not accurately predict urine culture contamination, but may predict urinalysis performance in predicting bacteriuria. Acad Emerg Med 2016;23:323–30.

123. Hooton TM, Scholes D, Stapleton AE, et al. A prospective study of asymptomatic bacteriuria in sexually active young women. N Engl J Med 2000;343(14): 992–7.

124. Nicolle LE. Urinary tract infections in long-term-care facilities. Infect Control Hosp Epidemiol 2001;22:167–75.

125. Nicolle LE. Asymptomatic bacteriuria in the elderly. Infect Dis Clin North Am 1997;11:647–62.

126. Burke JP. Antibiotic resistance—squeezing the balloon? JAMA 1998;280: 1270–1.

127. Abrutyn E, Mossey J, Berlin JA, et al. Does asymptomatic bacteriuria predict mortality and does antimicrobial treatment reduce mortality in elderly ambulatory women? Ann Intern Med 1994;120:827–33.

128. Fiorante S, Fernandez-Ruiz M, Lopez-Medrano F, et al. Acute graft pyelonephritis in renal transplant recipients: incidence, risk factors and long-term outcome. Nephrol Dial Transplant 2011;26:1065–73.

129. Fiorante S, Lopez-Medrano F, Lizasoain M, et al. Systematic screening and treatment of asymptomatic bacteriuria in renal transplant recipients. Kidney Int 2010;78:774–81.

130. Mody L, Juthani-Mehta M. Urinary tract infections in older women: a clinical review. JAMA 2014;311(8):844–54.

131. Cunha B. Therapeutic approach to treating urinary tract infections. In: Cuhna B, editor. Urinary tract infections: current issues in diagnosis and treatment. Antibiotics for Clinicians. 1998;2(suppl 2):35–40.
132. Vazquez JC, Abalos E. Treatments for symptomatic urinary tract infections during pregnancy. Cochrane Database Syst Rev 2011;(1):CD002256.
133. Wing DA, Fassett MJ, Getahun D. Acute pyelonephritis in pregnancy: an 18-year retrospective analysis. Am J Obstet Gynecol 2014;210(3):219.e1-6.
134. Bartlett JG. A call to arms: the imperative for antimicrobial stewardship. Clin Infect Dis 2011;53(Suppl 1):S4–7.
135. Gross PA, Patel B. Reducing antibiotic overuse: a call for a national performance measure for not treating asymptomatic bacteriuria. Clin Infect Dis 2007;45: 1335–7.
136. Kelley D, Aaronson P, Poon E, et al. Evaluation of an antimicrobial stewardship approach to minimize overuse of antibiotics in patients with asymptomatic bacteriuria. Infect Control Hosp Epidemiol 2014;35(2):193–5.
137. Tambyah PA, Maki DG. Catheter-associated urinary tract infection is rarely symptomatic: a prospective study of 1,497 catheterized patients. Arch Intern Med 2000;160:678–82.
138. Juthani-Mehta M, Quagliarello V, Perrelli E, et al. Clinical features to identify urinary tract infection in nursing home residents: a cohort study. J Am Geriatr Soc 2009;57:963–70.
139. Nicolle LE. Urinary tract infections in the elderly. Clin Geriatr Med 2009;25: 423–36.
140. Nicolle LE. Symptomatic urinary tract infection in nursing home residents. J Am Geriatr Soc 2009;57:1113–4.
141. Ninan S, Walton C, Barlow G. Investigation of suspected urinary tract infection in older people. BMJ 2014;349:g4070.

Emergency Department Approach to the Patient with Suspected Central Nervous System Infection

Rupal Jain, MD[a], Wan-Tsu W. Chang, MD[b],*

KEYWORDS

- Central nervous system infection • Meningitis • Encephalitis • Brain abscess
- Shunt infection • Lumbar puncture • Cerebrospinal fluid

KEY POINTS

- The emergency physician (EP) should have a structured approach to the clinical evaluation of patients with suspected central nervous system (CNS) infection, directed toward early initiation of antimicrobial agents.
- In certain patients who are at high risk of herniation, head computed tomographic scan must first be obtained to evaluate for mass lesions or cerebral edema before a lumbar puncture is performed.
- As critically ill patients with suspected CNS infections board in the emergency department for a long period of time, the EP should be familiar with managing systemic and neurologic complications of CNS infection.

INTRODUCTION

Infections in the central nervous system (CNS) can be sudden, catastrophic, and potentially lethal. In some cases, the CNS is the main target. In others, the CNS is a secondary target. Infections in the CNS can be caused by bacteria, viruses, fungi, and parasites. The main CNS infections that are covered in this article are meningitis, encephalitis, brain abscess, and ventricular shunt infections.

The following 4-question approach to the clinical evaluation of a patient with suspected CNS infection can aid the emergency physician (EP) in identifying the likely infection and tailoring further diagnostic and therapeutic strategies (**Fig. 1**).

The authors have declared that they have no financial conflicts of interest.
[a] Department of Emergency Medicine, University of Maryland Medical Center, University of Maryland School of Medicine, 110 South Paca Street, 6th Floor, Suite 200, Baltimore, MD 21201, USA; [b] Department of Emergency Medicine, University of Maryland School of Medicine, 110 South Paca Street, 6th Floor, Suite 200, Baltimore, MD 21201, USA
* Corresponding author.
E-mail address: wchang1@som.umaryland.edu

Emerg Med Clin N Am 36 (2018) 711–722
https://doi.org/10.1016/j.emc.2018.06.004
0733-8627/18/© 2018 Elsevier Inc. All rights reserved.

emed.theclinics.com

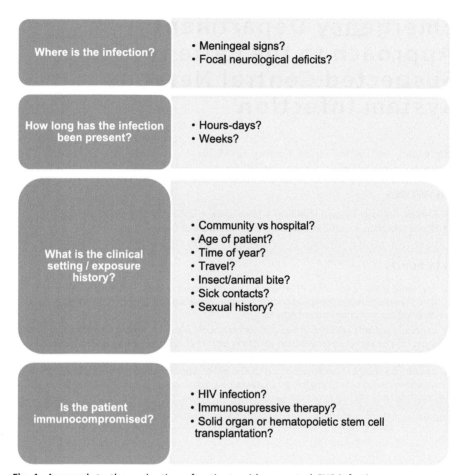

Fig. 1. Approach to the evaluation of patients with suspected CNS infection.

Where Is the Infection?

It is often impossible to distinguish between meningitis, encephalitis, and brain abscess with absolute certainty based on clinical presentation. Theoretic teaching relies on classic clinical triads. The classic triad of meningitis is fever, altered mental status, and neck stiffness. The classic triad of encephalitis is fever, altered mental status, and headache. The classic triad of brain abscess is fever, headache, and focal neurologic deficit. There is significant clinical overlap between these prototypical triads, making classic presentations unreliable. In a patient with suspected CNS infection, the clinical signs and symptoms may suggest whether the infection involves the meninges (meningitis), parenchyma (encephalitis, brain abscess), or both (meningoencephalitis). In meningitis, an increase of inflammatory cells within the cerebrospinal fluid (CSF) and resultant irritation of the meninges elicit a protective reflex to prevent stretching of the inflamed and hypersensitive nerve roots. This reflex is detectable clinically as nuchal rigidity (resistance to passive neck flexion), Kernig sign (contraction of hamstrings in response to knee extension while the hip is flexed), or Brudzinski sign (flexion of hips and knees in response to passive neck flexion while the patient is lying supine). Although the sensitivity of these 3 classic meningeal signs is low (30%, 5%, and 5%, respectively), their higher specificity may alert the EP when meningitis is present.[1]

On the other hand, when fever and focal neurologic signs and symptoms predominate, parenchymal CNS inflammation and infection should be considered. Signs and symptoms may include acute change in mental status, seizure, focal neurologic deficits, or personality changes.

Although these distinctions may be helpful in providing a framework for patients who present with features of CNS infection that localize mostly to the meninges or mostly to the parenchyma, most patients will have features of both, termed meningoencephalitis. It is also important to note that in advanced stages of meningitis as well as parenchymal pathologic conditions, such as encephalitis and brain abscess, developing cerebral edema can culminate in common signs of increased intracranial pressure, such as altered level of consciousness, headache, vomiting, and cranial nerve abnormality.

How Long Has the Infection Been Present?

Getting a sense of the temporal course and chronicity of illness can help identify CNS infection. For example, depending on the duration of symptoms, meningitis can be classified as acute or chronic. Acute meningitis (hours-days) is usually caused by bacterial infection and is considered an emergency because of the high likelihood of rapid clinical deterioration. Chronic meningitis (lasting for 4 weeks or more) is more likely due to viral infection, tuberculosis, Lyme disease, syphilis, or fungal infection, especially *Cryptococci*.

What Is the Clinical Setting and What Is the Exposure History?

Recognizing the clinical setting (community vs hospital acquired, age of patient, time of year) and unique exposure history (travel, insect/animal bite, sick contacts, sexual history) may help identify suspected pathogens and lay the groundwork for diagnostic workup and initiating empiric treatment. Community-acquired meningitis comprises mostly pneumococcal and meningococcal meningitis. Hospital-acquired meningitis, or postneurosurgical meningitis, should cover for methicillin-resistant *Staphylococcus aureus* and *Pseudomonas* meningitis. Certain pathogens are more likely to cause meningitis in certain age groups. Specifically, group B streptococcus and *Escherichia coli* are virulent pathogens that should be considered only in meningitis of newborns. Newborns and adults older than age 50 are also at an increased risk for *Listeria monocytogenes*. The time of year is also an important factor, especially with encephalitis. Generally, mosquito-borne encephalitis occurs from early summer to early fall, whereas tick-borne encephalitis occurs from spring to early fall.

Similarly, certain historic data and context can help increase the suspicion of CNS infection caused by a specific pathogen. For example, closed environments, such as army barracks or college dormitories, can harbor outbreaks of meningococcal meningitis. History of a penetrating head trauma, injection drug use, or endocarditis increases risk of meningitis due to *S aureus*. A recent tick bite may suggest Lyme disease, and a mosquito bite may suggest West Nile virus. Travel to Arizona, for example, may raise suspicion of meningitis secondary to *Coccidioides*. Unprotected sexual intercourse may increase the risk of human immunodeficiency virus (HIV) acute retroviral syndrome with meningitis, or neurosyphilis. Conversely, history of immunization will decrease risk of meningitis due to *Haemophilus influenzae* in children and pneumococcal pneumonia in the elderly.

Is the Patient an Immunocompromised Host?

CNS infection occurs when the virulence of an organism exceeds host immune capacity. Therefore, although certain organisms are less likely to be a pathogen in immunocompetent hosts, they can cause infection in patients with defective immune systems. Examples include toxoplasmosis, cryptococcal meningitis, and tuberculous meningitis.

PATHOPHYSIOLOGY AND EPIDEMIOLOGY

Of the CNS infections, meningitis is generally associated with the highest morbidity and mortality. Meningitis refers to inflammation of the meninges, often due to infection caused by bacteria, viruses, and fungi. These pathogens gain access to the CNS by direct contiguous spread from nearby infections, such as otitis media and sinusitis, hematogenous seeding from concurrent distant infection, or direct inoculation from surgery or trauma. Because of the introduction of conjugated vaccines against H influenzae type B (Hib), *Streptococcus pneumoniae*, and *Neisseria meningitidis*, the 3 most common pathogens of bacterial meningitis, there has been a decline in the incidence of community-acquired meningitis in Western countries. However, in developing countries and sub-Saharan Africa, also referred to as the meningitis belt, the incidence of meningitis is a significant problem.[2] Although Hib meningitis has been nearly eradicated after the introduction of the vaccine, due to changing serotypes, the incidence of pneumococcal meningitis worldwide in all age groups has only decreased by 25%.[3] Bacterial meningitis remains an important CNS infectious disease with high morbidity and mortality despite conjugate vaccine campaigns and modern antibiotics.

The incidence of viral meningitis depends on the age and vaccination status of the population. The most common pathogen, enterovirus, is responsible for 75,000 cases of viral meningitis per year in the United States, with most infections occurring in the summer and fall.[4] With the increasing population of immunocompromised patients, there has also been an overall increase in the incidence of fungal meningitis.

Although meningitis is pathophysiologically distinct from encephalitis, there is significant clinical overlap. Encephalitis refers to inflammation of the brain parenchyma. Examples include viral causes, such as herpes simplex virus (HSV) and varicella zoster virus, bacterial causes, such as *Mycobacterium tuberculosis*, and immune causes such as acute disseminated encephalomyelitis or antibody-associated encephalitis (voltage-gated potassium channel and NMDA receptor). Although one study suggests 85% of cases are of unknown cause; prompt diagnosis and distinction between the various etiologies are essential to guide treatment of this rare entity with unfortunate high mortality.[5]

A brain abscess is a focal infection in brain parenchyma that is caused by bacteria. Although healthy brain parenchyma is mostly resistant to bacterial infection, scar tissue from prior infarction, trauma, or surgery can serve as a nidus for infection, allowing early cerebritis to transform into a collection of pus encapsulated by a membrane. The incidence of brain abscesses has been estimated at 0.3 to 1.3 per 100,000 people per year but can be considerably higher in certain risk groups, such as immunocompromised patients.[6] Most commonly, infection reaches brain parenchyma via direct or indirect spread from paranasal sinuses, ears, and teeth. Despite these potential sources, 20% to 30% of case are considered "cryptic" abscess, in which no source can be identified.[7] The causative organism, when identified, is predominantly *Streptococcus* and *Staphylococcus* species. Over the last 30 years, neuroimaging techniques, stereotactic biopsy, and the introduction of new antibiotics have improved the case fatality rate from 40% to 10%, and the rate of patients with full recovery has increased from 33% to 70%.[6]

DIAGNOSTIC EVALUATION

The initial step in diagnosing a CNS infection is recognizing the potential for CNS infection based on clinical evaluation. In fact, when the diagnosis of meningoencephalitis is presumed, blood cultures should be obtained and antibiotics should be initiated empirically without delay. Distinguishing CNS infections on the basis of clinical presentation is difficult. Lumbar puncture (LP) can aid in the diagnosis of meningitis, but can be challenging because of patient factors, including obesity, anticoagulant use, and altered mental status. LP may also be unsafe for evaluation of parenchymal brain infections.

In 1909, Harvey Cushing[8] first described the risk of cerebral herniation and death when patients with unequal pressures between intracranial compartments underwent LP. The risk of transtentorial herniation or tonsillar herniation is higher in patients with a history or physical examination findings consistent with increased intracranial pressure. Neuroimaging, such as a head computed tomography (CT), can exclude mass lesions or radiologic evidence of increased intracranial pressure, which may increase risk of herniation with LP. According to the 2004 Infectious Diseases Society of America (IDSA) guidelines, LP should be delayed in order to first perform a head CT scan in a patient with suspected bacterial meningitis who has the following[9]:

- Immunocompromised state (eg, HIV infection, immunosuppressive therapy, solid organ or hematopoietic stem cell transplantation)
- History of CNS disease (eg, mass lesion, stroke, focal infection)
- New onset seizure within 1 week of presentation
- Papilledema
- Abnormal level of consciousness
- Focal neurologic deficit

However, even with a normal CT scan, clinical signs of "impending" herniation are the best predictors of when to delay or avoid LP, that is, deteriorating level of consciousness, particularly a Glasgow Coma Scale less than 11; brainstem signs including pupillary changes, posturing, or irregular respirations; or a very recent seizure. Other relative contraindications to LP include known spinal epidural abscess, thrombocytopenia, or another bleeding diathesis.[10]

Lumbar Puncture

The most useful diagnostic information is found in examination of the CSF, which allows for diagnosis of meningitis, identifying the causative organism, and performing in vitro susceptibility testing. The opening pressure of LP can provide additional diagnostic information, because bacterial and fungal meningitis can increase opening pressure from the normal range of 7 to 18 cm H_2O.[11] Of note, the measurement is only meaningful if the patient is lying extended in the lateral decubitus position, and therefore, the needle must be safely held in situ as the patient's legs are straightened from curled position. CSF analysis will include Gram stain and culture, cell count, and determination of protein and glucose concentration. Typical CSF findings for bacterial, viral, and fungal meningitis are displayed in **Table 1**. Additional tests may include viral cultures for patients with suspected viral meningitis, India ink stain for fungal antigens in patients with suspected cryptococcal meningitis, antibody for Borrelia in suspected Lyme meningitis, acid fast staining in suspected tuberculous meningitis, and Wright or Giemsa stain for suspected toxoplasmosis. Although viral cultures have variable sensitivity and may take 5 to 7 days for results, polymerase chain reaction testing has a high sensitivity and specificity and currently can be used to more accurately

Table 1
Typical cerebrospinal fluid findings in meningitis

Parameter	Normal	Bacterial	Viral[a]	Fungal[a]
CSF opening pressure	<170 mm	Elevated	Normal	Normal or elevated
Cell count	<5 cells/mm^3	>1000/mm^3	<1000/mm^3	<500/mm^3
Cell predominance	—	Neutrophils	Lymphocytes	Lymphocytes
CSF glucose	>0.66 × Serum	Low	Normal	Low
CSF protein	<45 mg/dL	Elevated	Normal	Elevated

[a] Findings may not be adequate to rule out bacterial disease in an individual patient.
  Data from Fitch MT, Abrahamian FM, Moran GJ, et al. Emergency department management of meningitis and encephalitis. Infect Dis Clin North Am 2008;22(1):33–52; and Tintinalli JE, Stapczynski JS. Tintinalli's emergency medicine: a comprehensive study guide. 7th edition. New York: McGraw-Hill; 2011.

define infection from enterovirus, HSV-1, Epstein-Barr virus, cytomegalovirus as well as possibly neurosyphilis and tuberculous meningitis.[12–14]

Cerebrospinal fluid lactate
Lactate within the CSF is produced by anaerobic metabolism of bacteria and is not influenced by serum concentration, unlike CSF glucose. Therefore, it was postulated as a possible marker for bacterial anaerobic metabolism and therefore possibly has advantages in differentiating bacterial meningitis from aseptic meningitis. Derived from a meta-analysis completed in 2011, CSF lactate has a sensitivity of 93% and specificity of 96% in distinguishing between bacterial and aseptic meningitis. Furthermore, this diagnostic performance is confirmed in both adults and children. This meta-analysis also established that, similar to other CSF markers, lactate is less sensitive if patients receive antibiotics before CSF sampling.[15]

Neuroimaging

Computed tomography
As previously discussed, head CT scan can be used before LP to rule out circumstances that may lead to brain herniation. Given that it is more readily available, head CT scan may be the initial radiologic test, which supplements clinical suspicion of CNS infection. The CT scan often underestimates extent of parenchymal involvement, however occasionally may demonstrate areas of ischemia due to secondary vasculitis, a complication in up to 20% of meningitis cases.[16] Contrast-enhanced CT may rarely show beginning meningeal enhancement, which becomes more prominent in later stages of meningitis. Similarly, with contrast enhancement, CT may demonstrate host response, such as capsule or granuloma formation, in parenchymal CNS infections, such as brain abscess or toxoplasmosis. This ringlike contrast enhancement may be subtle or completely absent in immunocompromised patients due to poor host defense mechanisms.[17] Although CT alone is unreliable in identifying CNS infection, it is useful as an initial neuroradiologic test, which assesses for safety of performing LP and identifying pathologic conditions of the base of the skull, including sinus fractures, inner ear infections, or mastoiditis, which may lead to expedited therapeutic intervention or surgical consultation.

MRI
Head MRI scan is superior in detecting CNS infections. MRI is not routinely necessary in cases of acute bacterial meningitis, although MRI may better detect early and subtle abnormalities, such as vasculitis accompanying meningitis. Also, meningeal enhancement of the basal cisterns on precontrast T1-weighted images may be highly

suggestive of tuberculous meningitis.[18] The pattern of parenchymal lesions on MRI may raise suspicion to the underlying CNS infectious organism and can therefore guide laboratory testing and treatment. MRI is especially useful in detecting necrotizing viral encephalitis, because the associated cytotoxic cortical edema can be detected within the initial 48 hours of presentation on T2-weighted or fluid-attenuated inversion recovery (FLAIR) images.[19] MRI is the most sensitive way to diagnose pyogenic ventriculitis, a clinically indolent and uncommon complication of meningitis or when an abscess ruptures into the ventricle. High periventricular signal, ependymal enhancement, and irregular intraventricular debris are signs of pyogenic ventriculitis, which is managed with high-dose antibiotics for a protracted period and/or administration of antibiotics via reservoir to the ventricle.

TREATMENT
Meningoencephalitis

When CNS infection is suspected and bacterial meningitis is considered, empiric treatment occurs simultaneously with diagnostic maneuvers. Clinical findings do not reliably distinguish between bacterial, viral, fungal meningitis, infectious encephalitis, or other noninfectious neoplastic or inflammatory process. Although laboratory and neuroimaging data can support the process of arriving at the correct diagnosis, given that bacterial meningitis has high mortality and high frequency of neurologic sequelae and morbidity, the highest priority is the prompt initiation of bactericidal antibiotics with adequate CNS penetration. Delays due to attaining neuroimaging before LP or due to transferring a patient to another hospital resulted in higher risk of adverse outcome.[20] Another retrospective study determined that there was a positive association between delays in administering antibiotics greater than 6 hours after arriving to the emergency department and death.[21]

Empiric treatment of meningoencephalitis is based on the likelihood of certain pathogens. S pneumoniae and N meningiditis are responsible for 80% of all cases of community-acquired bacterial meningitis.[22,23] **Table 2** lists recommendations for empiric treatment of bacterial meningitis, accounting for special populations in which ampicillin should be added to cover for L monocytogenes.

Adjunctive dexamethasone therapy
Adjuvant treatment with anti-inflammatory agents such as dexamethasone is postulated to provide a mortality benefit due to the reduction of CSF from bacterial lysis

---

Table 2
Infectious Diseases Society of America recommendations for empiric treatment of bacterial meningitis based on patient age

Age	Common Bacterial Pathogens	Antimicrobial Therapy
<1 mo	Streptococcus agalactiae, E coli, L monocytogenes, Klebsiella species	Ampicillin + Cefotaxime or aminoglycoside
1–23 mo	S pneumoniae, N meningitidis, S. agalactiae, H influenzae, Ecoli	Vancomycin + 3rd-generation cephalosporin
2–50 y	N meningitidis, S pneumoniae	Vancomycin + 3rd-generation cephalosporin
>50 y	S pneumoniae, N meningitidis, L monocytogenes, aerobic gram-negative bacilli	Vancomycin + Ampicillin + 3rd-generation cephalosporin

From Tunkel AR, Hartman BJ, Kaplan SL, et al. Practice guidelines for the management of bacterial meningitis. Clin Infect Dis 2004;39(9):1267–84.

induced by antibiotics. A prospective randomized double-blind, multicenter placebo-controlled trial involving 301 adult patients with suspected acute bacterial meningitis in combination with cloudy CSF, positive Gram stain, and CSF leukocytosis of more than 1000/mL[3] demonstrated that early treatment with dexamethasone improves outcomes and does not increase clinically significant adverse events such as gastrointestinal bleeding. In subgroup analysis, specifically adult patients with pneumococcal meningitis, patient mortality decreased from 34% to 14% as a result of reduced mortality from systemic complications.[24] As implicated by this study and subsequent systematic reviews, patients with acute bacterial meningitis should receive 10 mg of dexamethasone before or with the first dose of antibiotics to reduce hearing loss and neurologic sequelae.[25]

When viral meningitis is presumed, a broad range of approaches may be considered, including hospital admission for empiric antibiotic therapy until cultures result or discharge home with 24-hour follow-up. Although there are no established treatments for viral meningoencephalitis, acyclovir is commonly added to empiric treatment of meningoencephalitis because it has been shown by clinical trial to improve mortality in treatment of herpes simplex encephalitis. Therefore, in those with suspected encephalitis, due to relatively low-risk profile, empiric therapy is recommended, specifically, acyclovir 10 mg/kg every 8 hours for a 14- to 21-day course. Prognosis of viral meningoencephalitis depends on the specific etiologic virus as well as the host.

Of the pathogens that cause encephalitis, most are viruses. Despite availability of several tests, the infectious cause for most patients with encephalitis remains unknown.

Chemoprophylaxis for high-risk contacts

High-risk contacts of patients with documented meningococcal disease are generally considered to be individuals who have greater than 8 hours of contact in close proximity or if exposed to oral secretions of the patient within the past 7 days. Examples include household contacts, roommates or those living in dormitories or military barracks, intimate contacts, and health care personnel who intubate the patient without wearing a mask. In this situation, high-risk adult contacts should be given rifampin 10 mg/kg every 12 hours orally for 2 days, or a single dose of ciprofloxacin 500 mg orally or ceftriaxone 250 mg intramuscularly once in addition to close home surveillance and strict return precautions over the next 10 days.[26] Postexposure vaccination is less likely to be effective given that greater than half of secondary cases in household contacts occur in less than 5 days, and vaccination immunity is not effective for 5 to 7 days.[27]

Cerebral Abscess

The management of cerebral abscess will be determined by collaboration between infectious disease specialist, neurologist, and neurosurgeon. Treatment will largely be driven by stereotactic needle aspiration, which will allow both therapeutic drainage as well as diagnostic information, which will guide antimicrobial therapy. In the emergency department, however, immediate treatment of cerebral abscess may include initiation of empiric antimicrobial therapy in the critically ill, in conjunction with recommendations from neurosurgery colleagues. Although initial antimicrobial coverage can be chosen based on the likely pathogens at the suspected site of entry, that is, paranasal sinuses, ears, hematogenous spread, penetrating trauma, or postoperative, if the source is unknown, broad-spectrum antibiotics including anaerobic coverage can be initiated in the emergency department. Duration of antibiotics is usually 4 to

8 weeks, based on retrospective data; however, duration of therapy should be guided by clinical course and follow-up imaging studies.[28] Surgical excision is a more radical approach; however, it is first-line treatment in traumatic brain abscesses in order to remove bone fragments and foreign material, encapsulated fungal brain abscesses, multiloculated abscesses, or after incision and drainage if no clinical improvement after 1 week.[29,30]

Shunt Infection

As with any implanted foreign body, secondary infection is a serious complication of cerebral shunts. In adults, shunt infections manifest with fever and progressive altered mental status. Commonly in pediatrics, shunt infections manifest as altered mental status and abdominal complaints. The most commonly isolated microorganisms are *S aureus* and coagulase-negative *Staphylococcus*. There have also been increasing polymicrobial infections as well as gram-negative bacilli infections. Given the increase in oxacillin-resistant *Staphylococcus* infections and polymicrobial infections, the recommended empiric antibiotics are vancomycin and an agent to cover health care–associated gram-negative bacilli (ceftazidime, cefepime, or meropenem).[31] Treatment can involve various modalities, with the most recommended treatment being removal of the infected shunt with placement of an external ventricular drainage or serial taps and concomitant administration of antibiotics. A new shunt can be placed when CSF sterility is achieved. Less favorable is removal of infected shunt with immediate replacement and concomitant administration of antibiotics. The use of antibiotics alone results in the least favorable outcome.[32]

COMPLICATIONS

Because critically ill patients with suspected CNS infections board in the emergency department for longer periods of time, the EP should be familiar with managing complications of CNS infections. Given the substantial mortality and morbidity of CNS infections, patients with suspected CNS infection may need to be admitted to an intensive care unit in order to provide management of systemic and neurologic complications. Systemic complications include septic shock, disseminated intravascular coagulation, and acute respiratory distress syndrome. Neurologic complications include secondary insults to the brain, such as increased intracranial pressure, seizures, and ischemia. Systemic complications, rather than neurologic complications, are more likely to cause death in certain subgroups of patients such as the elderly.[33,34]

Sepsis

Sepsis occurs as a consequence of bacteremia, which frequently accompanies bacterial CNS infections, such as meningitis. In particular, meningococcal disease can cause significant system complications, including purpura fulminans, disseminated intravascular coagulation, and acute respiratory distress syndrome. Waterhouse-Friderichsen syndrome, or bilateral adrenal hemorrhage, is a fatal complication that can occur in a patient with overwhelming meningococcal sepsis. Many patients have a mixed picture with evidence of impaired central nervous function due to the direct infectious and inflammatory response within CNS due to infection as well as impaired function due to encephalopathy, which occurs secondary to profound shock.

Cerebral Edema and Hydrocephalus

Raised intracranial pressure is often the major underlying reason for alterations in mental status. Severe increases in intracranial pressure can cause papilledema, cranial nerve palsy, bradycardia with hypertension (Cushing reflex), coma, and herniation of cerebellar tonsils, leading to death. This increased pressure is due to vasogenic edema from increased permeability of the blood-brain barrier and cytotoxic edema from neuroinflammatory cells releasing cytotoxins. Especially in fungal and tuberculous meningitis, CSF absorption by arachnoid villi in the subarachnoid space is also impaired, leading to hydrocephalus. In these patients, hydrocephalus can be managed medically with osmotic agents but may also require surgical intervention with lumbar or ventricular drains.

Seizure

Seizures can occur in the setting of parenchymal inflammation. Once empiric treatment is begun, management of patients with suspected CNS infection will include monitoring for seizures. Although electroencephalography (EEG) is not routinely used in meningoencephalitis, EEG monitoring can be useful in patients with a history of seizures or in patients with a fluctuating mental status concerning for subclinical seizures. Antiepileptic medications are not recommended for routine prophylaxis.

Stroke and Intracranial Hemorrhage

CNS infections can have cerebrovascular sequelae, including stroke, formation of a mycotic aneurysm, arterial stenosis, and intracerebral hemorrhage. Possible mechanisms behind these vascular complications are immune-mediated vasospasm, invasion of the vessel wall by inflammatory cells, and endothelial dysfunction. Mortality is high with these vascular complications, and patients who present with neurologic deficits have worse outcomes.[16]

SUMMARY

Infections of the CNS are the responsibility of the EP to expeditiously recognize, diagnose, and treat to improve long-term morbidity and mortality. In the emergency department, once CNS infection is suspected, empiric treatment is initiated simultaneously with diagnostic maneuvers that aim to locate the infection and determine causative organism. LP remains the hallmark diagnostic study in order to obtain Gram stain and cultures that will guide antimicrobial management. However, the EP must remember that neuroimaging must precede LP in the patient who has an immunocompromised state, history of CNS focal disease, new onset seizure, papilledema, abnormal level of consciousness, or focal neurologic deficit. Bactericidal antibiotics with adequate CNS penetration and broad-spectrum coverage are standard, along with empiric treatment if suspecting HSV encephalitis. In the critically ill patients who board in the emergency department, the EP must monitor for complications of CNS infection, including decreased level of consciousness, cerebral edema, hydrocephalus, seizure, stroke, or intracranial hemorrhage.

REFERENCES

1. Thomas KE, Hasbun R, Jekel J, et al. The diagnostic accuracy of Kernig's sign, Brudzinski's sign, and nuchal rigidity in adults with suspected meningitis. Clin Infect Dis 2002;35(1):46–52.
2. Brouwer MC, Tunkel AR, van de Beek D. Epidemiology, diagnosis, and antimicrobial treatment of acute bacterial meningitis. Clin Microbiol Rev 2010;23(3):467–92.
3. McIntyre PB, O'Brien KL, Greenwood B, et al. Effect of vaccines on bacterial meningitis worldwide. Lancet 2012;380(9854):1703–11.

4. Desmond RA, Accortt NA, Talley L, et al. Enteroviral meningitis: natural history and outcome of pleconaril therapy. Antimicrob Agents Chemother 2006;50(7): 2409–14.

5. Granerod J, Ambrose HE, Davies NWS, et al. Causes of encephalitis and differences in their clinical presentations in England: a multicentre, population-based prospective study. Lancet 2010;10(12):835–44.

6. Brouwer MC, Coutinho JM, van de Beek D. Clinical characteristics and outcome of brain abscess. Neurology 2014;82(9):806–13.

7. Mathisen GE, Johnson JP. Brain abscess. Clin Infect Dis 1997;25(4):763–81.

8. Cushing H. Some aspects of the pathological physiology of intracranial tumors. Boston Med Surg J 1909;161(3):71–80.

9. Tunkel AR, Hartman BJ, Kaplan SL, et al. Practice guidelines for the management of bacterial meningitis. Clin Infect Dis 2004;39(9):1267–84.

10. Engelborghs S, Niemantsverdriet E, Struyfs H, et al. Consensus guidelines for lumbar puncture in patients with neurological diseases. Alzheimers Dement (Amst) 2017;8:111–26.

11. Reichman EF, Polglaze K, Euerle B. Neurological and neurosurgical procedures: lumbar puncture. Emergency medicine procedures. New York: McGraw Hill; 2013. p. 747–61.

12. Jeffery KJ, Read SJ, Peto TE, et al. Diagnosis of viral infections of the central nervous system: clinical interpretation of PCR results. Lancet 1997;349(9048):313–7.

13. Cinque P, Scarpellini P, Vago L, et al. Diagnosis of central nervous system complications in HIV-infected patients: cerebrospinal fluid analysis by the polymerase chain reaction. AIDS 1997;11(1):1–17.

14. Tanel RE, Kao S-Y, Niemiec TM, et al. Prospective comparison of culture vs genome detection for diagnosis of enteroviral meningitis in childhood. Arch Pediatr Adolesc Med 1996;150(9):919–24.

15. Sakushima K, Hayashino Y, Kawaguchi T, et al. Diagnostic accuracy of cerebrospinal fluid lactate for differentiating bacterial meningitis from aseptic meningitis: a meta-analysis. J Infect 2011;62(4):255–62.

16. Hayes L, Malhotra P. Central nervous system infections masquerading as cerebrovascular accidents: case series and review of literature. IDCases 2014;1(4): 74–7.

17. Ramsey RG, Geremia GK. CNS complications of AIDS: CT and MR findings. AJR Am J Roentgenol 1988;151(3):449–54.

18. Good CD, Jäger HR. Contrast enhancement of the cerebrospinal fluid on MRI in two cases of spirochaetal meningitis. Neuroradiology 2000;42(6):448–50.

19. Maschke M, Kastrup O, Forsting M, et al. Update on neuroimaging in infectious central nervous system disease. Curr Opin Neurol 2004;17(4):475–80.

20. Aronin SI, Peduzzi P, Quagliarello VJ. Community-acquired bacterial meningitis: risk stratification for adverse clinical outcome and effect of antibiotic timing. Ann Intern Med 1998;129(11):862–9.

21. Proulx N, Fréchette D, Toye B, et al. Delays in the administration of antibiotics are associated with mortality from adult acute bacterial meningitis. QJM 2005;98(4): 291–8.

22. van de Beek D, de Gans J, Spanjaard L, et al. Clinical features and prognostic factors in adults with bacterial meningitis. N Engl J Med 2004;351(18):1849–59.

23. Schuchat A, Robinson K, Wenger JD, et al. Bacterial meningitis in the United States in 1995. Active surveillance team. N Engl J Med 1997;337(14):970–6.

24. de Gans J, van de Beek D, European Dexamethasone in Adulthood Bacterial Meningitis Study Investigators. Dexamethasone in adults with bacterial meningitis. N Engl J Med 2002;347(20):1549–56.

25. Brouwer MC, McIntyre P, de Gans J, et al. Corticosteroids for acute bacterial meningitis. Cochrane Database Syst Rev 2010;(9):CD004405.

26. Centers for Disease Control and Prevention (CDC). Control and prevention of meningococcal disease: recommendations of the advisory committee on immunization practices (ACIP). MMWR Morbs Mortal Wkly Rep 1997;46(RR-5):1–51.

27. Munford RS, Taunay Ade E, de Morais JS, et al. Spread of meningococcal infection within households. Lancet 1974;303(7869):1275–8.

28. Helweg-Larsen J, Astradsson A, Richhall H, et al. Pyogenic brain abscess, a 15 year survey. BMC Infect Dis 2012;12:332–41.

29. Mampalam TJ, Rosenblum ML. Trends in the management of bacterial brain abscesses: a review of 102 cases over 17 years. Neurosurgery 1988;23(4):451–8.

30. Sharma BS, Gupta SK, Khosla VK. Current concepts in the management of pyogenic brain abscess. Neurol India 2000;48(2):105–11.

31. Dawod J, Tager A, Darouiche RO, et al. Prevention and management of internal cerebrospinal fluid shunt infections. J Hosp Infect 2016;93(4):323–8.

32. Schreffler RT, Schreffler AJ, Wittler RR. Treatment of cerebrospinal fluid shunt infections: a decision analysis. Pediatr Infect Dis J 2002;21(7):632–6.

33. Weisfelt M, van de Beek D, Spanjaard L, et al. Clinical features, complications, and outcome in adults with pneumococcal meningitis: a prospective case series. Lancet Neurol 2006;5(2):123–9.

34. Flores-Cordero JM, Amaya-Villar R, Rincón-Ferrari MD, et al. Acute community-acquired bacterial meningitis in adults admitted to the intensive care unit: clinical manifestations, management and prognostic factors. Intensive Care Med 2003; 29(11):1967–73.

Skin and Soft Tissue Infections in the Emergency Department

Amelia Breyre, MD, Bradley W. Frazee, MD*

KEYWORDS

- Abscess • Cellulitis • Necrotizing fasciitis • MRSA

KEY POINTS

- Purulent skin infections are often caused by methicillin-resistant *Staphylococcus aureus*.
- State-of-the-art treatment of skin abscesses combines thorough surgical drainage and adjunctive antibiotics that cover methicillin-resistant *S aureus*, such as trimethoprim-sulfamethoxazole.
- Nonpurulent cellulitis is a predominantly streptococcal disease and initial empiric antibiotics need not cover methicillin-resistant *S aureus*.
- Emergency physicians need be vigilant for rare, but potentially lethal, necrotizing skin and soft tissue infections.

INTRODUCTION

Skin and soft tissue infections (SSTIs) result in more than 14 million ambulatory visits and more than 6 million emergency department (ED) visits in the United States annually.[1,2] SSTIs are among the most common form of infection encountered in EDs. The term SSTI encompasses several distinct types of infections, with a broad spectrum of severity, ranging from routine to rapidly life threatening. This article focuses on the 3 most important clinical types of SSTI—abscess and purulent cellulitis, nonpurulent cellulitis and necrotizing soft tissue infections (NSTI). We also briefly review impetigo. Infections related to bite wounds and water exposure, with their unusual bacteriology, are not addressed in detail.

    SSTIs can be classified several different ways. We prefer the classification scheme proposed by the Infectious Disease Society of America (IDSA) because it suggests a useful clinical diagnostic approach – in which the first step is to "look for pus" (**Fig. 1**)—dividing SSTIs according to presence or absence of purulence. If there is purulence,

Disclosure Statement: No commercial or financial conflicts of interest. No funding sources.
Department of Emergency Medicine, Highland Hospital, 1411 East 31st Street, Oakland, CA 94602, USA
* Corresponding author.
E-mail address: bradf_98@yahoo.com

Emerg Med Clin N Am 36 (2018) 723–750
https://doi.org/10.1016/j.emc.2018.06.005
0733-8627/18/© 2018 Elsevier Inc. All rights reserved.

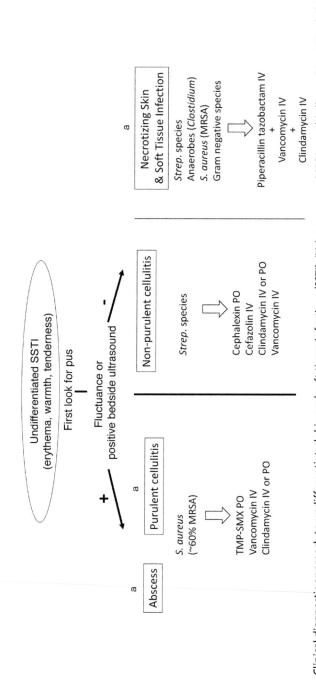

Fig. 1. Clinical diagnostic approach to undifferentiated skin and soft tissue infections (SSTI). IV, intravenous; MRSA, methicillin-resistant *Staphylococcus aureus*; PO, per os; TMP-SMX, trimethoprim-sulfamethoxazole. [a] Surgical disease.

the causative bacteria is likely *Staphylococcus aureus*. Establishing good drainage, usually with an incision and drainage procedure, is required and antibiotics with activity against methicillin-resistant *S aureus* (MRSA) are generally indicated. If there is no pus, the diagnostic considerations are nonpurulent cellulitis and NSTI. Nonpurulent cellulitis is usually caused by a β-hemolytic streptococcal species, thus beta-lactam antibiotics (which do not cover MRSA) can be used. If a necrotizing infection is suspected, the etiology may be polymicrobial and broad-spectrum antibiotics should be administered. In addition, prompt surgical intervention is indicated. **Table 1** presents a selected list of antibiotics recommended by the IDSA for each of the major SSTI categories. For *Staphylococcus* and *Streptococcus* infections the duration of therapy is 5 to 10 days, depending on the clinical circumstances and response to treatment.[3]

SSTIs can also be classified by the level of skin involved. The epidermis is the most superficial layer overlying the dermis; it is thin and avascular. Erysipelas is a form of nonpurulent cellulitis limited to the epidermis and impetigo is an infection that affects only the keratin cells of this layer. The dermis is a thicker layer containing hair follicles, sebaceous glands, and sweat glands; folliculitis is an infection confined to hair follicles. Hair follicles also represent the portal of entry for spontaneous *S aureus* furuncles. The hypodermis lies between the dermis and underlying muscle and fascia and contains adipose tissue. Furuncles are an infection originating in hair follicles that produce a localized subcutaneous abscess within the hypodermis. Carbuncles, which are a coalescence of multiple furuncles, tend to extend deeper into the hypodermis. The fascia is the connective tissue layer that lies below the hypodermis; necrotizing fasciitis is an infection of this layer.

The US Food and Drug Administration uses the term "acute bacterial skin and skin structure infection" to specifically classify SSTIs for the purpose of clinical trials evaluating antibiotic efficacy. This scheme differentiates minor and major cutaneous abscesses that are smaller or larger than 75 cm^2, respectively. The US Food and Drug Administration intentionally excludes less serious infections such as impetigo and more complex infections such as deep and necrotizing infections from clinical trials.[4] Another clinically useful scheme is to classify SSTIs based on severity of local and systemic symptoms, with the corresponding recommended management **(Table 2)**.[5,6]

MICROBIOLOGY

The majority of community-onset SSTIs encountered in the ED are caused by either *S aureus* or one of the β-hemolytic streptococcal species.[7,8] However, there are numerous important pathogens that cause SSTIs in special circumstances, such as nosocomial wound infections and infections after animal bites and water exposure. **Table 3** summarizes the special types of SSTI in which the bacteriology includes pathogens other than *S aureus* and β-hemolytic streptococcal spp. These more esoteric infections are not covered further in this review.

Staphylococcus aureus

S aureus is a gram-positive coccus that grows in clusters and is part of the normal human microbiota. It is frequently found on the nasal mucosa, the skin (especially of the axilla and groin), and in the gastrointestinal tract. Classically, it is associated with localized pus-producing lesions, such as furuncles, abscesses, and carbuncles. *S aureus* produces several molecules that recruit neutrophils, cause host cell lysis, and are involved in the formation of the fibrin capsule surrounding abscesses.[9]

Table 1
Antimicrobial therapy for purulent cellulitis, nonpurulent cellulitis and NSTI

Infection Category and Responsible Pathogen	Antibiotic	Dosage, Adults	Comments
Impetigo (*Staphylococcus* and *Streptococcus*)	Mupirocin ointment	Apply to lesions bid	For limited number of lesions
	Retapmulin ointment	Apply lesions bid	For limited number of lesions
	Dicloxacilin	250 mg qid po	—
	Cephalexin	250 mg qid po	
	Clindamycin	300–400 mg qid po	
	Trimethoprim-sulfamethoxazole	1–2 double strength tablets bid po	Bactericidal; limited published efficacy data
Abscess and purulent cellulitis (MRSA, MSSA)	Vancomycin	30 mg/kg/d in 2 divided doses IV	For penicillin allergic patients; parenteral drug of choice for MRSA
	Clindamycin	600 mg every 8 h IV or 300–450 mg qid po	Bacteriostatic; potential for cross-resistance and emergence of resistance in erythromycin-resistant strains; inducible resistance in MRSA
	Doxycycline, minocycline	100 mg bid po 100 mg bid po	—
	Linezolid	600 mg every 12 h IV or 600 mg bid po	Bacteriostatic. Expensive
Severe, known MSSA SSTI	Nafcillin or oxacillin	1-2g every 4 h IV	Parental drug of choice; inactive against MRSA
Nonpurulent cellulitis (Beta-hemolytic streptococcus, MSSA)	Cephalexin	500 mg every 6 h po	—
	Cefazolin	1 g every 8 h IV	
	Clindamycin	600–900 mg every 8 h IV	
	Nafcillin	1-2g every 4-6h IV	
	Penicillin VK	250–500 mg every 6 h po	
NSTI (GAS, *Clostridium* spp., MRSA, Gram-negative rods, Others)	Piperacillin Tazobactam	4.5 g every 6 h IV	—
	Azetreonam	2g every 6 h IV	For penicillin allergies
	Vancomycin +	15–20 mg/kg IV every 12 h IV	—
	Clindamycin	600–900 mg every 8 h IV	

Abbreviations: bid, twice a day; IV, intravenous; MRSA, methicillin-resistant *Staphylococcus aureus*; MSSA, methicillin-susceptible *Staphylococcus aureus*; NSTI, necrotizing soft tissue infection; po, per os; qid, 4 times a day.

Data from Stevens D, Bisno A, Chambers HF, et al. Practice Guidelines for the Diagnosis and Management of Skin and Soft Tissue Infections: 2014 Update by the Infectious Diseases Society of America. IDSA Guidelines. 2014(59):210–210.

Table 2
SSTI severity classification

Class	Description	Management
1	Afebrile and healthy, other than acute SSTI	If required, incision and drainage. If required, oral antimicrobials as an outpatient
2	Febrile and ill appearing, but no unstable comorbidities (eg, diabetes) that may complicate or delay resolution	Can be treated with oral antibiotics or outpatient IV therapy and may require a short period of observation in hospital
3	Appear toxic and unwell (fever, tachycardia, tachypnea and/or hypotension)	Likely to require inpatient treatment with parenteral antibiotics
4	Sepsis syndrome or life threatening infection (eg, necrotizing fasciitis)	Likely to require admission to intensive care facility for surgical assessment and parenteral antimicrobial agents

Abbreviations: IV, intravenous; SSTI, skin and soft tissue infection.
Data from Eron LJ, Lipsky BA, Low DE, et al. Managing skin and soft tissue infections: expert panel recommendations on key decision points. J Antimicrob Chemother 2003;52(suppl_1):i3–17; and Dryden MS. Skin and soft tissue infection: microbiology and epidemiology. Int J Antimicrob Agents 2009;34 Suppl 1:S2–7.

The worldwide emergence of community-associated MRSA (CA-MRSA) in the late 1990s and early 2000s led to a dramatic increase in purulent SSTIs and forced a change in the empiric antibiotics used to treat these infections. The predominant clonal type of CA-MRSA in the United States is named USA300; this strain invariably produces Panton-Valentine leukocidin, an exotoxin lethal to leukocytes, and was largely responsible for the explosive emergence of CA-MRSA across the country

Table 3
Microbiology of special types of SSTI

Condition	Possible Pathogens
Fresh or salt water exposure	Vibrio vulnificus, Aeromonas hydrophilia, Erysipelothrix rhusiopathiae, Mycobacterium marinum, others
Human bites	Eikenella corrodens, Fusobacterium nucleatum, Streptococcus anginosus, Staphylococcus aureus
Cat bites	Pasteurella multocida, Streptococcus spp, S aureus, Fusobacterium spp, Bacteroides spp, others; Bartonella henselae (cat scratch disease)
Dog bites	Pasteurella multocida, Streptococcus spp, S aureus, Fusobacterium spp, Bacteroides spp; Capnocytophaga (may cause overwhelming sepsis in susceptible patients)
Diabetic foot	S aureus (including MRSA), β-hemolytic streptococcal spp, Pseudomonas aeruginosa, Enterococcus spp., Escherichia coli, other Enterobacteriaciae spp., oral anaerobic spp, B spp., Clostridium spp.
Injection drug use	S aureus (including MRSA), Streptococcus spp, oral anaerobic spp, Clostridium perfringens, Clostridium sordellii, and Clostridium novyi
Perirectal abscess	S aureus, Streptococcus spp, E coli, other Enterobacteriacea spp, Bacteroides fragilis, other anaerobic spp

Abbreviations: MRSA, methicillin-resistant Staphylococcus aureus; SSTI, skin and soft tissue infection.

during the early 2000s. By 2004, CA-MRSA was responsible for roughly 60% of purulent SSTIs in US EDs.[10,11]

S aureus and CA-MRSA ecology have a bearing on clinical management. Because CA-MRSA colonizes the axilla, groin, and gastrointestinal tract; detection of colonization and subsequent decolonization strategies cannot be solely aimed at the anterior nares.[12] Because S aureus is uniquely able to survive on fomites, infection control measures should include disinfecting high-touch household surfaces and linen. Finally, the purulent nature of S aureus infections seems to allow transmission from person to person by even brief direct contact with the draining lesion.[13]

β-Hemolytic Streptococcal Species

The β-hemolytic streptoccocci species are gram-positive cocci that grow in chains. These species are also part of the normal human skin microbiota. In contrast with S aureus, a hallmark clinical feature of streptococcal SSTIs is lack of purulence, though serous fluid-filled blisters can be seen when inflammation is intense. Streptococcus pyogenes, also known as group A Streptococcus is the most common and renowned, but other species—groups G, D, and B—are increasingly recognized as etiologies of nonpurulent cellulitis. S pyogenes is one of the preeminent human pathogens, responsible for a range of clinical infections including not only impetigo, lymphantigitis, erysipelas, cellulitis, and necrotizing fasciitis, but also pharyngitis, scarlet fever, pneumonia, streptococcal toxic shock syndrome, and the notorious sequelae of infection, rheumatic fever and glomerulonephritis.[14]

Impetigo

Epidemiology and microbiology Impetigo is caused by both S aureus and S pyogenes. Infection is preceded by colonization of the unbroken skin. CA-MRSA has been implicated in some cases of bullous impetigo. Colonization precedes infection by an average interval of 10 days.[15] The peak incidence of impetigo is in children between ages 2 and 5, although it may also occur in older children or adults. Risk factors for impetigo include poor hygiene and disruption of the epidermal layer by mosquito bites, abrasions, and eczema.[14]

Clinical features There are 2 major types of impetigo: nonbullous and bullous. Nonbullous impetigo is the more common form. It presents as a yellowish crust on the face, arms, or legs. Impetigo begins as a papule, briefly progresses to a vesicle, and then becomes a pustule surrounded by an area of erythema (**Fig. 2**A). The pustule gives rise to the characteristic thick, golden crust over a period of 4 to 6 days (**Fig. 2**B). Sores are not painful but may be pruritic. Fever is rare, but regional lympadenopathy may be present. Touching the sores may result in spread of the infection. Bullous impetigo is a staphylococcal disease typically more common in children less than 2 years of age. It is characterized by painless fluid-filled bullae, predominantly on the arms, legs, and trunks. After the bullae break, they may form yellow scabs. The term ecthyma refers to a form of chronic S pyogenes and S aureus infection that is considered by some investigators to be a form of impetigo. The infection penetrates deeper into the dermis forming ulcers covered with a crust or eschar that tend to scar (**Fig. 2**C). Poststreptococcal glomerulonephritis is a possible sequela of streptococcal impetigo.[14,16]

Diagnosis The diagnosis of impetigo is made by visual recognition. Gram stain and culture, which differentiate staphylococcal from streptococcal infection, are optional. Assays of antistreptolysin O are not useful in the diagnosis or management of impetigo because antistreptolysin O response is weak in patients with streptococcal impetigo.

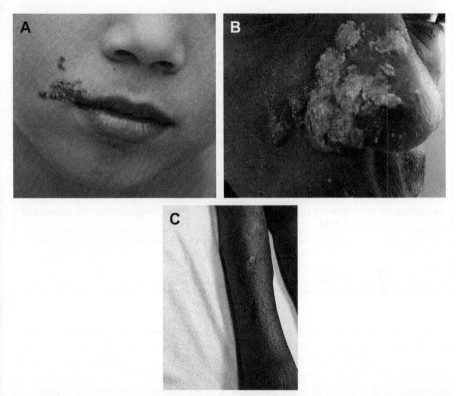

Fig. 2. (*A*) Impetigo with red sores around nose and mouth with honey-crusted lesions. (*B*) Ecthyma, a deeper form of impetigo that extends into the dermis. Pustules erode into ulcers with adherent crust. (*C*) Scarring caused by ecthyma. ([*A*] *From* Wikimedia Commons. Available at: https://commons.wikimedia.org/w/index.php?curid=53728118. Accessed February 15, 2018.)

This serologic test may, however, be useful in patients who are suspected of having poststreptococcal glomerulonephritis.[14]

Treatment and prophylaxis Impetigo treatment involves removing the crust and washing the affected area with soap and water followed by some type of antibiotic. A topical antibiotic with reliable antistaphylococcal activity is often sufficient. Muporicin is the most widely recommended topical agent. For more widespread lesions, oral antistaphylococcal (but not necessarily anti-MRSA) antibiotics may be used, such as cephalexin and dicloxacillin. However, there is a lack of data on the treatment of extensive impetigo and it remains unclear whether oral antibiotics are superior to topical antibiotics.[17] Good personal hygiene can prevent the spread of impetigo to susceptible individuals.

Abscess

Epidemiology and microbiology Cutaneous abscesses are focal collections of pus located within the dermis and hypodermis, which typically present as "painful, tender and fluctuant red nodules, often surmounted by a pustule and surrounded by a rim of erythematous swelling," according to the IDSA. The definitions and terminology of common types of abscesses and other purulent infections are listed in **Table 4**.[18]

Table 4
Purulent skin and soft tissue infection definitions

Condition	Description
Cutaneous abscess (skin abscess)	Subcutaneous collection of pus, with a wide spectrum of size and severity.
Folliculitis	Inflammation and infection of hair follicles resulting in tiny, papular abscesses
Furuncle	Small, spontaneous (no evident portal of entry), cutaneous abscess, that develops around a hair follicle, resulting in purulence extending below the epidermis. Commonly called a "boil." Patients may report a "spider bite."
Carbuncle	Coalescence of multiple furuncles, typically involving the deep subcutaneous tissues; often occur at the base of the neck.
Paronychia	Abscess at the base of a finger or toe nail, trapped below the eponychial fold.
Hidradenitis suppurativa	An often inherited form of acute and chronic inflammation of sebaceous and apocrine glands that causes follicular occlusion; abscesses appear purulent but are sterile.
Purulent cellulitis	Erythema, induration, and warmth that extends from a purulent focus.

The etiology of uncomplicated skin abscesses has been investigated in multiple large studies since the early 2000s and the findings are consistent. *S aureus* is isolated in about 60% to 75% of cases, of which 50% to 70% is MRSA. MRSA is now considered to be endemic in all regions of the United States.[11,19–21] Coagulase-negative staphylococcus is the next most common species isolated, followed by a variety of β-hemolytic streptococcal species that together account for only about 5% of positive cultures. Of note, about 10% of cultures show no growth. Injection drug use (IDU)-related cutaneous abscesses may be polymicrobial and contain oral streptococci and anaerobes, because saliva is so often used to dissolve the drug and clean needles and syringes.[22] Although *S aureus* is still commonly isolated from perianal abscesses, gram-negative bacteria and anaerobes may be more common in these abscesses.[23] Likewise, Bartholin gland abscesses are most often caused by *S aureus*, but may also be due to gram-negative and anaerobic bacteria and occasionally *Chlamydia trachomatis* or *Neisseria gonorrheoea*.[24,25]

Risk factors for recurrent abscesses include IDU; shaving of legs, axilla, and pubic hair; and colonization or prior infection with CA-MRSA. In a recent study of patients with culture-confirmed purulent SSTI, 70% were colonized with *S aureus* in their anterior nares[26] (the epidemiology of *S aureus* is discussed further in Microbiology, elsewhere in this article).

Clinical features Cutaneous abscesses are easily recognized by their appearance. The erythema, swelling, and induration have a circular shape often associated with a small point of necrosis or signs of spontaneous drainage. There may or may not be significant purulent cellulitis extending radially from the purulent focus. (This is in contrast with nonpurulent cellulitis, which is often circumferential around a limb.) Fluctuance is a classic hallmark of abscesses; however, it is frequently absent in the early stages of formation and in the case of a deep subcutaneous abscess. In fact, cutaneous abscesses located where adipose of the hypodermis is particularly thick, like the gluteal and thigh region, may have minimal external signs. **Fig. 3** demonstrates a variety of presentations of cutaneous abscesses.

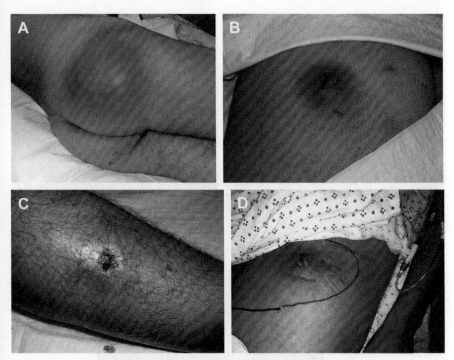

Fig. 3. (*A*) Injection drug use–related abscess. Injection of drugs subcutaneously, known as "skin popping," can result in large abscesses where the patient injects drugs, such as in the buttocks and deltoids. (*B*) Furuncle, a simple cutaneous skin abscess. (*C*) Furuncle after spontaneous drainage, with shallow ulcer and eschar, often mistaken by the patient as a spider bite. (*D*) A deep abscess within the adipose of the thigh, with only a small point of purulence and limited cellulitis evident.

Diagnosis Careful palpation for fluctuance represents the first-line "diagnostic test" for a cutaneous abscess and in many cases is all that is required. Ultrasound examination may be a useful adjunct to the physical examination when fluctuance is absent or difficult to localize. Abscess cavities usually appear hypoechoic or anechoic on ultrasound examination and acoustic enhancement may be seen deep to the pus collection. In addition, for deep or intramuscular abscesses, ultrasound examination can be invaluable in identifying the best location for incision (**Fig. 4**). A metaanalysis of 8 small studies demonstrated the effectiveness of point-of-care ultrasound examination in differentiating between abscess and cellulitis. The pooled sensitivity and specificity for identifying abscesses were 96.2% and 82.9%, respectively.[27] In our experience, the distinction between an abscess with irregular margins and cellulitis is often not straightforward. A study by Squire and colleagues[28] demonstrated a sensitivity and specificity for identifying abscesses with ultrasound examination alone of only 86% and 70%, respectively, but found that diagnostic performance was improved when clinical impression and ultrasound findings were used together. These results are more in line with our impression of ultrasound examination's usefulness for diagnosing cutaneous abscesses.

A computed tomography scan may be used for deep subcutaneous or intramuscular abscesses, although it is rarely needed. Its greatest usefulness may be to evaluate for abscesses around the perineum (scrotum, rectum) and in the neck. Cultures

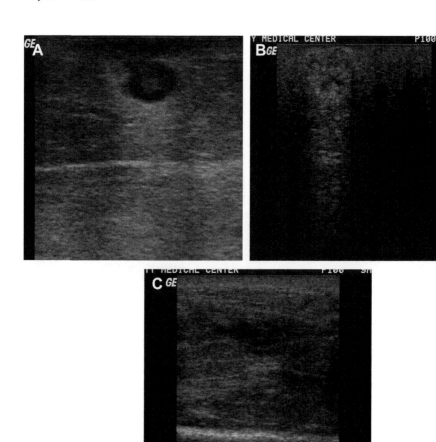

Fig. 4. (*A*) Ultrasound image of spherical cutaneous abscess demonstrating acoustic enhancement. (*B*) Ultrasound image of superficial cutaneous abscess with isoechoic cavity and acoustic enhancement. (*C*) Deep intramuscular deltoid abscess, with muscular fascia in the near field and cortex of the humerus in the far field.

are usually not necessary, because the bacteriology has been well-established and MRSA is endemic. The IDSA recommends Gram staining and culture of the pus for recurrent abscesses.[3]

Treatment and prevention The IDSA strongly recommends incision and drainage for treatment of carbuncles, abscesses, and large furuncles.[3] Incision and drainage traditionally involves a single, linear incision followed by blunt dissection. Needle aspiration has been shown to be generally inferior to incision and drainage for drainage of cutaneous abscesses.[29] However, needle aspiration may be preferred on the face when cosmesis is a major consideration.

Irrigation of the abscess cavity after incision and drainage is routinely used by some practitioners. We do not recommend this practice in part because it may aerosolize *S aureus*-laden liquid onto nearby surfaces. There is a recent trial comparing irrigation with no irrigation in 187 uncomplicated abscesses that found no difference in 30-day reintervention.[30]

Packing the abscess cavity with one-quarter to one-half inch of gauze after incision and drainage, another widely accepted routine practice, also seems to be unnecessary, at least for small abscesses. Three studies have been conducted comparing packing with no packing in small abscesses in children and young adults.[31–33] All found no difference in the need for repeat incision and drainage or additional antibiotics. Not surprisingly, patients in the packing groups experienced more pain, required greater analgesic use, and were more likely to return to the ED within 48 hours. Two patients in the no packing group had recurrent gluteal abscesses, which suggests that for deeper abscesses there is still a need to promote adequate abscess drainage in some way.

The loop drainage technique, in which a loop of rubber material is placed through the abscess cavity after incision and drainage, seems to be the new state-of-the-art for promoting ongoing drainage (**Fig. 5**).[34] Most of the data are retrospective, but a recent prospective trial comparing loop drainage with incision and drainage without packing found better resolution with loop drainage.[35,36] In addition, it is likely less painful than packing, may reduce scarring because 2 smaller incisions can be made, and requires fewer if any return visits, because patients can cut the loop and remove it painlessly themselves once drainage stops. Most important in our view, the sturdy rubber drains allow the patient to immediately begin soaking and washing the incised abscess.

Whether or not adjuvant antibiotics (in addition to incision and drainage) are needed for uncomplicated cutaneous abscesses has been a longstanding debate. The 2014 IDSA SSTI guidelines emphasize the primary role of incision and drainage, recommending that antibiotics be reserved for large or complicated abscesses, defined as those with fever or other systemic inflammatory response syndrome signs, greater than 5 cm of surrounding cellulitis, or occurring in an immunocompromised host.[3] However, since the publication of these guidelines, 2 high-quality randomized trials have been published examining use of off-patent oral antibiotics for uncomplicated cutaneous abscesses.[20,37] Both trials found a clinically small but consistent benefit from antibiotics. In the study by Talan and colleagues, treatment failure occurred in 19.5% of the trimethoprim-sulfamethoxazole (TMP-SMX) group versus 26.4% with placebo, for an absolute risk reduction of 6.9% (number needed to treat of 14). Daum and colleagues[20] reported an absolute reduction in treatment failure of 14% (number needed to treat of 7) with clindamycin and 13% with TMP-SMX. MRSA was isolated in 45% to 49% of cases. The results of these trials seem to put the debate to rest, supporting the routine use of adjunctive TMP-SMX or clindamycin for 7 days (see **Table 1** for additional treatment options). However, we believe there is still room for a less sweeping approach, in particular respecting the wishes of patients who may be disinclined to take antibiotics when the benefit is small. Keep in mind that treatment failure still occurred in approximately 20% of patients assigned to antibiotics. This finding underscores the importance of good aftercare and follow-up instructions that anticipate treatment failure. Treatment failure in the case of an uncomplicated abscess typically means the drainage or purulent cellulitis fails to resolve completely or a new abscess springs up. In such cases, one simply needs to make sure that any sequestered purulence is again unroofed and able to drain and that the area is scrubbed with soap and water. At that point, antibiotics should be prescribed if not prescribed initially; if antibiotics have already been prescribed, confirm whether the patient was actually taking them.[38,39]

Early and frequent washing of the abscess cavity with soapy water has not been formally studied, but it is likely beneficial in promoting resolution. Patients should be

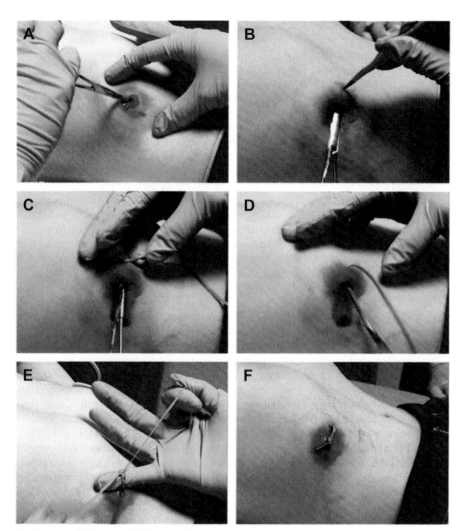

Fig. 5. Loop drainage technique. (*A*) Step 1. Prepare the area and administer local anesthesia. Make a central incision and use a hemostat to break up loculations within the abscess. The abscess may be irrigated now or after the vessel loop is placed. (*B*) Step 2. Use the hemostat to tent the skin near the farthest edge of the abscess cavity, and make a second incision over the tip of the hemostat. (*C*) Step 3. Once the second incision is made, push the hemostat through the new incision, and use it to grab the vessel loop and pull it through the abscess cavity. (*D*) Step 4. Pull vessel loop through the abscess cavity. (*E*) Step 5. Tie the vessel loop, using a finger or hemostat to keep it loose over the surface of the skin. (*F*) Step 6. Appearance of final vessel loop placement. (*From* Ladde JG, Baker S, Rodgers CN, et al. The LOOP technique: a novel incision and drainage technique in the treatment of skin abscesses in a pediatric ED. Am J Emerg Med 2015;33(2):271–6.)

empowered to do this as part of routine discharge instructions. It is a more realistic recommendation when there is a loop drain in place rather than packing. Discharge instructions aimed at reducing recurrences and spread of S *aureus* within households are listed in **Box 1**.[40]

Box 1
Discharge instructions after abscess incision and drainage

Keep draining wounds covered with a clean bandage.

Wash hands frequently especially after touching infected wounds or soiled bandages.

Launder clothing that is contaminated by drainage.

Do not share contaminated items like towel, clothing, bedding, or razors.

While there is drainage, avoid activities that involve skin to skin contact.

Clean contaminated environment surfaces with bleach, detergent, or disinfectant that specifies activity against *S aureus* on the label.

From Wallin TR, Hern HG, Frazee BW. Community-associated methicillin-resistant Staphylococcus aureus. Emerg Med Clin North Am 2008;26(2):431–55, ix.

If incision and drainage is successful, the need for admission is rare. Exceptions include the following:

- Abscesses requiring drainage in the operating room,
- Fever,
- Significant surrounding cellulitis requiring parenteral antibiotics,
- Evidence of severe sepsis suggesting bacteremia, and
- Immunocompromised patients (including AIDS, end-stage renal disease, and poorly controlled diabetes mellitus).

Purulent cellulitis
Purulent cellulitis, also known as culturable cellulitis, is associated with a purulent focus such as an abscess, a pustule, ulcer, or purulent wound. As demonstrated in a study by Miller and colleagues[7] and emphasized in the 2014 IDSA guidelines, cellulitis with purulence indicates that the pathogen is very likely *S aureus*, with approximately 60% being MRSA. Recommended antibiotics are oral TMP-SMX or intravenous vancomycin; clindamycin (oral or intravenous) is second line (see **Table 1**).

It is very important for physicians to understand the distinction between purulent and nonpurulent cellulitis and the implications regarding etiology and antibiotic choice. In many cases, purulent cellulitis will simply be regarded as the usual rim of erythema and induration radiating from a cutaneous abscess (**Fig. 6**A, B). In some cases, however, the extent of cellulitis may seem to be out of proportion to a trivial-seeming purulent focus or the purulence may be occult (**Fig. 6**C). In such cases, it is the responsibility of the physician to search for the purulent focus, drain purulence when it is found, obtain a culture if the patient is going to be admitted, and select appropriate antibiotics. In cases where it is unclear if cellulitis is associated with pus, an ultrasound examination can be invaluable. Tayal and colleagues[41] demonstrated that ultrasound examination altered management by revealing unsuspected pus in up to 48% of patients clinically suspected of having just cellulitis with no need for incision and drainage.

Nonpurulent cellulitis
Epidemiology and microbiology Nonpurulent cellulitis typically occurs when there is a breakdown in the physical skin barrier, immune system, and/or circulatory system. Thus, diabetes mellitus, obesity, venous insufficiency, impaired lymphatic drainage (eg, trauma or prior surgery), IDU, and old age are all major risk factors.[42–44] The

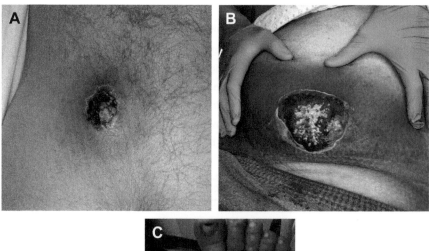

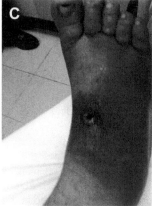

Fig. 6. (*A*) Abscess with caseating pus and eschar, accompanied by a rim of purulent cellulitis radiating symmetrically from the purulent focus (culture-proven methicillin-resistant *Staphylococcus aureus*). (*B*) Carbuncle on the abdominal wall with purulent cellulitis. (*C*) Small cutaneous abscess with prominent purulent cellulitis.

bacteriology of nonpurulent cellulitis is difficult to determine, because blood and tissue (punch biopsy) cultures are rarely positive. In studies using mostly serologic methods, β-hemolytic streptococcus species are implicated in most cases of nonpurulent cellulitis.[8] This includes not only *S pyogenes*, but also group C or G streptococci.[45] In a systematic literature review of 1578 cases of cellulitis, 7.9% were accompanied by positive blood cultures, of which 19% grew *S pyogenes*, 38% other β-hemolytic streptococci, 14% *S aureus*, and 28% gram-negative species.[46] The high proportion of gram-negative bacteria in this study was likely due to the inclusion of immunocompromised patients. In contrast, and underscoring the importance of correctly classifying cellulitis as purulent versus nonpurulent, in a review of studies of unselected cellulitis, positive punch biopsy cultures grew *S aureus* in 51% and *S pyogenes* in 27%.[47] However, cultures that grow MRSA are almost invariably linked to pus, an ulcer, a wound, or other purulent drainage.[48]

Clinical features Clinical findings in nonpurulent cellulitis include local pain, tenderness, swelling, and erythema. The process may extend rapidly to involve large areas of skin (**Fig. 7**). Systemic manifestation such as fever, lymphangitis, or

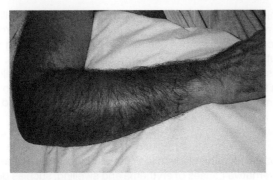

Fig. 7. Nonpurulent cellulitis of the upper arm.

bacteremia may be associated. In lower extremity cellulitis, it is recommended to examine the interdigital spaces between the toes for fissures or maceration, which may represent a portal of entry for bacteria and indicate a fungal coinfection requiring treatment.

Erysipyelas A distinctive subtype of nonpurulent cellulitis, erysipelas, is an infection that is limited to the epidermis. Classically, erysipelas is distinguished by acute onset, high fever, and a clear line of demarcation between involved and uninvolved tissue. It most often occurs on the lower extremity (**Fig. 8**). Lesions are a brilliant salmon red color. Facial erysipelas may be preceded by streptococcal sore throat and classically has a butterfly-shaped distribution.[14] The IDSA does not make a distinction between erysipelas and nonpurulent cellulitis.[3]

Diagnosis Correct diagnosis of nonpurulent cellulitis can be challenging. Miscategorization of cellulitis as nonpurulent when it is actually purulent (and potentially caused by MRSA) can lead to inappropriate treatment. In purulent cellulitis, fluctuance may be absent or underappreciated, especially early in the infection. In a treatment trial by Moran and colleagues[49] that sought to enroll only cases of nonpurulent cellulitis, approximately 10% of subjects subsequently developed an abscess, the majority owing to CA-MRSA.

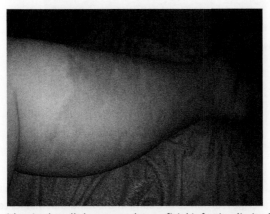

Fig. 8. Erysipelas with raised, well-demarcated superficial infection limited to the epidermis.

In addition, noninfectious processes are often misdiagnosed as cellulitis. Weng and colleagues[50] estimated that 30% of patients admitted for cellulitis were misdiagnosed. There are many common mimics of nonpurulent cellulitis, including chronic venous insufficiency, gout, large local reactions (allergic) to bee stings (**Fig. 9**), and contact dermatitis. Others potential mimics that are less commonly mistaken for cellulitis include deep vein thrombosis, fungal infection, drug rash, vasculitis, malignancy (lymphantitis, carcinomatosa), and herpes zoster. The most important and life-threatening mimic of cellulitis is NSTI.

Although imaging generally is not used to make the diagnosis of cellulitis, it is reasonable to use point-of-care ultrasound examination to evaluate undifferentiated erythematous processes, particularly to look for occult abscess. Ultrasound examination may reveal alternative causes of erythema and swelling, such as deep vein thrombosis, superficial thrombophlebitis, bursitis, and acute arthritis (septic joint).[41,51] Ultrasound findings in cellulitis are those of subcutaneous edema, with hyperechoic fat lobules and adjacent hypoechoic interlobular septae giving rise to a "cobblestone" appearance (**Fig. 10**).

The IDSA recommends that all patients with a soft tissue infection accompanied by signs of systemic toxicity (fever, hypotension, tachycardia) have blood cultures and laboratory tests performed. These include complete blood count with differential, serum chemistries, creatine phosphokinase, and C-reactive protein and lactate levels.[3] Marked leukocytosis, hyponatremia, and elevated creatine phosphokinase should raise the concern for an NSTI.

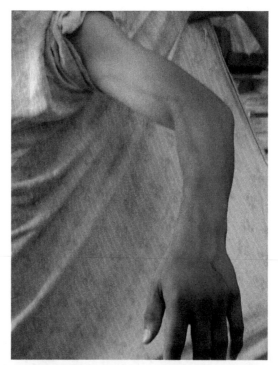

Fig. 9. Large local allergic reaction to bee sting in the hand that mimics cellulitis, including the ascending red streaking characteristic of lymphangitis.

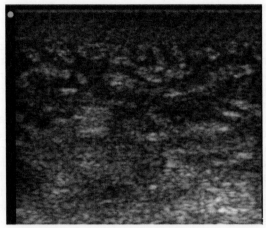

Fig. 10. Ultrasound image of nonpurulent cellulitis demonstrates characteristic cobblestone appearance, which is a result of hyperechoic fat lobules separated by hypoechoic fluid-filled areas.

Treatment and prevention For uncomplicated nonpurulent cellulitis, empiric therapy must cover *Streptococcus* species. If there is no purulence, staphylococcal coverage is not needed. Two trials of antibiotic therapy for uncomplicated cellulitis found no difference in clinical resolution between treatment with cephalexin plus TMP-SMX (MRSA coverage) compared with cephalexin alone.[49,52]

For cases of cellulitis without systemic signs of infection, the IDSA recommends 5 days of antibiotic therapy covering streptococci, with close follow-up. The duration of therapy should be extended if infection has not improved in that time. Options include cephalexin, dicloxacillin, clindamycin, and penicillin. We recommend that emergency physicians avoid penicillin because it does not cover MSSA, which may be responsible for up to 27% of nonpurulent cellulitis.[8] For nonpurulent cellulitis with systemic signs of infection such as a high fever, intravenous antibiotics are indicated. Options include cefazolin, ceftriaxone, and clindamycin. In addition, patients with cellulitis should generally be admitted for infections involving the hand if there is concern for compliance with outpatient therapy or if the patient is immunocompromised (eg, poorly controlled diabetes, infected with the human immunodeficiency virus, and end-stage renal disease).

In apparently nonpurulent cellulitis, initial MRSA coverage should be considered in the setting of a traumatic wound and in patients with a history of MRSA infection or IDU. In addition, if the cellulitis does not respond to initial empiric antistreptococcal treatment, MRSA coverage can be added. But more important in such cases, a search should be undertaken for an undrained purulent focus. Options for oral MRSA therapy include addition of TMP-SMX or doxycycline to the beta-lactam, or switching to clindamycin.

Elevation of the extremity is considered an important component of cellulitis treatment. Evidence of an underlying fungal infection, such as interdigital fissures, scales, and maceration, should be treated with a topical azole drug. Other underlying predisposing conditions such as edema, eczema, venous insufficiency, diabetes mellitus, and obesity should be identified and treated accordingly. The IDSA recommends considering prophylactic antibiotics in patients with 3 or more episodes of cellulitis annually despite efforts to treat predisposing factors. Options include penicillin or erythromycin for a duration of up to 1 year.[3]

NECROTIZING SOFT TISSUE INFECTIONS

The term necrotizing fasciitis was first used in 1952,[53] but fasciitis is now understood to be only one aspect of NSTIs, a broad infection category characterized by rapid bacterial spread and necrosis of subcutaneous fat, muscle, and fascia. Subtypes of NSTIs include synergistic necrotizing cellulitis, clostridial gas gangrene and myonecrosis, spontaneous streptococcal myositis with streptococcal toxic shock, and others. By definition, these infections require prompt surgical exploration and debridement for definitive diagnosis and cure. This definition is problematic for acute care providers. It means there are just 2 ways the diagnosis of an NSTI is reached: (1) the diagnosis is suspected, the patient is taken for surgical exploration and necrosis is found, in which case the patient may survive after debridement, and (2) the diagnosis of NSTI is not initially entertained and, despite antibiotics and resuscitation, the patient deteriorates and dies. It should be clear that these infections are among the most difficult and high-stakes problems in emergency medicine, and require close teamwork with surgical colleagues.

Epidemiology, Microbiology, and Pathophysiology

NSTIs are uncommon. Globally the annual incidence ranges from 1.69 to 15.5 cases per 100,000 persons.[48,54–56] NSTI mortality rates average 20% to 30% in the literature, but range widely depending on the pathogen(s) involved, underlying host factors, and how quickly the diagnosis is recognized.[57–59]

It is classically taught that NSTIs occur in the wake of devitalized tissue, such as in the postoperative or battlefield setting. More often, however, NSTIs occur after a minor wound or trauma, and can even develop without any evident portal of entry in otherwise healthy patients. Most cases are associated with at least one of the following risk factors: IDU, recent surgery or other trauma, diabetic foot infection (especially ulcers), peripheral artery disease, malnutrition, or alcoholism. IDU is the most common identified risk factor for community-acquired NSTI (ie, presenting to the ED) in the United States. In large, recent studies from the western United States, IDU accounted for 50% to 88% of cases and these studies showed a dramatic increase in the incidence of NSTIs in the 1990s linked to the arrival of black tar heroin from Mexico.[60,61]

NSTIs are divided into 2 broad categories: polymicrobial infection (type I) and monomicrobial infection (type II). The proportion of cases that are polymicrobial can vary according to the study setting. In a cohort of 115 cases of necrotizing fasciitis, a single organism was identified in 61% of cases, multiple organisms in 17% of cases, and no microorganism in 17% of cases.[59] Polymicrobial infections can include a variety of bacteria, including streptococcal species, *Enterobacteriaceae* (gram-negative rods), clostridial species, nonclostridial anaerobes, nonclostridial anaerobes such as *B spp* and *Peptosptreptococcus spp, Staphylococcus species,* and *E spp.*[62]

Monomicrobial infections classically are caused by group A *Streptococcus*, previously called streptococcal gangrene. This infection may occur in any age group and in healthy patients. For example, it can be a complication of varicella infection in previously healthy children. *Vibrio vulnificus* and *Aeromonas hydrophilia* cause monomicrobial NSTIs after exposure to salt water and fresh water, respectively. *Clostridium perfringens* is found in both monomicrobial and polymicrobial infections. *Clostridium sordelli* NSTI occurs in IDUs and in the postpartum setting.[63] Additionally, CA-MRSA has been implicated as a cause of monomicrobial necrotizing fasciitits.[16]

NSTIs occurring in certain high-risk anatomic areas have been given eponyms. Fournier's gangrene is an NSTI of the genitourinary region. Ludwig's angina is an

NSTI that begins in the floor of the mouth. Both have the potential to spread rapidly along adjacent fascial planes. A summary of terms commonly encountered to categorize NSTI is listed in **Table 5**.

The pathophysiology of NSTIs differs depending on the inciting mechanism and etiologic pathogen. When a wound provides the portal of entry for bacteria or Clostridial spores, inflammation and necrosis spread from the skin and immediate subcutaneous tissue eventually to deeper muscle and fascia. When the inciting mechanism is the seeding of injured muscle by GAS bacteremia, inflammation and necrosis spreads from the muscle (at which point pain and hypotension may be the only signs) to the skin, eventually producing visible necrosis and bullae.[64] Vascular occlusion is a key component of NSTI pathophysiology. C perfringens and GAS produce exotoxins, or virulence factors, that contribute to lethality. For example, the C perfringens alpha-toxin is involved in platelet destruction, hemolysis, and increased capillary permeability, and produces direct cardiotoxic effects, contributing to massive circulatory collapse. S pyogenes produces myriad virulence factors, such as streptococcal pyrogenic exotoxins, which can evade normal immune defenses, act as superantigens, and trigger massive cytokine release ("cytokine storm") culminating in streptococcal toxic shock syndrome.[65] **Fig. 11** presents a simplified taxonomy and pathophysiology of NTSI.

Clinical Features

Classic NSTI skin findings—frequently absent at the time of ED presentation—include bullae, crepitus, necrosis, and cutaneous sensory deficit (from cutaneous nerve necrosis; **Fig. 12**A, B). The presence of any of these "hard findings" on physical examination should be considered evidence of an NSTI until proven otherwise. However, the most common presenting signs and symptoms are nonspecific and include fever, pain, tenderness, local swelling, and erythema.[59] A lack of hard findings early in the course of the disease makes diagnosis challenging. Massive "woody" soft tissue swelling, referred to as the Michelin Man sign, has been described, and likely is associated with C sordelli and C novyii infections among IDUs[60] (**Fig. 12**C).

A systematic review of 9 studies including 1463 NSTI cases reported a 71% initial misdiagnosis rate.[66] Contributing to this difficulty, only 40% of patients were febrile at presentation and 21% were hypotensive. Severe C sordelli infections classically

---

Table 5
Types of NSTI

Type	Description
Gas Gangrene	Associated with contamination of traumatic or surgical wounds by the toxin-producing anaerobe *Clostridium perfringens*, typically involves deep muscle tissue and spreads along facial planes.
Fournier's gangrene	Typically polymicrobial NSTI of the perianal and perineal region, more common in men.
Ludwig's angina	Typically polymicrobial odontogenic infection involving the floor of the mouth, with potential to spread via fascial planes to the neck and mediastinum.
Type 1, polymicrobial	Polymicrobial (synergistic) infection, often involving oral and bowel flora. Includes Fournier's gangrene and Ludwig's angina.
Type 2, monomicrobial	Typified by GAS and *Vibrio vulnificus*. GAS disease is classically associated with trivial injury and produces streptococcal toxic shock syndrome.

Abbreviations: GAS, group A *streptococcus*; NSTI, necrotizing soft tissue infection.

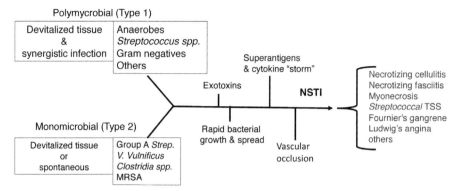

Fig. 11. Necrotizing skin and soft tissue infection (NSTI) simplified taxonomy and patho-physiology. MRSA, methicillin-resistant *Staphylococcus aureus*; TSS, toxic shock syndrome.

produces no fever.[67] Gastrointestinal symptoms may predominate and be misleading early in cases of streptococcal toxic shock.[64] Myositis may present as isolated, severe deep muscle pain; in such cases, an elevated creatine phosphokinase, mysteriously rising serum lactate, or small hemorrhagic bullae may be the first clues to a serious infection.

One way for emergency physicians to keep from missing NSTIs is to use a pattern recognition approach, which emphasizes diagnostic sensitivity. Just as a "thunder-clap headache" automatically triggers concern for subarachnoid hemorrhage, certain presentation patterns should trigger consideration of NSTI every time they are encountered. These include the following:

- Diabetic foot infection (**Fig. 12**D);
- Perineal infections, especially in men (Fournier's gangrene);

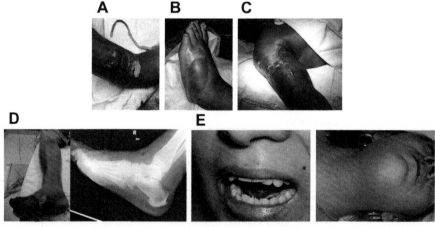

Fig. 12. (*A*) Necrotizing skin and soft tissue infection (NSTI) of the arm, demonstrating skin necrosis, open bullae, and weeping of dishwater-like fluid. (*B*) NSTI with large hem-orrhagic bullous. (*C*) NSTI owing to injection drug use showing bullae, skin necrosis, and severe, diffuse soft tissue edema spreading to the trunk (Michelin man sign). (*D*) NSTI in the setting of a diabetic foot ulcer and peripheral arterial disease; on a plain radiograph, tissue gas is evident superior to the ankle. (*E*) Ludwig's angina with characteristic swelling of the floor of the mouth. ([*B*] *Courtesy of* B. Frazee, MD, Oakland, CA.)

- Odontogenic infections involving extension into the floor of the mouth (Ludwig's angina; **Fig. 12**E);
- Any skin infection or poorly differentiated soft tissue complaint in an IDU; and
- Unexplained, severe deep muscle pain.

Diagnosis

Laboratory testing may be useful in distinguishing NSTIs from other SSTIs, particularly from nonpurulent cellulitis. Wall and colleagues[68] found that among patients with undifferentiated SSTIs, the combination of a white blood cell count of greater than 15.4 per mm^3 and sodium of less than 135 mmol/L identified NSTIs with a positive and negative predictive value of 26% and 99%, respectively. Extreme leukocytosis (>30,000 per mm^3), termed a leukemoid reaction, is a hallmark of infection with some *Clostridium* species. This finding in the setting of a skin or soft tissue complaint should be considered an NSTI until proven otherwise. Elevated creatine phosphokinase can suggest infection involving deep muscle or fascia.[64] Wong and colleagues[69] derived the Laboratory Risk Indicator for Necrotizing Fasciitis score based on 6 laboratory tests including white blood cell count, sodium and C-reactive protein (**Table 6**). A score of 6 or higher is considered moderate to high risk for NSTI. Numerous subsequent studies have sought to validate this clinical decision rule, with varying success.[70–72] The Laboratory Risk Indicator for Necrotizing Fasciitis score may be a useful tool in determining when to pursue further imaging and surgical consultation.[72]

Numerous imaging modalities have been evaluated for their ability to distinguish NSTI from other less serious SSTIs. Plain radiographs may demonstrate subcutaneous gas in a stippled pattern (**Fig. 13**) in roughly 25% of NSTIs.[66] Computed tomography scanning has emerged as the initial imaging modality of choice in most cases. It can delineate the extent of inflammation and identify asymmetric thickening of the deep fascia and fluid adjacent to fascia, and is likely more sensitive than plain radiography for detecting tissue gas (**Fig. 14**). MRI has performance characteristics similar to the computed tomography scan, but its clinical usefulness is limited because it is generally too time consuming for a disease that demands prompt diagnosis.[51,73] In contrast, ultrasound examination in the ED can be used to evaluate hemodynamically unstable patients at the bedside. Specific ultrasound findings in NSTI include tissue

Table 6
Laboratory Risk Indicator for Necrotizing Fasciitis score

Variable	Range	Points
C-reactive protein (mg/L)	≥150	4
White blood cell count (per mm^3)	15–25	1
	>25	2
Hemoglobin (g/dL)	11.0–13.5	1
	<11	2
Na (mmol/L)	<135	2
Creatinine (mg/dL)	>1.6	2
Glu (mg/dL)	>180	1

A score of greater than 6 should prompt further evaluation (imaging) and surgical consultation.
Data from Wong C, Khin L, Heng K, et al. The LRINEC (Laboratory Risk Indicator for Necrotizing Fasciitis) score: a tool for distinguishing necrotizing fasciitis from other soft tissue infections. Crit Care Med 2004;32(7):1535–41.

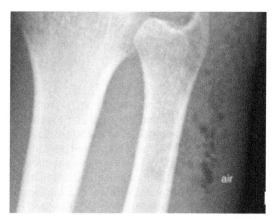

Fig. 13. Radiograph of necrotizing skin and soft tissue infection demonstrating air in the soft tissue. (*Data from* Chen K, Lin AC, Chong C, et al. An overview of point-of-care ultrasound for soft tissue and musculoskeletal applications in the emergency department. J Intensive Care 2016;4(55):1–11.)

gas, irregular fascia thickening, and perifascial fluid (**Fig. 15**). One study reported that the finding of a perifascial fluid stripe of 4 mm or more had a sensitivity and specificity 88.2% and 93.3%, respectively.[74] In our experience, however, severe swelling is often the only finding on ultrasound examination, which may be difficult to distinguish from cellulitis.

Although a positive result from a noninvasive diagnostic test is useful in confirming the need for immediate operation, a negative result generally cannot be relied on to exclude the diagnosis of NSTI. Surgical exploration and debridement remains the definitive diagnostic test for NSTI, as well as the definitive treatment.[3] The gold standard is a constellation of surgical findings that includes nonbleeding tissue,

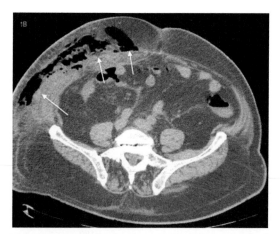

Fig. 14. Computed tomography scan of a necrotizing skin and soft tissue infection that demonstrates involvement of the deep muscular fascia. The arrows demonstrate the presence of air collections. (*From* Carbonetti F, Cremona A, Guidi M, et al. A case of postsurgical necrotizing fasciitis invading the rectus abdominis muscle and review of the literature. Case Rep Med 2014;2014:479057.)

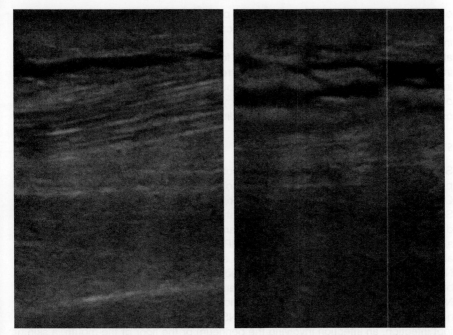

Fig. 15. Ultrasound image of a necrotizing skin and soft tissue infection with anechoic (*black*) fluid tracking along the echogenic (*bright white*) deep fascial plane (*left*). Thickened irregular fascia with anechoic fluid tracking is seen along the fascial plane (*right*). (*From* Oelze L, Wu S, Carnell J. Emergency ultrasonography for the early diagnosis of necrotizing fasciitis: a case series from the ED. Am J Emerg Med 2013;31(3):632.e6; with permission.)

nonadherent muscular fascia on blunt dissection, greyish appearance of the fascia, and so-called dishwater pus. A Gram stain of the surgical specimen can be used to guide empiric antibiotic treatment.[64]

Treatment

Prompt surgical debridement is considered the cornerstone of effective treatment. Numerous studies have shown improved survival among patients taken to surgery within 24 hours after admission as compared with those where surgery was delayed.[75,76] Survival is further increased when surgical intervention occurs within 6 hours.[77] Surgical treatment involves wide debridement down to bleeding, viable-appearing tissue. Repeated inspection and debridement during the hospitalization is often necessary.[64]

The most critical aspect of supportive care is evidence-based, early goal-directed treatment of sepsis, emphasizing timely crystalloid resuscitation, tissue perfusion monitoring, and the use of norepinephrine when indicated. Analgesic requirements may be substantial and a multimodal approach is recommended that minimizes hypotension and depressed respiratory drive.

Because the bacterial etiology is almost never known at the time NSTI is first suspected in the ED, broad empiric antimicrobial coverage is required, targeting GAS, *Clostridium* species, gram-negative bacteria and MRSA. Survival is likely inversely correlated with how soon antibiotics are started, as it is in septic shock, although this factor has not been studied for NSTIs.[78] There is limited research to guide the optimal specific regimen; we recommend piperacillin/tazobactam, vancomycin, and clindamycin.[3] Clindamycin is included because it may reduce exotoxin production in clostridial and GAS disease, and may downmodulate host cytokine response, although current IDSA guidelines reserve it for confirmed streptococcal and clostridial infections. Clindamycin and metronidazole reduced mortality compared with penicillin in a *C perfringens* gas gangrene mouse model.[3,79] For suspected *Aeromonas hydrophila*, the recommended treatment is doxycycline plus either ciprofloxacin or ceftriaxone, and for *Vibrio vulnificus* it is doxycycline plus either ceftriaxone or cefotaxime.[3]

SUMMARY

SSTIs are among the most common infections encountered in the ED and emergency physicians should be expert in their diagnosis and management. The emergence of CA-MRSA at the turn of the millennium greatly increased the incidence of purulent SSTIs and forced a change in antibiotic treatment. The first step in approaching an undifferentiated skin infection should be to carefully assess for purulence, which generally indicates a staphylococcal (often MRSA) infection. Drainage is required for abscesses and adjuvant antibiotics active against MRSA provide additional benefit. Nonpurulent cellulitis can be reliably treated with beta-lactam antibiotics alone. Antibiotic choice is best guided by a hospital antibiogram, if available. Potentially deadly NSTIs require prompt recognition and surgical treatment, yet they are difficult to diagnose. A prudent approach is to consider NSTI every time one encounters a diabetic foot infection, an infection involving the perineum or the floor of the mouth, a skin or soft tissue complaint in an IDU, or any patient with unexplained severe muscle compartment pain.

REFERENCES

1. Hersh AL, Chambers HF, Maselli JH, et al. National trends in ambulatory visits and antibiotic prescribing for skin and soft-tissue infections. Arch Intern Med 2008;168(14):1585–91.

2. Center for Disease Control. National Hospital Ambulatory Medical Care Survey: 2008 Emergency Department Summary Tables. Available at: https://www.cdc.gov/nchs/data/ahcd/nhamcs_emergency/2011_ed_web_tables.pdf. Published 2011. Accessed February 1, 2018.

3. Stevens DL, Bisno AL, Chambers HF, et al. Practice guidelines for the diagnosis and management of skin and soft tissue infections: 2014 update by the infectious diseases society of America. Clin Infect Dis 2014;59(2):e10–52.

4. US Food and Drug Administration. Guidance for industry acute bacterial skin and skin structure: developing drugs for treatment. Available at: https://www.fda.gov/downloads/Drugs/Guidances/ucm071185.pdf. Published October 2013. Accessed February 1, 2018.

5. Eron LJ, Lipsky BA, Low DE, et al. Managing skin and soft tissue infections: expert panel recommendations on key decision points. J Antimicrob Chemother 2003;52(suppl_1):i3–17.

6. Dryden MS. Skin and soft tissue infection: microbiology and epidemiology. Int J Antimicrob Agents 2009;34(Suppl 1):S2–7.

7. Miller LG, Daum RS, Creech CB, et al. Clindamycin versus trimethoprim-sulfamethoxazole for uncomplicated skin infections. N Engl J Med 2015; 372(12):1093–103.

8. Jeng A, Beheshti M, Li J, et al. The role of beta-hemolytic streptococci in causing diffuse, nonculturable cellulitis: a prospective investigation. Medicine 2010;89(4): 217–26.

9. Kobayashi SD, Malachowa N, DeLeo FR. Pathogenesis of Staphylococcus aureus abscesses. Am J Pathol 2015;185(6):1518–27.

10. Frazee BW, Lynn J, Charlebois ED, et al. High prevalence of methicillin-resistant Staphylococcus aureus in emergency department skin and soft tissue infections. Ann Emerg Med 2005;45(3):311–20.

11. Moran GJ, Krishnadasan A, Gorwitz RJ, et al. Methicillin-resistant S. aureus infections among patients in the emergency department. N Engl J Med 2006;355(7): 666–74.

12. Albrecht VS, Limbago BM, Moran GJ, et al. staphylococcus aureus colonization and strain type at various body sites among patients with a closed abscess and uninfected controls at U.S. emergency departments. J Clin Microbiol 2015; 53(11):3478–84.

13. Miller LG, Diep BA. Clinical practice: colonization, fomites, and virulence: rethinking the pathogenesis of community-associated methicillin-resistant Staphylococcus aureus infection. Clin Infect Dis 2008;46(5):752–60.

14. Stevens DL, Bryant AE. Impetigo, Erysipelas and Cellulitis. In: Ferretti JJ, Stevens DL, Fischetti VA, editors. Streptococcus pyogenes: Basic Biology to Clinical Manifestations [Internet]. Oklahoma City (OK): University of Oklahoma Health Sciences Center; 2016. Available at: http://www.ncbi.nlm.nih.gov/books/NBK333408/.

15. Fermry P, Dajani AS, Wannamaker LW, et al. Natural history of impetigo. I. Site sequence of acquisition and familial patterns of spread of cutaneous streptococci. J Clin Invest 1972;51:2851–62.

16. Torok ME, Conlon CP. Skin and soft tissue infections. Medicine 2009;37(11): 603–9.

17. Koning S, van der Sande R, Verhagen AP, et al. Interventions for impetigo. Cochrane Database Syst Rev 2012;(1):CD003261.

18. Kujath P, Kujath C. Complicated skin, skin structure and soft tissue infections - are we threatened by multi-resistant pathogens? Eur J Med Res 2010;15(12):544–53.

19. Talan DA, Krishnadasan A, Gorwitz RJ, et al. Comparison of Staphylococcus aureus from skin and soft-tissue infections in US emergency department patients, 2004 and 2008. Clin Infect Dis 2011;53(2):144–9.

20. Daum RS, Miller LG, Immergluck L, et al. A placebo-controlled trial of antibiotics for smaller skin abscesses. N Engl J Med 2017;376(26):2545–55.

21. Talan DA, Mower WR, Krishnadasan A. Trimethoprim-sulfamethoxazole for uncomplicated skin abscess. N Engl J Med 2016;375:284–6.

22. Jenkins TC, Knepper BC, Jason Moore S, et al. Microbiology and initial antibiotic therapy for injection drug users and non-injection drug users with cutaneous abscesses in the era of community-associated methicillin-resistant Staphylococcus aureus. Acad Emerg Med 2015;22(8):993–7.

23. Ulug M, Gedik E, Girgin S, et al. The evaluation of bacteriology in perianal abscesses of 81 adult patients. Braz J Infect Dis 2010;14(3):225–9.

24. Bhide A, Nama V, Patel S, et al. Microbiology of cysts/abscesses of Bartholin's gland: review of empirical antibiotic therapy against microbial culture. J Obstet Gynaecol 2010;30(7):701–3.

25. Kessous R, Aricha-Tamir B, Sheizaf B, et al. Clinical and microbiological characteristics of Bartholin gland abscesses. Obstet Gynecol 2013;122(4):749.

26. Ellis MW, Schlett CD, Millar EV, et al. Prevalence of nasal colonization and strain concordance in patients with community-associated Staphylococcus aureus skin and soft-tissue infections. Infect Control Hosp Epidemiol 2014;35(10):1251–6.

27. Barbic D, Chenkin J, Cho DD, et al. In patients presenting to the emergency department with skin and soft tissue infections what is the diagnostic accuracy of point-of-care ultrasonography for the diagnosis of abscess compared to the current standard of care ? A systematic review and meta-a. BMJ Open 2017;7: e013688.

28. Squire BT, Fox JC, Anderson C. ABSCESS: applied bedside sonography for convenient evaluation of superficial soft tissue infections. Acad Emerg Med 2005;12(7):601–6.

29. Gaspari RJ, Resop D, Mendoza M, et al. A randomized controlled trial of incision and drainage versus ultrasonographically guided needle aspiration for skin abscesses and the effect of methicillin-resistant Staphylococcus aureus. Ann Emerg Med 2011;57(5):483–91.e1.

30. Chinnock B, Hendey G. Irrigation of cutaneous abscesses does not improve treatment success. Ann Emerg Med 2016;2016(67):3.

31. O'Malley GF, Dominici P, Giraldo P, et al. Routine packing of simple cutaneous abscesses is painful and probably unnecessary. Acad Emerg Med 2009;16(5): 470–3.

32. Leinwand M, Downing M, Slater D, et al. Incision and drainage of subcutaneous abscesses without the use of packing. J Pediatr Surg 2013;48(9):1962–5.

33. Kessler DO, Krantz A, Mojica M. Randomized trial comparing wound packing to no wound packing following incision and drainage of superficial skin abscesses in the pediatric emergency department. Pediatr Emerg Care 2012;28(5):514–7.

34. Ladde JG, Baker S, Rodgers CN, et al. The LOOP technique: a novel incision and drainage technique in the treatment of skin abscesses in a pediatric ED. Am J Emerg Med 2015;33(2):271–6.

35. Ozturan IU, Dogan NO, Karakayali O, et al. Comparison of loop and primary incision & drainage techniques in adult patients with cutaneous abscess: a preliminary, randomized clinical trial. Am J Emerg Med 2017;35(6):830–4.

36. Gottlieb M, Peksa GD. Comparison of the loop technique with incision and drainage for soft tissue abscesses: a systematic review and meta-analysis. Am J Emerg Med 2018;36(1):128–33.

37. Talan DA, Mower WR, Krishnadasan A. trimethoprim-sulfamethoxazole for uncomplicated skin abscess. N Engl J Med 2016;375:285–6.

38. Frazee B. Antibiotics for simple skin abscesses: the new evidence in perspective. Emerg Med J 2018;35(4):277–8.

39. Vermandere M, Aertgeerts B, Agoritsas T, et al. Antibiotics after incision and drainage for uncomplicated skin abscesses: a clinical practice guideline. BMJ 2018;360:k243.

40. Wallin TR, Hern HG, Frazee BW. Community-associated methicillin-resistant Staphylococcus aureus. Emerg Med Clin North Am 2008;26(2):431–55, ix.

41. Tayal VS, Hasan N, Norton HJ, et al. The effect of soft-tissue ultrasound on the management of cellulitis in the emergency department. Acad Emerg Med 2006;4:348.

42. Lentnek AL, Giger O, O'Rourke E. Group A beta-hemolytic streptococcal bacteremia and intravenous substance abuse. A growing clinical problem? Arch Intern Med 1990;150(1):89–93.

43. Simon MS, Cody RL. Cellulitis after axillary lymph node dissection for carcinoma of the breast. Am J Med 1992;93(5):543–8.

44. Teerachaisakul M, Ekataksin W, Durongwatana S, et al. Risk factors for cellulitis in patients with lymphedema: a case-controlled study. Lymphology 2013;46(3): 150–6.

45. Bruun T, Oppegaard O, Kittang BR, et al. Etiology of cellulitis and clinical prediction of streptococcal disease: a prospective study. Open Forum Infect Dis 2016; 3(1):ofv181.

46. Gunderson CG, Martinello RA. A systematic review of bacteremias in cellulitis and erysipelas. J Infect 2012;64(2):148–55.

47. Chira S, Miller LG. Staphylococcus aureus is the most common identified cause of cellulitis: a systematic review. Epidemiol Infect 2010;138(3):313–7.

48. Chambers HF. Cellulitis, by any other name. Clin Infect Dis 2013;56:1763–4.

49. Moran GJ, Krishnadasan A, Mower WR, et al. Effect of cephalexin plus trimethoprim-sulfamethoxazole vs cephalexin alone on clinical cure of uncomplicated cellulitis: a randomized clinical trial. JAMA 2017;317(20):2088–96.

50. Weng QY, Raff AB, Cohen JM, et al. Costs and consequences associated with misdiagnosed lower extremity cellulitis. JAMA Dermatol 2016. [Epub ahead of print].

51. Mehta P, Morrow M, Russell J, et al. Magnetic resonance imaging of musculoskeletal emergencies. Semin Ultrasound CT MR 2017;38(4):439–52.

52. Pallin DJ, Binder WD, Allen MB, et al. Clinical trial: comparative effectiveness of cephalexin plus trimethoprim-sulfamethoxazole versus cephalexin alone for treatment of uncomplicated cellulitis: a randomized controlled trial. Clin Infect Dis 2013;56(12):1754–62.

53. Wilson B. Necrotizing fasciitis. Am Surg 1952;18(4):416–31.

54. Das D, Baker M, Venugopal K. Increasing incidence of necrotizing fasciitis in New Zealand: a nationwide study over the period 1990 to 2006. J Infect 2011; 63(6):429–33.

55. Khamnuan P, Chongruksut W, Jearwattanakanok K, et al. Necrotizing fasciitis: epidemiology and clinical predictors for amputation. Int J Gen Med 2015;8: 195–202.

56. Glass GE, Sheil F, Ruston J, et al. Necrotising soft tissue infection in a UK metropolitan population. Ann R Coll Surg Engl 2015;97(1):46–51.

57. Nelson GE, Pondo T, Toews KA, et al. Epidemiology of Invasive Group A Streptococcal Infections in the United States, 2005-2012. Clin Infect Dis 2016;63(4): 478–86.

58. Stevens DL, Tanner M, Winship J, et al. Severe group A streptococcal infections associated with a toxic shock-like syndrome and scarlet fever toxin A. N Engl J Med 1989;321:1–7.

59. Wang J-M, Lim H-K. Necrotizing fasciitis: eight-year experience and literature review. Braz J Infect Dis 2014;18(2):137–43.

60. Gonzales y Tucker RD, Frazee B. View from the front lines: an emergency medicine perspective on clostridial infections in injection drug users. Anaerobe 2014; 30:108–15.

61. Chen JL, Fullerton KE, Flynn NM. Necrotizing fasciitis associated with injection drug use. Clin Infect Dis 2001;33(1):6–15.

62. Brook I, Frazier EH. Clinical and microbiological features of necrotizing fasciitis. J Clin Microbiol 1995;33(9):2382–7.

63. Aldape MJ, Bryant AE, Stevens DL, et al. Clostridium sordellii infection: epidemiology, clinical findings, and current perspectives on diagnosis and treatment. Clin Infect Dis 2006;43(11):1436–46.

64. Stevens DL, Bryant AE. Necrotizing soft-tissue infections. N Engl J Med 2017; 377(23):2253–65.
65. Low DE. Toxic shock syndrome: major advances in pathogenesis, but not treatment. Crit Care Clin 2013;29(3):651–75.
66. Goh T, Goh LG, Ang CH, et al. Early diagnosis of necrotizing fasciitis. Br J Surg 2014;101(1):e119–25.
67. Kimura AC, Higa J, Levin R, et al. Outbreak of necrotizing fasciitis due to Clostridium sordellii among black-tar heroin users. Clin Infect Dis 2004;38(9):e87–91.
68. Wall DB, Klein SR, Black S, et al. A simple model to help distinguish necrotizing fasciitis from nonnecrotizing soft tissue infection. J Am Coll Surg 2000;19(3): 227–31.
69. Wong C, Khin L, Heng K, et al. The LRINEC (Laboratory Risk Indicator for Necrotizing Fasciitis) score: a tool for distinguishing necrotizing fasciitis from other soft tissue infections. Crit Care Med 2004;32(7):1535–41.
70. Narasimhan V, Ooi G, Weidlich S, et al. Laboratory Risk Indicator for Necrotizing Fasciitis score for early diagnosis of necrotizing fasciitis in Darwin. ANZ J Surg 2018;88(1–2):E45–9.
71. Neeki MM, Dong F, Au C, et al. Evaluating the laboratory risk indicator to differentiate cellulitis from necrotizing fasciitis in the emergency department. West J Emerg Med 2017;2017(18):4.
72. Bechar J, Sepehripour S, Hardwicke J, et al. Laboratory risk indicator for necrotising fasciitis (LRINEC) score for the assessment of early necrotising fasciitis: a systematic review of the literature. Ann R Coll Surg Engl 2017;99(5):341–6.
73. Malghem J, Lecouvet FE, Omoumi P, et al. Necrotizing fasciitis: contribution and limitations of diagnostic imaging. Joint Bone Spine 2013;80(2):146–54.
74. Yen ZS, Wang H, Ma H, et al. Ultrasonographic screening of clinically-suspected necrotizing fasciitis. Acad Emerg Med 2002;9(12):1448–51.
75. McHenry CR, Piotrowski JJ, Petrinic D, et al. Determinants of mortality for necrotizing soft-tissue infections. Ann Surg 1995;221(5):558–65.
76. Freischlag JA, Ajalat G, Busuttil RW. Treatment of necrotizing soft tissue infections. The need for a new approach. Am J Surg 1985;149(6):751–5.
77. Hadeed GJ, Smith J, O'Keeffe T, et al. Early surgical intervention and its impact on patients presenting with necrotizing soft tissue infections: a single academic center experience. J Emerg Trauma Shock 2016;9(1):22–7.
78. Gaieski DF, Fau MM, Band RA, et al. Impact of time to antibiotics on survival in patients with severe sepsis or septic shock in whom early goal-directed therapy was initiated in the emergency department. Crit Care Med 2010;38(4):1045–53.
79. Stevens DL, Maier KA, Mitten JE. Effect of antibiotics on toxin production and viability of Clostridium perfringens. Antimicrob Agents Chemother 1987;31(2): 213–8.

Musculoskeletal Infections in the Emergency Department

Daniel C. Kolinsky, MD[a], Stephen Y. Liang, MD, MPHS[b,c],*

KEYWORDS

- Osteomyelitis • Spondylodiscitis • Spinal epidural abscess
- Posttraumatic osteomyelitis • Septic arthritis • Periprosthetic joint infection
- Emergency department

KEY POINTS

- Patients with musculoskeletal infections can have heterogeneous presentations, as the signs and symptoms are often occult and nonspecific.
- *Staphylococcus aureus* is the most common microorganism associated with bone and joint infections.
- Definitive diagnosis requires sampling of affected tissue for Gram stain and microbiologic culture.
- The mainstay of treatment for bone and joint infections is antibiotic therapy, but surgical consultation for irrigation and/or debridement may be necessary in certain clinical situations.

INTRODUCTION

Bone and joint infections are a relatively uncommon cause of musculoskeletal complaints among patients seeking care in the emergency department (ED). Atypical and nonspecific presentations can be misleading, and definitive diagnosis of infection challenging, often requiring invasive and time-consuming procedures. This review outlines the clinical signs and symptoms that should lead emergency physicians to consider a musculoskeletal infection, the diagnostic workup, and key therapeutic interventions when the clinical suspicion for infection is high. The approach to

Disclosure Statement: S.Y. Liang reports no conflicts of interest in this work. S.Y. Liang is the recipient of a KM1 Comparative Effectiveness Research Career Development Award (KM1CA156708-01) and received support through the Clinical and Translational Science Award (CTSA) program (UL1RR024992) of the National Center for Advancing Translational Sciences as well as the Barnes-Jewish Patient Safety & Quality Career Development Program, which is funded by the Foundation for Barnes-Jewish Hospital.
a Department of Emergency Medicine, Southeast Louisiana Veterans Health Care System, 2400 Canal Street, New Orleans, LA 70119, USA; b Division of Emergency Medicine, Washington University School of Medicine, 4523 Clayton Avenue, Campus Box 8072, St Louis, MO 63110, USA; c Division of Infectious Diseases, Washington University School of Medicine, 4523 Clayton Avenue, Campus Box 8051, St Louis, MO 63110, USA
* Corresponding author. 4523 Clayton Avenue, Campus Box 8051, St Louis, MO 63110.
E-mail address: syliang@wustl.edu

Emerg Med Clin N Am 36 (2018) 751–766
https://doi.org/10.1016/j.emc.2018.06.006
0733-8627/18/© 2018 Elsevier Inc. All rights reserved.

osteomyelitis, spondylodiscitis, spinal epidural abscess, antibiotic prophylaxis for an open fracture, septic arthritis, and periprosthetic joint infection in the ED will serve as the primary FOCI.

OSTEOMYELITIS

Osteomyelitis is an inflammatory reaction of the bone due to infection, most often bacterial in nature. Infection can involve the bone marrow, cortex, periosteum, or surrounding soft tissues, leading to destruction of any or all of these anatomic structures.[1] In a US population-based study conducted in Olmstead County, Minnesota, the overall incidence of osteomyelitis increased from 11.4 cases per 100,000 person-years in the period from 1969 to 1979 to 24.4 per 100,000 person-years in the period from 2000 to 2009.[2] Although rates remained stable among children and adults younger than 50 years, incidence nearly tripled among those 60 years or older, fueled by a significant rise in diabetes-related osteomyelitis over the past 4 decades.

Osteomyelitis develops from 1 of 3 mechanisms of pathogenesis: bacteremia leading to hematogenous seeding of bone, contiguous spread of infection from adjacent soft tissue to bone, or direct inoculation of microorganisms into bone. Hematogenous osteomyelitis results either from the introduction of microorganisms into the bloodstream (eg, via injection drug use or an infected central venous catheter) or an infection elsewhere that has now been complicated by bloodstream involvement (eg, endocarditis, urinary tract infection). Osteomyelitis due to contiguous spread occurs most frequently in the setting of skin breakdown (eg, diabetic foot ulcer, vascular ulcer, or pressure-related decubitus ulcer) and soft tissue infection extending to underlying bone. Infected joints, both native (septic arthritis) or prosthetic, and other infected orthopedic devices can likewise involve adjacent bone. Osteomyelitis from direct inoculation classically arises in the setting of an open fracture or surgery. Patients with osteomyelitis will often have one or more pathologic risk factors associated with these mechanisms (**Table 1**). *Acute* osteomyelitis progresses over days to weeks and is characterized by inflammation of viable bone. In contrast, *chronic* osteomyelitis evolves over weeks, months, or even years and is distinguished by progression to osteonecrosis with the formation of sequestrum, often in the setting of recurrent or refractory infection.

Several classification systems exist to categorize osteomyelitis. The Waldvogel classification system differentiates osteomyelitis by mechanism of pathogenesis, focusing on hematogenous seeding, contiguous spread, and vascular insufficiency.[3]

Table 1 Risk factors for development of osteomyelitis	
Mechanism of Pathogenesis	**Risk Factor**
Hematogenous seeding	Injection drug use
	Central venous catheter or other long-term vascular device
	Urinary tract infection
	Immunosuppression (including chronic corticosteroid use)
Contiguous spread from adjacent tissues	Extremes of age
	Diabetes mellitus
	Vascular insufficiency
	Abscess/cellulitis/infected ulcer
Direct inoculation	Prior orthopedic surgery or indwelling orthopedic hardware
	Trauma (open fracture)
	Human/animal bite

The Cierney-Mader classification system organizes osteomyelitis by the extent of host anatomic involvement, physiologic status, and comorbid factors that may influence clearance of infection.[4]

The causative pathogen associated with osteomyelitis is determined by the risk profile of the patient (eg, age, comorbid diseases, immune status, exposure, or travel history) and the suspected mechanism of pathogenesis.[5] *Staphylococcus aureus* remains the most common microorganism isolated across all forms of osteomyelitis.[6] Coagulase-negative staphylococci are often associated with osteomyelitis due to prosthetic joint and other orthopedic hardware infections.[5] *Streptococcus* species, gram-negative bacteria, and anaerobes are also frequently encountered, particularly in polymicrobial infections associated with a diabetic foot ulcer, vascular ulcer, or pressure-related decubitus ulcer.[1,6] Infections due to gram-negative bacteria, including *Pseudomonas aeruginosa* and *Escherichia coli*, are often seen in the elderly.[7] *P aeruginosa* is frequently associated with health care–associated osteomyelitis.[1] *Salmonella* is a well-recognized cause of osteomyelitis in patients with sickle cell anemia.[5] Immunocompromised patients are at risk for infection due to a wide range of unusual microorganisms, including *Bartonella henselae*,[8] *Mycobacterium avium* complex,[9] and fungi (*Aspergillus, Candida*).[10]

Clinical Presentation and Physical Examination

Osteomyelitis can present clinically in a myriad of ways. Reasons prompting ED evaluation may be as obvious as a gaping wound with exposed bone or as cryptic as a fever of unknown origin.[11] Infections can be as insidious and misleading as a solitary draining sinus tract.[1] Nonhealing wounds or chronic, recurrent soft tissue infections may portend a deeper bone infection. The presenting complaint often will be related to localized pain at the site of the infection. This may be accompanied by warmth, swelling, or erythema.[12] Patients with diabetes mellitus may lack these signs or symptoms due to underlying vascular disease and/or preexisting neuropathy.[13] Oftentimes, the patient may lack systemic symptoms, such as fever, chills, fatigue, irritability, or malaise.

The most common anatomic locations of osteomyelitis correlate with their mechanism of pathogenesis. Hematogenous osteomyelitis usually occurs in the metaphyseal region of long bone (eg, femur, tibia) in children and the spine in adults.[7] Contiguous spread of an adjacent infection to bone is most often seen in the lower extremities, namely the feet, where diabetic and vascular ulcers are likely to develop.[14] Osteomyelitis from direct inoculation occurs in traumatized long bones as well as adjacent to large joints (eg, hip, knee) associated with recently implanted prosthetic hardware.

The utility of the physical examination in diagnosing osteomyelitis is variable, ranging from equivocal to all but confirmatory. Acute infection classically includes any combination of the 4 cardinal signs of inflammation: rubor (redness), calor (heat), dolor (tenderness), or tumor (swelling).[12] In other cases, a draining sinus tract may be the only outward indication of a deeper bone infection. Physical findings associated with a chronic wound suggesting an underlying osteomyelitis can include nonpurulent drainage, friable or discolored granulation tissue, undermining of the wound edges, and/or foul odor.[12] Hematogenous osteomyelitis, especially of the spine, may present solely with tenderness to palpation of the affected bone.

In diabetic and other patients with chronic wounds, certain physical examination findings specific to and highly suggestive of osteomyelitis are easily identified at the bedside. Visible bone exposed in the wound or ulcer bed has a positive likelihood ratio (LR) of 9.2 (95% confidence interval [CI], 0.6–146.0) for predicting osteomyelitis.[13] Exploration of the wound or ulcer bed with a sterile surgical probe contacting bone (a positive probe-to-bone test) has a positive LR of 6.4 (95% CI 3.6–11.0).[13] An ulcer area larger than 2 cm^2 has a positive LR of 7.2 (95% CI 1.1–49.0).[13]

Diagnostic Evaluation

Clinical suspicion for osteomyelitis based on history and physical examination should lead to formal diagnosis with comprehensive laboratory testing, dedicated imaging, and tissue sampling. Due to the nonspecific constellation of signs and symptoms often associated with osteomyelitis, emergency physicians must have a high index of suspicion for this disease.

Initial laboratory testing in the ED should include a complete blood count (CBC), erythrocyte sedimentation rate (ESR), and C-reactive protein (CRP) at a minimum. If the patient has systemic symptoms to suggest active bacteremia, blood cultures should be obtained. Patients with osteomyelitis may or may not have a leukocytosis.[6] Inflammatory markers are often elevated acutely and can be helpful in trending response to treatment later on.[1] An ESR ≥70 mm/h is suggestive of osteomyelitis with a positive LR of 11.0 (95% CI 1.6–79.0).[13] Superficial wound cultures obtained in the ED have little diagnostic benefit, as they correlate poorly with pathogens isolated from the bone.[13] In diabetic foot ulcers, wound cultures correlate with microbiologic findings in bone culture in only 19% to 36% of cases.[15–17]

Initial imaging should consist of plain radiography of the region of interest. Although plain films may not demonstrate bony changes of acute osteomyelitis until after 2 to 3 weeks of infection, they help rule out other potential pathology (eg, fracture)[5] and provide a baseline for future comparison. One meta-analysis of diabetic foot osteomyelitis found a sensitivity of 54% and specificity of 68% when plain radiographs were used to establish the diagnosis.[18] Radiographs may show cortical bone deformity and/or destruction, at times with adjacent soft tissue swelling, joint space widening or narrowing, or periosteal reaction.[13,19] They may also reveal indirect signs of infection, such as subcutaneous gas or radio-opaque foreign bodies that could serve as a nidus of infection. Computed tomography (CT) can demonstrate periosteal reaction, cortical/medullary bone destruction, and/or adjacent soft tissue infection in greater detail. MRI is the most sensitive (90%) and specific (83%) imaging modality available for diagnosing osteomyelitis, often as early as 3 to 5 days after initial onset of infection.[20,21] It can also identify early bone edema, cortical destruction, soft tissue infection, and/or sinus tract development.

Definitive diagnosis of osteomyelitis is made by bone biopsy with histopathology and microbiologic culture. Isolation of the infecting microorganism from bone followed by antibiotic susceptibility testing are important in directing treatment.

Management

Limited well-designed prospective randomized clinical trials exist to guide the management of patients with osteomyelitis. Treatment recommendations are based on experimental animal models, retrospective studies, and expert opinion.[12] Eradicating a deep-seated infection of the bone can be difficult and successful treatment of osteomyelitis often requires a combination of medical and surgical therapies.

The first determination an emergency physician must make in caring for a patient with osteomyelitis is to decide whether antibiotic therapy needs to be initiated in the ED. If the patient is hemodynamically stable and without signs of systemic illness, consider delaying empiric antibiotic therapy until a bone biopsy can be obtained to optimize culture yield and better guide long-term antibiotic therapy tailored to the patient's infection. However, if the patient is unstable or has signs of sepsis, empiric antibiotic therapy in the ED is justified.[12] If hematogenous osteomyelitis or active bacteremia is suspected, blood cultures should be obtained before antibiotic administration to aid in the isolation of a causative microorganism.

Empiric antibiotic therapy should include broad coverage of gram-positive (eg, S aureus, Streptococcus spp.) and gram-negative bacteria, including antibiotic-resistant organisms (eg, methicillin-resistant S aureus [MRSA]) depending on patient risk factors and any prior history of a resistant infection. If a polymicrobial infection is suspected, usually in the setting of a chronic wound, anaerobic coverage should be added. Gram-positive coverage is most commonly achieved with vancomycin; alternatives include daptomycin or linezolid. Gram-negative coverage, including that of P aeruginosa, can be achieved with cefepime or meropenem. If cefepime is used, metronidazole should be added for anaerobic coverage; meropenem has intrinsic activity against anaerobes. Use of vancomycin in combination with piperacillin-tazobactam for empiric therapy should be avoided whenever possible to limit the risk of nephrotoxicity.[22]

The indications for surgical treatment of osteomyelitis will depend on many factors, including the anatomic location, duration of symptoms, mechanism of pathogenesis, and patient comorbidities. The main objectives of surgical intervention include source control (eg, debridement of infected tissues, removal of infected orthopedic prostheses or other hardware), management of wounds and dead space (eg, flap coverage), and stabilization of any infected and unstable bone that cannot be resected.[7] Chronic osteomyelitis requires surgical debridement, as antibiotics have limited ability to penetrate devascularized or necrotic bone (eg, sequestrum). In patients with osteomyelitis and vascular insufficiency, revascularization procedures may be necessary to ensure adequate delivery of systemic antibiotic therapy to the site of infection.

With regard to disposition, patients with acute osteomyelitis should generally be admitted to facilitate bone biopsy, determine any need for surgical intervention, and initiate long-term intravenous antibiotic therapy (usually lasting 6 weeks) in consultation with an infectious disease specialist. Patients with chronic osteomyelitis who have already been cultured, are on appropriate antibiotics, and are without signs of systemic infection or instability may be considered for outpatient treatment provided adequate follow-up is available.

SPONDYLODISCITIS (VERTEBRAL OSTEOMYELITIS)

Spondylodiscitis is an infection of the intervertebral disc (discitis) and adjacent vertebrae (osteomyelitis). Commonly referred to as vertebral osteomyelitis, spondylodiscitis has an annual incidence of 2.4 to 4.8 cases per 100,000 persons.[23,24]

Infection primarily arises as a sequela of bacteremia (eg, urinary tract infection, endocarditis, infected central venous catheter, injection drug use) with subsequent hematogenous seeding of the spine. Spondylodiscitis typically affects 2 contiguous vertebrae and the intervertebral disc space between them.[7] The most common site of infection is the lumbar spine (58%), followed by the thoracic (30%) and cervical spine (11%).[25] Diabetes mellitus, immunocompromised state, systemic steroid use, chronic kidney disease requiring hemodialysis, liver disease, malignancy, bacteremia/endocarditis, previous back surgery, and injection drug use are established risk factors for this infection.[26,27] Spondylodiscitis can also result from contiguous spread of an infection involving adjacent structures (eg, aorta, esophagus, colon).[28–30] Direct inoculation of the spine with microorganisms leading to spondylodiscitis can occur in the setting of spine surgery and has been reported rarely after epidural corticosteroid injections as well as penetrating trauma.[31–33]

S aureus remains the predominant causative microorganism associated with spondylodiscitis, although Streptococcus species are also common, particularly among the elderly and those with diabetes mellitus.[25,34] Infection with *P aeruginosa* is frequently associated with injection drug use. Other bacteria including *Mycobacterium tuberculosis* and *Brucella* also can cause spondylodiscitis and should be considered based on exposure and travel history.[35,36]

Clinical Presentation and Physical Examination

Diagnosing spondylodiscitis can be especially challenging, as the disease is rare and clinical presentations are nonspecific and highly variable. More than 90% of patients will complain of localized back or neck pain that is often worse at night and not alleviated by rest or analgesics.[37–39] Anywhere from 35% to 60% of patients will present with fever.[25,40] In one study, only a quarter of patients had neurologic symptoms, such as a sensory deficit, muscle weakness/paralysis, radiculopathy, or sphincter dysfunction due to spinal cord compression.[41]

When infection due to spondylodiscitis spreads to adjacent structures, more salient findings are also possible (**Table 2**). Infection of the cervical spine can spread to the retropharyngeal space leading to abscess formation.[42] In addition to paraspinal abscesses, thoracic spine infections can be accompanied by a reactive pleural effusion or empyema.[43] Lumbar spine infections can precipitate abscesses of the psoas muscle.[44]

Diagnosis is frequently delayed by up to 2 to 4 months after symptom onset.[45] In one study, more than a third of patients with vertebral osteomyelitis were initially misdiagnosed,[46] highlighting the underrecognition of this infection in clinical practice. Atypical presentations and late diagnoses are particularly common among patients older than 65 years, and a low threshold should exist to further investigate new or worsening back pain in this high-risk population.[47]

Diagnostic Evaluation

The diagnostic workup for spondylodiscitis is similar to that of nonaxial osteomyelitis. Typical laboratory tests should include a CBC, ESR, and CRP. Up to 40% of patients with vertebral osteomyelitis may have a normal white blood cell (WBC) count.[48] A high ESR or CRP in a patient with back pain has a sensitivity of 94% to 100% for the disease.[48,49] As vertebral osteomyelitis is often hematogenous in origin, multiple sets of blood cultures should be obtained. Blood cultures are positive in 58% of cases and approximately 25% to 59% of positive blood cultures accurately identify the causative microorganism responsible for the spine infection.[25,50,51]

As part of an initial evaluation, plain radiographs may demonstrate narrowing of the disk space and destruction of the vertebral endplates or vertebral body as well as alternative etiologies for back pain (eg, compression fracture, metastatic disease).[52] However, their sensitivity for detecting osteomyelitis or an isolated discitis is poor.[37,52] MRI remains the preferred imaging modality for early diagnosis of spondylodiscitis, as it is both highly sensitive (93%–96%) and specific (92.5%–97.0%).[53,54] More than half of patients with spondylodiscitis will have characteristic radiographic

Table 2
Sequelae of vertebral osteomyelitis

Region	Spread of Infection	Symptoms
Cervical	Retropharyngeal abscess	Sore throat, painful swallowing, change in voice
Thoracic	Reactive pleural effusion, empyema, paraspinal abscess	Cough, shortness of breath, chest pain, flank pain
Lumbar	Psoas muscle abscess	Abdominal or flank pain, pain on extension or internal rotation of hip (positive psoas sign)

findings of the disease on MRI within 2 weeks after onset of infection, followed by another 20% over the following 2 weeks.[55] CT is helpful in identifying cortical destruction and adjacent soft tissue infection when MRI is contraindicated.

Definitive diagnosis of spondylodiscitis is made by bone biopsy with multiple specimens submitted for microbiologic culture and pathologic review.[7] CT-guided bone biopsy has a sensitivity of 50%.[56]

Management

The mainstay of treatment for spondylodiscitis is medical management with long-term antibiotic therapy for at least 6 weeks.[57] If the patient is hemodynamically stable and has a normal neurologic examination, consider withholding antibiotic therapy until blood cultures and a bone biopsy can be obtained to guide antibiotic selection. If the patient is clinically unstable or has signs of sepsis, empiric antibiotic coverage for S aureus (including MRSA), streptococci, and gram-negative bacilli can be achieved with a combination of vancomycin and a third-generation or fourth-generation cephalosporin, ideally after blood cultures have been obtained.

Consultation with a spine surgeon and infectious disease specialist is advised, along with hospital admission, to facilitate further evaluation and treatment. Surgical debridement may be necessary in the setting of epidural or paravertebral abscess formation, evolving neurologic deficits, or spinal instability.[7,57]

SPINAL EPIDURAL ABSCESS

Spinal epidural abscess (SEA) is a collection of pus located in the spinal canal between the dura mater and overlying vertebral column. Although SEA can develop independently of spondylodiscitis, it often occurs as direct complication. In one study, a third of spondylodiscitis cases were accompanied by a secondary SEA.[58] Overall, SEA remains uncommon, with an estimated incidence of 1.8 per 100,000 persons per year.[59] As with spondylodiscitis, S aureus is the predominant causative microorganism, although infections involving other gram-positive and gram-negative bacteria are also possible.[60]

Clinical Presentation and Physical Examination

Patients with SEA can present to the ED anywhere along a continuum of disease with a wide range of clinical signs and symptoms (Table 3). When each symptom is considered in isolation, back pain is present in three-quarters of patients, fever in nearly half of patients, neurologic abnormalities in a third of patients, and paralysis in a fifth of patients.[61–64] The classic triad of fever, back pain, and neurologic deficits is exhibited by only a minority of patients with SEA.[60] A high index of clinical suspicion followed by timely diagnosis of SEA is essential to prevent complications of cord compression and irreversible sensory loss or paralysis.

Diagnostic Evaluation

The initial evaluation of SEA in the ED should mirror that of spondylodiscitis. The presence of leukocytosis is neither sensitive nor specific for the diagnosis.[60] Although elevated ESR and CRP are sensitive, neither is specific to the disease. Blood cultures are positive in approximately 60% of patients with SEA.[65,66]

Although plain radiography and noncontrast CT cannot directly visualize SEA, both may provide indirect evidence of its presence, usually in the form of a concomitant spondylodiscitis.[67,68] MRI and CT myelography are highly sensitive (>90%) in diagnosing SEA.[61,69] MRI is the imaging modality of choice, as it is noninvasive and

Table 3	
Stages of clinical progression in spinal epidural abscess	
Stage	**Clinical Findings**
1	Back pain at the level of the affected spine, fever, tenderness
2	Radicular pain, nuchal rigidity/neck stiffness, reflex changes
3	Motor weakness, sensory deficit, and bladder and bowel dysfunction
4	Paralysis

From Heusner AP. Nontuberculous spinal epidural infections. N Engl J Med 1948;239(23):845–54; and Peterson JA, Paris P, Williams AC. Acute epidural abscess. Am J Emerg Med 1987;5(4):287–90.

facilitates assessment of surrounding structures for spread of infection (eg, paraspinal abscess) and evaluation for spinal cord compression.[60]

Lumbar puncture is not recommended, as Gram stain and cerebrospinal fluid culture are not sensitive enough to detect the presence of SEA and may inadvertently introduce infection into the central nervous system.[60]

Management

Whereas spondylodiscitis is often managed medically with long-term antibiotic therapy alone, SEA frequently requires a combined medical and surgical approach, particularly when the cervical or thoracic spine is involved and spinal canal narrowing with cord compression can progress rapidly to neurologic dysfunction.[38] Consultation with a spine surgeon is paramount to consider surgical drainage of the abscess, debridement of adjacent infected tissue, preservation of the local blood supply to promote tissue healing, and maintenance of spinal stability.[70] Empiric antibiotic therapy with a combination of vancomycin and a third-generation or fourth-generation cephalosporin is reasonable until cultures of the abscess or blood permit tailored coverage for a prolonged course, best determined in concert with an infectious disease specialist.

ANTIBIOTIC PROPHYLAXIS FOR OPEN FRACTURE

Osteomyelitis can complicate up to a quarter of open fractures due to direct inoculation of bacteria into bone, either from the patient's skin flora or the external environment.[6,71] The risk of posttraumatic osteomyelitis hinges on the severity of the fracture and any associated soft tissue defect, vascular compromise, or gross wound contamination, as well as surgical debridement and postinjury antibiotic prophylaxis.[71–76]

In the ED, any gross contaminant should be removed from the wound followed by copious irrigation with normal saline.[77] The wound should be covered with a sterile dressing pending evaluation by an orthopedic surgeon and formal irrigation and surgical debridement in the operating room. Antibiotic prophylaxis should be administered systemically, preferably within 6 hours of the injury. Current guidelines from the Eastern Association for the Surgery of Trauma (EAST), the Surgical Infection Society, and US Department of Defense recommend specific antibiotic regimens based on fracture severity as defined by Gustilo-Anderson classification[78–80] (**Table 4**). Although gram-positive coverage is universally endorsed, EAST guidelines also recommend gram-negative coverage (historically with an aminoglycoside) for type III open fractures.[79] In situations in which fecal or clostridial contamination (eg, farmyard injury) is suspected, the same guidelines also suggest the addition of high-dose penicillin.

Table 4
Antibiotic prophylaxis for open fracture by Gustilo-Anderson classification

Type	Description	Infection Rate[71–73]	Antibiotic
I	Open fracture with wound ≤1 cm and clean	0%–2%	Cefazolin 2 g IV[a,b]
II	Open fracture with wound >1 cm without extensive soft tissue injury, flap, or avulsion	2%–10%	
III	Open segmental fracture with wound >10 cm with extensive soft tissue injury or traumatic amputation	10%–50%	Cefazolin 2 g IV[a] + gentamicin 5 mg/kg IV (adjusted body weight)[c]

Abbreviation: IV, intravenous.
[a] If actual body weight ≥120 kg, consider 3 g.
[b] If penicillin allergy, may substitute with vancomycin 15 mg/kg IV (actual body weight).
[c] Antibiotic prophylaxis directed against gram-negative bacteria (including *Pseudomonas aeruginosa*) remains controversial.[78–80] Institution-specific protocols and/or infectious disease consultation can help guide safe and appropriate gram-negative coverage, particularly in the setting of impaired renal function.
From Hoff WS, Bonadies JA, Cachecho R, et al. EAST practice management guidelines work group: update to practice management guidelines for prophylactic antibiotic use in open fractures. J Trauma 2011;70(3):751–4.

SEPTIC ARTHRITIS

Septic arthritis is an infection of the joint. Worldwide, the annual incidence of septic arthritis ranges from 5 to 12 per 100,000 persons.[81–83] In the United States, more than 16,000 ED visits in 2012 involved a primary diagnosis of septic arthritis, comprising 0.01% of all ED visits during that year.[84]

Most cases of septic arthritis stem from hematogenous seeding of a joint in the setting of bacteremia. Less frequently, overlying soft tissue infections can spread contiguously to the joint. Direct inoculation of bacteria into a joint can occur through a traumatic arthrotomy, open fracture or dislocation, arthrocentesis, or intra-articular injection resulting in infection. Common risk factors for developing septic arthritis include older age, diabetes mellitus, rheumatoid arthritis, joint surgery, prosthetic joint, skin infection, and injection drug use.[81–83,85]

As with other musculoskeletal infections, *S aureus* and *Streptococcus* species are the most frequent causative microorganisms associated with septic arthritis.[83,86] Infections due to gram-negative bacilli are more common among the elderly (ie, in the setting of an underlying urinary tract infection), as well as those who inject drugs.[86,87] Disseminated *Neisseria gonorrhoeae* infection can present as septic arthritis, usually in young sexually active adults. *Candida* septic arthritis may be encountered in patients with impaired or normal immune systems.[88]

Clinical Presentation and Physical Examination

Joint pain with associated warmth, swelling, and restricted movement is the primary presenting feature of septic arthritis.[89,90] Large joints, such as the knee and hip, are most commonly involved, although smaller joints also can become infected. Fever may be present but is not diagnostic.[89,91] Examination of the affected joint is often notable for an effusion with associated erythema, warmth, and tenderness. Range of motion of the joint may be limited and painful. Many of these signs and symptoms can be muted in the setting of immunosuppression and fail to distinguish septic arthritis from other noninfectious forms of arthritis. Unrecognized, septic arthritis can progress to joint destruction, osteomyelitis, and sepsis, with an overall mortality approaching 10%.[91] Timely recognition of septic arthritis by the emergency physician is necessary to improve outcomes.

Diagnostic Evaluation

Although CBC, ESR, and CRP should be obtained, definitive diagnosis rests with performing an arthrocentesis of the affected joint. Fluoroscopic or ultrasound guidance by interventional radiology may be necessary to sample certain joints (eg, hip, sacroiliac joint). Synovial fluid should be submitted for cell count with differential, Gram stain, and microbiologic (aerobic and anaerobic) culture. The higher the synovial WBC count, the greater the likelihood of septic arthritis.[89,90] A synovial WBC count greater than 50,000 cells/mm^3 has a positive LR of 7.7 (95% CI 5.7–11.0); a synovial WBC count greater than 100,000 cells/mm^3 has a positive LR of 28.0 (95% CI 12.0–66.0).[89] A synovial WBC count with a differential of greater than 90% polymorphonuclear cells has an LR of 3.4 (95% CI 2.8–4.2) for septic arthritis.[89] At best, Gram stain has a sensitivity of 50% for detecting bacteria in synovial fluid, whereas that of synovial fluid culture approaches 80%.[89] If only 1 test can be sent due to a limited volume of synovial fluid, the culture should receive priority. Multiple sets of blood cultures also should be obtained when hematogenous septic arthritis is suspected to improve the chances of identifying a causative microorganism.

As far as imaging, plain radiography of the infected joint may reveal joint destruction or an associated osteomyelitis. CT and MRI can be helpful in evaluating for septic arthritis involving difficult-to-assess sites such as the hip or sacroiliac joint.

Management

Empiric antibiotic therapy for septic arthritis in the ED should cover gram-positive bacteria, including MRSA, with vancomycin being a reasonable initial choice. If the patient has risk factors for a gram-negative infection (eg, injection drug use, immunocompromised state, elderly), a third-generation or fourth-generation cephalosporin should be added. Ideally, antibiotic therapy should be started after synovial fluid sampling and blood culture collection. An orthopedic surgeon should be consulted to pursue irrigation and surgical drainage in the operating room or serial arthrocentesis. Patients with septic arthritis will generally require hospital admission and several weeks of antibiotic therapy.

PERIPROSTHETIC JOINT INFECTION

Anywhere from 0.5% to 2.0% of primary total hip or knee arthroplasty procedures are complicated by periprosthetic joint infection (PJI).[92–94] Infections arising within the first few months of joint implantation are more likely to be related to microorganisms acquired at the time of surgery (eg, S aureus), whereas late infections may be attributable to chronic infection with indolent microorganisms (eg, coagulase-negative staphylococci) or hematogenous seeding of bacteria from a distant site (eg, urinary tract, infected central venous catheter).[95,96] Risk factors for PJI include male gender, tobacco use, elevated body mass index (≥30 kg/m^2), diabetes mellitus, rheumatoid arthritis, corticosteroid use, previous joint surgery (including revision arthroplasty), and depression.[97]

Clinical Presentation and Physical Examination

Similar to patients with septic arthritis, those with PJI may present with warmth, swelling, and tenderness over the affected joint, with or without signs of surrounding soft tissue infection or systemic illness.[95,96] In late or chronic infections, pain at the site of the prosthetic may be the only complaint endorsed. A nonhealing or draining wound overlying or a draining sinus tract communicating deep to the prosthesis is concerning for infection, with the latter considered definitive evidence for PJI.[96]

Diagnostic Evaluation

Standard laboratory testing should include CBC, ESR, and CRP, although these tests are nonspecific for PJI.[96] If there is a strong clinical suspicion for PJI, diagnostic arthrocentesis of the affected joint should be pursued in consultation with an orthopedic surgeon and interventional radiologist (particularly in the case of a prosthetic hip).[96,98,99] Emergency physicians should recognize that parameters for diagnosing PJI on synovial fluid analysis differ significantly from that of septic arthritis involving a native joint.[95,96] As part of its definition for PJI, the International Consensus Group on Periprosthetic Joint Infection recommends a minimum synovial WBC count threshold of 10,000 cells/mm^3 as one of several criteria for acute PJI (<90 days since surgery) and 3000 cells/mm^3 for chronic PJI (>90 days).[100] Likewise, this definition suggests a minimum synovial fluid WBC differential of 90% polymorphonuclear cells as another criterion for acute PJI and 80% for chronic PJI.[100] Synovial fluid culture is moderately sensitive and highly specific for predicting PJI, with a positive LR of 15.3 (95% CI 10.6–22.1).[101] Superficial cultures should not be obtained from draining wounds or sinus tracts, as they correlate poorly with deep cultures obtained from the infected joint.[102]

Imaging as part of the ED evaluation for PJI should include plain radiographs of the affected joint to assess for osteolysis or hardware loosening that might suggest infection; there is no clearly defined role for CT or MRI in making the diagnosis.[95,103]

Although diagnostic workup in the ED may yield findings supportive of PJI, diagnosis remains clinical in many instances and may ultimately need intraoperative evaluation and tissue sampling by an orthopedic surgeon for confirmation.[96,98,103]

Management

In the absence of hemodynamic instability, sepsis, or a severe soft tissue infection, empiric antibiotic therapy in the ED can be withheld until synovial fluid culture is obtained in order to maximize their yield. Patients with PJI will require multidisciplinary care combining surgical debridement with or without removal of the infected prosthesis and appropriate long-term antibiotics.

SUMMARY

Clinical presentations of musculoskeletal infection in patients presenting to emergency care can range from chronic wounds and nonspecific bone or joint pain to functional debilitation, and even neurologic compromise when the spine is involved. Emergency physicians play a critical role in the early recognition, evaluation, and management of these infections. Appropriate collection of microbiologic cultures (eg, blood, synovial fluid) before empiric antibiotic therapy in the ED has significant implications for isolating causative microorganisms and guiding downstream treatment. Antibiotic therapy may even be safely withheld to pursue bone biopsy and culture if the patient is clinically stable. A low threshold should exist to seek orthopedic surgery and infectious disease consultation in patients presenting with bone and joint infections to the ED and many will require hospitalization for definitive care, combining medical and surgical approaches.

REFERENCES

1. Lew DP, Waldvogel FA. Osteomyelitis. Lancet 2004;364(9431):369–79.

2. Kremers HM, Nwojo ME, Ransom JE, et al. Trends in the epidemiology of osteomyelitis: a population-based study, 1969 to 2009. J Bone Joint Surg Am 2015; 97(10):837–45.
3. Waldvogel FA, Medoff G, Swartz MN. Osteomyelitis: a review of clinical features, therapeutic considerations and unusual aspects. 3. Osteomyelitis associated with vascular insufficiency. N Engl J Med 1970;282(6):316–22.
4. Cierny G 3rd, Mader JT, Penninck JJ. A clinical staging system for adult osteomyelitis. Clin Orthop Relat Res 2003;(414):7–24.
5. Chihara S, Segreti J. Osteomyelitis. Dis Mon 2010;56(1):5–31.
6. Schmitt SK. Osteomyelitis. Infect Dis Clin North Am 2017;31(2):325–38.
7. Lew DP, Waldvogel FA. Osteomyelitis. N Engl J Med 1997;336(14):999–1007.
8. Maman E, Bickels J, Ephros M, et al. Musculoskeletal manifestations of cat scratch disease. Clin Infect Dis 2007;45(12):1535–40.
9. Petitjean G, Fluckiger U, Schären S, et al. Vertebral osteomyelitis caused by non-tuberculous mycobacteria. Clin Microbiol Infect 2004;10(11):951–3.
10. Stratov I, Korman TM, Johnson PD. Management of Aspergillus osteomyelitis: report of failure of liposomal amphotericin B and response to voriconazole in an immunocompetent host and literature review. Eur J Clin Microbiol Infect Dis 2003;22(5):277–83.
11. Cunha BA. Fever of unknown origin: focused diagnostic approach based on clinical clues from the history, physical examination, and laboratory tests. Infect Dis Clin North Am 2007;21(4):1137–87, xi.
12. Lipsky BA, Berendt AR, Cornia PB, et al. 2012 Infectious Diseases Society of America clinical practice guideline for the diagnosis and treatment of diabetic foot infections. Clin Infect Dis 2012;54(12):e132–73.
13. Butalia S, Palda VA, Sargeant RJ, et al. Does this patient with diabetes have osteomyelitis of the lower extremity? JAMA 2008;299(7):806–13.
14. Caputo GM, Cavanagh PR, Ulbrecht JS, et al. Assessment and management of foot disease in patients with diabetes. N Engl J Med 1994;331(13):854–60.
15. Lavery LA, Sariaya M, Ashry H, et al. Microbiology of osteomyelitis in diabetic foot infections. J Foot Ankle Surg 1995;34(1):61–4.
16. Kessler L, Piemont Y, Ortega F, et al. Comparison of microbiological results of needle puncture vs. superficial swab in infected diabetic foot ulcer with osteomyelitis. Diabet Med 2006;23(1):99–102.
17. Senneville E, Melliez H, Beltrand E, et al. Culture of percutaneous bone biopsy specimens for diagnosis of diabetic foot osteomyelitis: concordance with ulcer swab cultures. Clin Infect Dis 2006;42(1):57–62.
18. Dinh MT, Abad CL, Safdar N. Diagnostic accuracy of the physical examination and imaging tests for osteomyelitis underlying diabetic foot ulcers: meta-analysis. Clin Infect Dis 2008;47(4):519–27.
19. Gold RH, Hawkins RA, Katz RD. Bacterial osteomyelitis: findings on plain radiography, CT, MR, and scintigraphy. AJR Am J Roentgenol 1991;157(2):365–70.
20. Pineda C, Vargas A, Rodriguez AV. Imaging of osteomyelitis: current concepts. Infect Dis Clin North Am 2006;20(4):789–825.
21. Kapoor A, Page S, Lavalley M, et al. Magnetic resonance imaging for diagnosing foot osteomyelitis: a meta-analysis. Arch Intern Med 2007;167(2):125–32.
22. Hammond DA, Smith MN, Li C, et al. Systematic review and meta-analysis of acute kidney injury associated with concomitant vancomycin and piperacillin/tazobactam. Clin Infect Dis 2017;64(5):666–74.

23. Grammatico L, Baron S, Rusch E, et al. Epidemiology of vertebral osteomyelitis (VO) in France: analysis of hospital-discharge data 2002-2003. Epidemiol Infect 2008;136(5):653–60.
24. Issa K, Diebo BG, Faloon M, et al. The epidemiology of vertebral osteomyelitis in the United states from 1998 to 2013. Clin Spine Surg 2018;31(2):E102–8.
25. Mylona E, Samarkos M, Kakalou E, et al. Pyogenic vertebral osteomyelitis: a systematic review of clinical characteristics. Semin Arthritis Rheum 2009; 39(1):10–7.
26. Kak V, Chandrasekar PH. Bone and joint infections in injection drug users. Infect Dis Clin North Am 2002;16(3):681–95.
27. Yoon SH, Chung SK, Kim KJ, et al. Pyogenic vertebral osteomyelitis: identification of microorganism and laboratory markers used to predict clinical outcome. Eur Spine J 2010;19(4):575–82.
28. McHenry MC, Rehm SJ, Krajewski LP, et al. Vertebral osteomyelitis and aortic lesions: case report and review. Rev Infect Dis 1991;13(6):1184–94.
29. Sreedharan L, Lakshmanan P, Shenfine J, et al. Thoracic vertebral osteomyelitis secondary to chronic esophageal perforation. Spine J 2009;9(4):e1–5.
30. Hopton B, Barron D, Ambrose S, et al. The flatulent spine: lumbar spinal infection secondary to colonic diverticular abscess: a case report and review of the literature. J Spinal Disord Tech 2008;21(7):527–30.
31. Simopoulos TT, Kraemer JJ, Glazer P, et al. Vertebral osteomyelitis: a potentially catastrophic outcome after lumbar epidural steroid injection. Pain Physician 2008;11(5):693–7.
32. Moudgal V, Singal B, Kauffman CA, et al. Spinal and paraspinal fungal infections associated with contaminated methylprednisolone injections. Open Forum Infect Dis 2014;1(1):ofu022.
33. Schwed AC, Plurad DS, Bricker S, et al. Abdominal hollow viscus injuries are associated with spine and neurologic infections after penetrating spinal cord injuries. Am Surg 2014;80(10):966–9.
34. Courjon J, Lemaignen A, Ghout I, et al. Pyogenic vertebral osteomyelitis of the elderly: characteristics and outcomes. PLoS One 2017;12(12):e0188470.
35. Colmenero JD, Jiménez-Mejías ME, Sánchez-Lora FJ, et al. Pyogenic, tuberculous, and brucellar vertebral osteomyelitis: a descriptive and comparative study of 219 cases. Ann Rheum Dis 1997;56(12):709–15.
36. Eren Gok S, Kaptanoğlu E, Celikbaş A, et al. Vertebral osteomyelitis: clinical features and diagnosis. Clin Microbiol Infect 2014;20(10):1055–60.
37. Hopkinson N, Stevenson J, Benjamin S. A case ascertainment study of septic discitis: clinical, microbiological and radiological features. QJM 2001;94(9):465–70.
38. Govender S. Spinal infections. J Bone Joint Surg Br 2005;87(11):1454–8.
39. An HS, Seldomridge JA. Spinal infections: diagnostic tests and imaging studies. Clin Orthop Relat Res 2006;444:27–33.
40. Priest DH, Peacock JE Jr. Hematogenous vertebral osteomyelitis due to *Staphylococcus aureus* in the adult: clinical features and therapeutic outcomes. South Med J 2005;98(9):854–62.
41. Butler JS, Shelly MJ, Timlin M, et al. Nontuberculous pyogenic spinal infection in adults: a 12-year experience from a tertiary referral center. Spine (Phila Pa 1976) 2006;31(23):2695–700.
42. Faidas A, Ferguson JV Jr, Nelson JE, et al. Cervical vertebral osteomyelitis presenting as a retropharyngeal abscess. Clin Infect Dis 1994;18(6):992–4.
43. Bass SN, Ailani RK, Shekar R, et al. Pyogenic vertebral osteomyelitis presenting as exudative pleural effusion: a series of five cases. Chest 1998;114(2):642–7.

44. van den Berge M, de Marie S, Kuipers T, et al. Psoas abscess: report of a series and review of the literature. Neth J Med 2005;63(10):413–6.
45. Gasbarrini AL, Bertoldi E, Mazzetti M, et al. Clinical features, diagnostic and therapeutic approaches to haematogenous vertebral osteomyelitis. Eur Rev Med Pharmacol Sci 2005;9(1):53–66.
46. Buranapanitkit B, Lim A, Geater A. Misdiagnosis in vertebral osteomyelitis: problems and factors. J Med Assoc Thai 2001;84(12):1743–50.
47. Amadoru S, Lim K, Tacey M, et al. Spinal infections in older people: an analysis of demographics, presenting features, microbiology and outcomes. Intern Med J 2017;47(2):182–8.
48. Siemionow K, Steinmetz M, Bell G, et al. Identifying serious causes of back pain: cancer, infection, fracture. Cleve Clin J Med 2008;75(8):557–66.
49. Jensen AG, Espersen F, Skinhøj P, et al. Bacteremic *Staphylococcus aureus* spondylitis. Arch Intern Med 1998;158(5):509–17.
50. Cheung WY, Luk KD. Pyogenic spondylitis. Int Orthop 2012;36(2):397–404.
51. Aagaard T, Roed C, Dragsted C, et al. Microbiological and therapeutic challenges in infectious spondylodiscitis: a cohort study of 100 cases, 2006-2011. Scand J Infect Dis 2013;45(6):417–24.
52. Zimmerli W. Clinical practice. Vertebral osteomyelitis. N Engl J Med 2010; 362(11):1022–9.
53. Khan IA, Vaccaro AR, Zlotolow DA. Management of vertebral diskitis and osteomyelitis. Orthopedics 1999;22(8):758–65.
54. Varma R, Lander P, Assaf A. Imaging of pyogenic infectious spondylodiskitis. Radiol Clin North Am 2001;39(2):203–13.
55. Cottle L, Riordan T. Infectious spondylodiscitis. J Infect 2008;56(6):401–12.
56. Nolla JM, Ariza J, Gómez-Vaquero C, et al. Spontaneous pyogenic vertebral osteomyelitis in nondrug users. Semin Arthritis Rheum 2002;31(4):271–8.
57. Berbari EF, Kanj SS, Kowalski TJ, et al. 2015 Infectious Diseases Society of America (IDSA) clinical practice guidelines for the diagnosis and treatment of native vertebral osteomyelitis in adults. Clin Infect Dis 2015;61(6):e26–46.
58. Hadjipavlou AG, Mader JT, Necessary JT, et al. Hematogenous pyogenic spinal infections and their surgical management. Spine (Phila Pa 1976) 2000;25(13): 1668–79.
59. Zimmerer SM, Conen A, Müller AA, et al. Spinal epidural abscess: aetiology, predisponent factors and clinical outcomes in a 4-year prospective study. Eur Spine J 2011;20(12):2228–34.
60. Darouiche RO. Spinal epidural abscess. N Engl J Med 2006;355(19):2012–20.
61. Rigamonti D, Liem L, Sampath P, et al. Spinal epidural abscess: contemporary trends in etiology, evaluation, and management. Surg Neurol 1999;52(2):189–96 [discussion: 197].
62. Akalan N, Ozgen T. Infection as a cause of spinal cord compression: a review of 36 spinal epidural abscess cases. Acta Neurochir (Wien) 2000;142(1):17–23.
63. Reihsaus E, Waldbaur H, Seeling W. Spinal epidural abscess: a meta-analysis of 915 patients. Neurosurg Rev 2000;23(4):175–204 [discussion: 205].
64. Schoenfeld AJ, Wahlquist TC. Mortality, complication risk, and total charges after the treatment of epidural abscess. Spine J 2015;15(2):249–55.
65. Danner RL, Hartman BJ. Update on spinal epidural abscess: 35 cases and review of the literature. Rev Infect Dis 1987;9(2):265–74.
66. Curry WT Jr, Hoh BL, Amin-Hanjani S, et al. Spinal epidural abscess: clinical presentation, management, and outcome. Surg Neurol 2005;63(4):364–71 [discussion: 371].

67. Khan SH, Hussain MS, Griebel RW, et al. Title comparison of primary and secondary spinal epidural abscesses: a retrospective analysis of 29 cases. Surg Neurol 2003;59(1):28–33 [discussion: 33].
68. Sendi P, Bregenzer T, Zimmerli W. Spinal epidural abscess in clinical practice. QJM 2008;101(1):1–12.
69. Hlavin ML, Kaminski HJ, Ross JS, et al. Spinal epidural abscess: a ten-year perspective. Neurosurgery 1990;27(2):177–84.
70. Grados F, Lescure FX, Senneville E, et al. Suggestions for managing pyogenic (non-tuberculous) discitis in adults. Joint Bone Spine 2007;74(2):133–9.
71. Patzakis MJ, Wilkins J. Factors influencing infection rate in open fracture wounds. Clin Orthop Relat Res 1989;(243):36–40.
72. Gustilo RB, Anderson JT. Prevention of infection in the treatment of one thousand and twenty-five open fractures of long bones: retrospective and prospective analyses. J Bone Joint Surg Am 1976;58(4):453–8.
73. Gustilo RB, Mendoza RM, Williams DN. Problems in the management of type III (severe) open fractures: a new classification of type III open fractures. J Trauma 1984;24(8):742–6.
74. Gosselin RA, Roberts I, Gillespie WJ. Antibiotics for preventing infection in open limb fractures. Cochrane Database Syst Rev 2004;(1):CD003764.
75. Penn-Barwell JG, Murray CK, Wenke JC. Early antibiotics and debridement independently reduce infection in an open fracture model. J Bone Joint Surg Br 2012;94(1):107–12.
76. Lack WD, Karunakar MA, Angerame MR, et al. Type III open tibia fractures: immediate antibiotic prophylaxis minimizes infection. J Orthop Trauma 2015;29(1):1–6.
77. Zalavras CG. Prevention of infection in open fractures. Infect Dis Clin North Am 2017;31(2):339–52.
78. Hauser CJ, Adams CA Jr, Eachempati SR, et al. Surgical Infection Society guideline: prophylactic antibiotic use in open fractures: an evidence-based guideline. Surg Infect (Larchmt) 2006;7(4):379–405.
79. Hoff WS, Bonadies JA, Cachecho R, et al. EAST practice management guidelines work group: update to practice management guidelines for prophylactic antibiotic use in open fractures. J Trauma 2011;70(3):751–4.
80. Murray CK, Obremskey WT, Hsu JR, et al. Prevention of infections associated with combat-related extremity injuries. J Trauma 2011;71(2 Suppl 2):S235–57.
81. Kaandorp CJ, Dinant HJ, van de Laar MA, et al. Incidence and sources of native and prosthetic joint infection: a community based prospective survey. Ann Rheum Dis 1997;56(8):470–5.
82. Geirsson AJ, Statkevicius S, Vikingsson A. Septic arthritis in Iceland 1990-2002: increasing incidence due to iatrogenic infections. Ann Rheum Dis 2008;67(5):638–43.
83. Kennedy N, Chambers ST, Nolan I, et al. Native joint septic arthritis: epidemiology, clinical features, and microbiological causes in a New Zealand population. J Rheumatol 2015;42(12):2392–7.
84. Singh JA, Yu S. Septic arthritis in emergency departments in the US: a national study of health care utilization and time trends. Arthritis Care Res (Hoboken) 2018;70(2):320–6.
85. Kaandorp CJ, Van Schaardenburg D, Krijnen P, et al. Risk factors for septic arthritis in patients with joint disease. A prospective study. Arthritis Rheum 1995;38(12):1819–25.
86. Ross JJ. Septic arthritis of native joints. Infect Dis Clin North Am 2017;31(2):203–18.

87. Peterson TC, Pearson C, Zekaj M, et al. Septic arthritis in intravenous drug abusers: a historical comparison of habits and pathogens. J Emerg Med 2014;47(6):723–8.
88. Gamaletsou MN, Rammaert B, Bueno MA, et al. Candida arthritis: analysis of 112 pediatric and adult cases. Open Forum Infect Dis 2016;3(1):ofv207.
89. Margaretten ME, Kohlwes J, Moore D, et al. Does this adult patient have septic arthritis? JAMA 2007;297(13):1478–88.
90. Carpenter CR, Schuur JD, Everett WW, et al. Evidence-based diagnostics: adult septic arthritis. Acad Emerg Med 2011;18(8):781–96.
91. Mathews CJ, Weston VC, Jones A, et al. Bacterial septic arthritis in adults. Lancet 2010;375(9717):846–55.
92. Tsaras G, Osmon DR, Mabry T, et al. Incidence, secular trends, and outcomes of prosthetic joint infection: a population-based study, Olmsted County, Minnesota, 1969-2007. Infect Control Hosp Epidemiol 2012;33(12):1207–12.
93. Bozic KJ, Grosso LM, Lin Z, et al. Variation in hospital-level risk-standardized complication rates following elective primary total hip and knee arthroplasty. J Bone Joint Surg Am 2014;96(8):640–7.
94. Marang-van de Mheen PJ, Bragan Turner E, Liew S, et al. Variation in prosthetic joint infection and treatment strategies during 4.5 years of follow-up after primary joint arthroplasty using administrative data of 41397 patients across Australian, European and United States hospitals. BMC Musculoskelet Disord 2017;18(1):207.
95. Luthringer TA, Fillingham YA, Okroj K, et al. Periprosthetic joint infection after hip and knee arthroplasty: a review for emergency care providers. Ann Emerg Med 2016;68(3):324–34.
96. Osmon DR, Berbari EF, Berendt AR, et al. Diagnosis and management of prosthetic joint infection: clinical practice guidelines by the Infectious Diseases Society of America. Clin Infect Dis 2013;56(1):e1–25.
97. Kunutsor SK, Whitehouse MR, Blom AW, et al. Patient-related risk factors for periprosthetic joint infection after total joint arthroplasty: a systematic review and meta-analysis. PLoS One 2016;11(3):e0150866.
98. Gomez-Urena EO, Tande AJ, Osmon DR, et al. Diagnosis of prosthetic joint infection: cultures, biomarker and criteria. Infect Dis Clin North Am 2017; 31(2):219–35.
99. Della Valle C, Parvizi J, Bauer TW, et al. American Academy of Orthopaedic Surgeons clinical practice guideline on: the diagnosis of periprosthetic joint infections of the hip and knee. J Bone Joint Surg Am 2011;93(14):1355–7.
100. Parvizi J, Gehrke T, International Consensus Group on Periprosthetic Joint Infection. Definition of periprosthetic joint infection. J Arthroplasty 2014;29(7):1331.
101. Qu X, Zhai Z, Wu C, et al. Preoperative aspiration culture for preoperative diagnosis of infection in total hip or knee arthroplasty. J Clin Microbiol 2013;51(11): 3830–4.
102. Tetreault MW, Wetters NG, Aggarwal VK, et al. Should draining wounds and sinuses associated with hip and knee arthroplasties be cultured? J Arthroplasty 2013;28(8 Suppl):133–6.
103. Ting NT, Della Valle CJ. Diagnosis of periprosthetic joint infection—an algorithm-based approach. J Arthroplasty 2017;32(7):2047–50.

Management of Patients with Sexually Transmitted Infections in the Emergency Department

SueLin M. Hilbert, MD[a], Hilary E.L. Reno, MD, PhD[b],*

KEYWORDS

- Gonorrhea • Chlamydia • Syphilis • Public health • Pelvic inflammatory disease

KEY POINTS

- Sexually transmitted infections (STI) are very common infections in the United States.
- Most patients with STIs are evaluated and treated in primary care settings; however, many also present to the emergency department (ED) for initial care.
- Management of STIs in the ED includes appropriate testing and treatment per Centers for Disease Control and Prevention Sexually Transmitted Diseases Treatment Guidelines.
- Although most patients with STIs are asymptomatic or may only exhibit mild symptoms, serious complications from untreated infection are possible.
- Pregnant women with STIs are particularly vulnerable to serious complications; therefore, empiric ED treatment combined with close follow-up care and referral to obstetrics are paramount.

INTRODUCTION
Epidemiology and National Trends

Sexually transmitted infections (STIs) are the most common infections in the United States and include human papilloma virus, Neisseria gonorrhoeae (GC), Chlamydia trachomatis (Ct), herpes simplex virus (HSV), syphilis, human immunodeficiency virus (HIV), and others. In recent years, STIs have been increasing at significant rates especially among adolescents, pregnant women, and high-risk groups such as men who have sex with men (MSM). Syphilis, once targeted for elimination, increased 17.6% from 2015 to 2016.[1] Congenital syphilis rates increased 38% from 2012 to 2014[2] followed by an additional 27.6% from 2015 to 2016.[1]

[a] Department of Emergency Medicine, Washington University in St. Louis, 660 S. Euclid Campus Box 8072, St. Louis, MO 63110, USA; [b] Division of Infectious Disease, Washington University in St. Louis, Campus Box 8051, 4523 Clayton Avenue, St Louis, MO 63110, USA
* Corresponding author.
E-mail address: hreno@wustl.edu

Emerg Med Clin N Am 36 (2018) 767–776
https://doi.org/10.1016/j.emc.2018.06.007
0733-8627/18/© 2018 Elsevier Inc. All rights reserved.
emed.theclinics.com

STIs are largely ambulatory illnesses, but the care of patients with STIs can often fall on emergency departments (ED) when health care access is limited or complications occur. Although most STIs are cared for in the primary care setting, 7% to 16% are managed in the ED.[3,4] Surveillance data indicate that STI visits to EDs are increasing[5] during the same time that public health funding has decreased and traditional sexually transmitted diseases (STD) clinics have closed. Health care access for patients at highest risk for STIs (ie, the young and healthy) can be challenging. In addition, although women may have access to health care via family planning, men are more likely than women to present to an ED for STI care.[3]

Role of the Emergency Department in the Care of Patients with Sexually Transmitted Infections

STIs are largely asymptomatic, and screening for STIs in an ED can be challenging while managing acute medical problems. ED providers are less likely to screen patients for STIs than providers in other health care settings[6] likely because of concerns about cost and test result follow-up. Most patients are evaluated and treated for STIs in the ED based on their symptoms and/or chief complaint, such as dysuria or vaginal/penile discharge. Considering the high rate of asymptomatic infections, however, it is likely that many infections go undiagnosed and therefore untreated. This is the concern for under treated STIs underscores the importance of knowing local disease prevalence, having a high index of clinical suspicion, and maintaining a low threshold to treat patients for STIs.

ED providers are likely to encounter patients presenting with symptoms such as vaginal or penile discharge or dysuria for which STIs are included in the differential. Testing for STIs even when test results are not immediately available is advised over syndromic management without testing.[7] Nucleic acid amplification tests (NAATs) are highly specific and sensitive and can direct postvisit management and improve patient health in the following ways:

- Patients who know they have tested positive for an STI in the ED may be less likely to acquire an STI in the future. In a study of adolescent women, those who were aware of their test results had a lower rate of return to the ED for subsequent STI diagnoses.[8]
- Many symptomatic STIs self-resolve without treatment, giving patients a false sense of security. Undiagnosed and untreated infections can still lead to permanent sequalae over time (eg, pelvic inflammatory disease [PID], infertility).
- For patients who have recurrent symptoms, testing is especially important in directing appropriate management, including consideration of drug-resistant infections or other STIs.
- When testing yields a specific STI diagnosis, patients can more accurately direct their partners to care. Expedited partner therapy (EPT), available in some states, requires diagnosis of an STI and is a method of reducing reinfection rates.[9]
- A diagnosis of STI may be an indication for preexposure prophylaxis (PrEP) to prevent HIV infection. Empiric STI treatment without testing can hamper referral for PrEP.
- Public health efforts to address STIs on a population level are best guided by epidemiologic data. STI treatment without testing impairs accurate determination of STI prevalence and incidence.

A comprehensive approach to patients with STIs in any setting is to conduct a sexual history test based on symptoms and physical examination and then treat the patient as indicated. A sexual history can be as simple as asking, "Tell me about your sex partners," and obtaining additional information as indicated. Counseling messages can be delivered directly to the patient and in discharge instructions. STI testing will confirm diagnoses and further direct care. Treatment in the ED is often limited unless findings supportive of STI are obvious; having reliable follow-up with patients ensures comprehensive care.

Gold-standard testing for most STIs, such as NAATs and cultures, often does not have sufficient turn-around times for practical diagnostic use in the ED. This is the delay in test results leads to a primarily syndromic approach to STI diagnosis and frequent empiric treatment. Overtreatment of STIs in the ED will occur, although rates of overtreatment are highly variable. In one study, patients who tested positive for chlamydia or gonorrhea were more likely to have received appropriate antibiotics than those patients who were negative for either, demonstrating that ED providers use symptoms and clinical findings to avoid overtreatment.[10] ED providers treat about 50% of patients with an STI at the time of visit.[10] Follow-up for these patients with an untreated STI is essential, and challenges can be met with focused follow-up planning.[11]

EDs should be aware of community and public health STI testing sites. Patients with an STI need testing for other STIs, including HIV, and should be referred for complete STI evaluation if this cannot be performed at their ED visit. These sites can also be a resource for follow-up testing and care. The Centers for Disease Control and Prevention (CDC) maintains a Web site that can direct patients to local clinics that offer STI testing (gettested.cdc.gov).

Diagnosis and Empiric Treatment

Resources for diagnosis, treatment, and management of STIs are available in a variety of formats. The CDC Division of STD Prevention produces provider and patient fact sheets as well as the CDC STD Treatment Guidelines. Consultation with STI experts is available via the National Network of STD Prevention Training Centers (https://www.stdccn.org/). A directed summary of treatment of STIs is included in **Table 1**.

Chlamydia

Ct is a sexually transmitted bacterium that is largely asymptomatic but can present with vaginal or urethral discharge, rectal discharge, dysuria, testicular pain, abdominal pain, or PID. Examination may show a watery urethral discharge in men or a clear endocervical discharge in women, but discharge appearance can vary. Resistance to treatment has not been observed with Ct (see **Table 1**).

Special attention should be paid to patients presenting with rectal pain or discharge who are suspected to have chlamydia. Some serotypes of Ct cause lymphogranuloma venerum (LGV), which has been increasingly reported in patients that participate in anal sex, specifically among MSM.[12] LGV acquired from receptive anal sex can present with proctocolitis, and the associated lymphadenopathy can cause discomfort, a rectal mass, or other symptoms. It should be managed with 3 weeks of doxycycline 100 mg orally twice a day and prompt follow-up care.

All patients with Ct need instructions to abstain from sex for 7 days after treatment and to seek retesting in 3 months (1 month if pregnant) along with prevention counseling. All sex partners in the previous 60 days should also be tested and treated. Some state laws allow for EPT, which is prescribing treatment to partners of patients with proven Ct via a prescription given to the patient for the partner. Large-scale randomized controlled trials have shown that EPT reduced rates of recurrent infections in patients, but EPT is often not available in the ED setting.[13]

Table 1
Treatment of sexually transmitted diseases

Disease	Recommended Regimen	Alternative Regimen and Notes
Genital ulcer disease		
Herpes simplex		
First episode	• Acyclovir 400 mg PO 3 times a day × 7–10 d OR • Valacyclovir 1 g PO 2 times a day × 7–10 d	
Recurrent episodes	• Acyclovir 400 mg PO 3 times a day × 5 d or 800 mg 2 times a day × 5 d OR • Valacyclovir 1 g PO once a day × 5 d or 500 mg PO 2 times a day × 3 d	
Syphilis		
Primary, secondary, or early syphilis	• Benzathine penicillin G 2.4 million U IM single dose	Penicillin-allergic: • Doxycycline 100 mg PO twice daily × 14 d
Syphilis of unknown duration or late syphilis	• Benzathine penicillin G 2.4 million U IM once weekly × 3 doses	Penicillin-allergic: • Doxycycline 100 mg PO twice daily × 28 d
Neurosyphilis or ocular syphilis	• Aqueous crystalline penicillin G 18–24 million U/d × 10–14 d	• Procaine penicillin 2.4 million U IM once daily + probenecid 500 mg PO 4 times daily × 10–14 d
Urethritis/cervicitis		
Gonorrhea (GC)	• Ceftriaxone 250 mg IM once + azithromycin 1 g PO once even if testing for *C trachomatis* is negative Given concern for antibiotic resistance, dual treatment is recommended	• Oral cephalosporin treatment is not recommended as long as ceftriaxone is available • Penicillin/cephalosporin allergic: Gentamycin 240 mg IM × 1 + azithromycin 2 g PO × 1
Disseminated gonococcal infection	• Ceftriaxone 1 g IV daily or cefotaxime 1 g IV every 8 h × 7 d	
Chlamydia	• Azithromycin 1 g PO single dose OR • Doxycycline 100 mg PO twice daily × 7 d	• Erythromycin base 500 mg PO 4 times a day × 7 d Retesting is recommended in 3 mo
Pelvic inflammatory disease		
Outpatient	• Ceftriaxone 250 mg IM once + doxycycline 100 mg PO twice daily × 14 d + consider metronidazole 500 mg orally twice daily × 14 d	• Cefoxitin 2 g IM + probenecid 1 g PO once can be substituted for ceftriaxone
Inpatient	• (Cefoxitin 2 g IV every 6 h or cefotetan 2 g IV every 12 h) + doxycycline 100 mg PO twice daily × 14 d + consider metronidazole 500 mg PO twice daily × 14 d	• Clindamycin 900 mg IV every 8 h + gentamicin 2 mg/kg loading dose, then 1.5 mg/kg every 8 h + doxycycline 100 mg PO twice daily × 14 d • Ampicillin-sulbactam 3 g IV every 6 h + doxycycline 100 mg PO twice daily × 14 d

(*continued on next page*)

Table 1 *(continued)*		
Disease	**Recommended Regimen**	**Alternative Regimen and Notes**
Vaginitis/vaginosis		
Trichomonas	• Metronidazole 2 g PO single dose OR • Tinidazole 2 g PO single dose	• Metronidazole 500 mg PO twice daily × 7 d
Trichomonas in pregnancy	• Metronidazole 2 g PO × 1 (not teratogenic)	
Bacterial vaginosis	• Metronidazole 500 mg PO twice daily × 7 d • Clindamycin cream 2% intravaginally at bedtime × 7 d • Metronidazole gel 0.75% intravaginal once a day for 5 d	• Tinidazole 2 g PO once daily × 2 d or 1 g PO once daily × 5 d • Clindamycin 300 mg PO twice daily × 7 d

See cdc.gov/std/ for the current STD treatment guidelines.
From Workowski KA, Bolan GA, Centers for Disease Control and Prevention. Sexually transmitted diseases treatment guidelines, 2015. MMWR Recomm Rep 2015 64(RR-03):1–137.

Gonorrhea

GC presents with symptoms similar to Ct, although urethral discharge in men traditionally is more mucopurulent than clear in appearance. As with chlamydia, symptoms can be subtle. Treatment is limited by drug resistance in GC, and dual therapy is needed. Both ceftriaxone and azithromycin are used to reduce the development of cephalosporin resistance in GC; however, outbreaks of cephalosporin- and azithromycin-resistant strains have been noted.[14,15] In patients with true cephalosporin allergy or severe penicillin allergy, the recommended regimen is gentamicin 240 mg intramuscularly (IM) × 1 plus azithromycin 2 g orally × 1 with follow-up. This regimen can induce nausea and gastrointestinal side effects, so patients should be counseled. Azithromycin should not be prescribed alone given growing concerns for azithromycin-resistant GC.

Follow-up for patients with GC is similar to patients with Ct. EPT is more challenging with GC given that IM ceftriaxone is the recommended treatment. Cefixime is an alternative oral treatment option but is less effective in pharyngeal infections.

GC can disseminate and present as a more significant illness. Disseminated gonorrhea presents with septic arthritis, polyarticular arthritis, and/or pustular skin lesions and fever. Patients are usually hospitalized and treated initially with intravenous (IV) ceftriaxone.

Trichomonas Vaginitis

Vaginal discharge is a common complaint in EDs. Vaginal discharge can indicate infection with chlamydia, gonorrhea, trichomonas, yeast, or bacterial vaginitis (BV), among other causes. Trichomonas vaginitis is frequently diagnosed in the ED.[16]

In the case of trichomonas and BV, the pelvic examination will show a white discharge. With trichomonas, discharge may be copious and malodorous and vaginal mucosa can be irritated. Testing vaginal discharge for pH is relatively low cost and is an important test in that most patients with trichomonas or BV will have a pH >4.5. Newer NAATs for Trichomonas perform well and are now recommended over the traditional wet mount examination for definitive diagnosis.[9]

Patients with trichomonas need similar prevention and follow-up instructions as other patients with STIs. Patients with BV should be referred to primary care or gynecology because the recurrence rate can be high.

Syphilis

Syphilis was called the great imitator by Sir William Osler and always requires a high level of suspicion for diagnosis. Primary syphilis is characterized by a painless ulcer with an indurated border known as a chancre. The chancre will resolve in 3 to 6 weeks without treatment. Secondary syphilis is characterized by a palmar/plantar rash, condyloma lata, and other findings. Patients are more likely to present for care with secondary syphilis than any other stage of syphilis. A familiarity with the stages of syphilis and the appearance and distribution of the rash of secondary syphilis is important. Other findings like arthralgias and elevated liver function tests can also be seen with secondary syphilis.

Ocular syphilis is another manifestation that may bring patients to the ED and can occur at any stage of syphilis. Ocular syphilis clusters were noted in the United States in 2012 and have been increasingly diagnosed.[17] Any patient with syphilis should be asked about eye or vision complaints. Eye pain and blurry vision are common. Ophthalmology evaluation may confirm uveitis or retinitis. Patients need testing and prompt treatment with IV penicillin as loss of vision can occur.[18]

Congenital syphilis is also increasing in the United States. All providers who see pregnant women should have familiarity with local syphilis rates, clinical examination findings of syphilis, and screening recommendations and recognize the importance of OB/GYN referral.

Herpes Simplex Virus

Primary HSV can present with systemic symptoms of fever, bilateral lymphadenopathy, and painful lesions. Lesions are blisterlike but will coalesce into a shallow ulcer after a few days. Testing with viral culture or polymerase chain reaction of lesions will indicate if HSV-1 or HSV-2 is the cause and can help direct follow-up care and counseling.

Oral antivirals are effective to reduce the number of symptomatic days. If swelling or pain is severe, IV acyclovir may be indicated with pain control. Referral to a primary care provider is needed for consideration of suppressive therapy that will reduce recurrences and reduce asymptotic shedding of HSV to reduce transmission to partners.

Pelvic Inflammatory Disease

PID is an infection in women of the upper reproductive tract and can lead to scarring and infertility when not treated or with multiple episodes. The presentation of PID includes abdominal pain, sometimes fever, and possibly vaginal discharge. On physical examination, mucopurulent cervical discharge and cervical motion tenderness or adnexal tenderness is indicative of PID.

If a patient can tolerate oral antibiotics, recommended ambulatory regimens can be prescribed (see **Table 1**). Management with hospitalization and IV antibiotics is indicated if patients are not tolerating PO, have a complication of PID (tuboovarian abscess), are pregnant, or have failed oral treatment. Surgical consultation may be necessary for the appropriate management of tubo-ovarian abscess (TOA).

SPECIAL POPULATIONS
Pediatrics

The presence of an STI in a pediatric patient should always raise concern of sexual abuse. Transmission from mother to child of GC, Ct, trichomonas, human papillomavirus (HPV), and HSV are all possible in the neonate and can present as nongenital infections, such as conjunctivitis, pneumonia, and, in the case of HSV, encephalitis. Cases of vertical transmission of these infections can be severe and life threatening.

Sexually active adolescents are at high risk for STIs due to several biologic, cognitive, and behavioral factors.[19] As with adult patients, infections in this population are often asymptomatic and follow-up is often poor, so providers should have a low threshold for empiric treatment. All 50 states allow minors to consent for testing and treatment of STIs.

Pregnant Women

Complications associated with STIs in pregnancy include preterm labor, premature rupture of membranes, low birth weight, stillbirth, and congenital infections in the newborn. Given these risks and the observation that gonorrhea and chlamydia in pregnant women are often unrecognized or untreated in the ED,[20] physicians should have a low threshold for empiric treatment, particularly of GC, Ct, and trichomonas.

The approach to diagnosis and treatment is essentially unchanged from nonpregnant patients, except to avoid tetracyclines in pregnant women. Special attention to PID management is needed; PID can occur in the first trimester and warrants OB/GYN consultation and admission. Testing is especially important for complete partner services and to reduce the risk of another STI during the pregnancy.

Any STI diagnosed in a pregnant woman is an indication and opportunity to confirm that they are engaged in regular prenatal care, and if not, to initiate a referral. New lesions suspicious for HSV should be cultured and patients started on acyclovir or valacyclovir with close follow-up, especially if late into the third trimester. Pregnant patients with syphilis need treatment and close follow-up. Those patients with a penicillin allergy should undergo desensitization therapy.

Men Who Have Sex with Men and Transgender Persons

Effective care of groups at high risk for STIs in the ED includes providing lesbian, gay, bisexual, and transgender (LGBT) affirming and respectful care. LGBT patients face discrimination in health care that can lead to avoidance of health care[21] and serious health issues. Transgender persons are especially at risk; in the Nation Transgender Health Survey, 33% of transgender persons reported experiencing discrimination in health care and 16% had experienced discrimination in an ED.[22]

Having a registration process that is affirming and inclusive will lead to greater trust in the medical system. One survey of patients found they would not be offended to be asked about sexual orientation/gender identity in health care settings.[23] During the provider-patient interaction, ask the patient what their preferred name and pronouns are. Do not assume. Apologize if mistakes are made. Asking sexual history questions in ED visits can be direct and at the same time respectful and inclusive. Avoid the traditional, "Do you have sex with men, women, or both?," in favor of "Can you tell me about your sex partners?" or "What is the gender of your sex partners?"

STI testing should follow CDC recommendations. Testing at all sites of sexual contact is very important. In the case of MSM, performing only urine/urethral testing can miss up to 80% of STIs.[9] Extragenital testing of pharyngeal and rectal sites with NAATs is therefore indicated. Check with local laboratories to determine which are able to perform these tests because they require special validation. For any patient uncomfortable with testing, self-collected NAATs perform well and can be considered for patient comfort.[24]

Sexual Assault Victims

Managing and counseling patients after sexual assault should include being familiar with STI prevalence and risk consistent with local disease patterns. Patients should be comanaged by professionals trained in assessing and counseling patients who have experienced an assault. Regarding STI testing, historically, there were often concerns regarding screening victims of sexual assault for STIs out of fear that positive test results could be presented as evidence to undermine a victim's credibility in court. CDC STD treatment guidelines note that the use of a victim's prior sexual history as evidence is strictly limited in all 50 states, and most states consider any aspect of the medical examination or treatment to have evidentiary privilege.[9] Testing at the initial encounter also allows for notification and treatment of recent consensual partners and continued public health monitoring of reportable conditions.

Although all screening and treatment decisions should be made on an individual basis, the CDC STD treatment guidelines recommend the following screening tests in adult and adolescent victims of sexual assault[9]:

○ NAATs at sites of penetration or attempted penetration for GC and Ct
○ NAATs from urine or vaginal specimen for trichomonas
○ Wet mount with pH and KOH testing for BV and candidiasis
○ Serum testing for HIV, hepatitis B, and syphilis

CDC STD treatment guidelines recommend the following for treatment and prophylaxis:

○ Considering the low rate of follow-up care among victims of sexual assault, single-dose empiric treatment is recommended whenever possible (ie, for chlamydia, gonorrhea, and trichomonas). See infection-specific treatment regimens in **Table 1**.
○ Emergency contraception.
○ Postexposure hepatitis B vaccination if the assailant is unknown or the victim has not been previously vaccinated.
○ If not already, female victims aged 9 to 26 years, male victims aged 9 to 21 years (MSM up to 26 years), should receive HPV vaccination.
○ HIV postexposure prophylaxis (PEP):
1. Considerations for starting PEP should take into account the following:
  • If the patient presents within 72 hours of the assault
  • Characteristics and HIV risk behavior of the assailant or assailants, if known (eg, MSM or injection drug use)
  • Local epidemiology of HIV/AIDS
  • Exposure characteristics of the assault:
    ○ Vaginal or anal penetration
    ○ Ejaculation on mucus membranes
    ○ Multiple assailants
    ○ Presence of mucosal lesions
    ○ Any other characteristics that may increase risk for HIV transmission
2. For specific regimen and to ensure close follow-up, consult with an Infectious Disease specialist
3. Dispense enough medications to last until the follow-up visit in 3 to 7 days
4. Draw baseline complete blood count and complete metabolic panel

SUMMARY

The management of STIs in the ED can be complex and challenging, and STI-related emergencies can occur with almost every STI. As STI rates increase across the United States, EDs will continue to provide invaluable care for patients with STIs. ED providers should be familiar with the prevalence and incidence of STIs in their community as well as current STI treatment guidelines. Rigorous follow-up care plans incorporating local STI clinics and other referral sites ensure appropriate retesting, counseling, and partner treatment and can help mitigate the risk of serious complications due to STIs in high-risk patient populations.

REFERENCES

1. Centers for Disease Control and Prevention. *Sexually Transmitted Disease Surveillance 2016.* Atlanta: U.S. Department of Health and Human Services; 2017.
2. Bowen V, Torrone E, Kidd S, et al. Increase in incidence of congenital syphilis - United States, 2012-2014. MMWR Morb Mortal Wkly Rep 2015;64(44):1241-5.
3. Brackbill RM, Sternberg MR, Fishbein M. Where do people go for treatment of sexually transmitted diseases? Fam Plann Perspect 1999;31(1):10-5.
4. Ware CE, Ajabnoor Y, Mullins PM, et al. A retrospective cross-sectional study of patients treated in US EDs and ambulatory care clinics with sexually transmitted infections from 2001 to 2010. Am J Emerg Med 2016;34(9):1808-11.
5. Pearson WS, Peterman TA, Gift TL. An increase in sexually transmitted infections seen in US emergency departments. Prev Med 2017;100:143-4.
6. Gift TL, Hogben M. Emergency department sexually transmitted disease and human immunodeficiency virus screening: findings from a national survey. Acad Emerg Med 2006;13(9):993-6.
7. Centers for Disease, Control and Prevention. Recommendations for the laboratory-based detection of Chlamydia trachomatis and Neisseria gonorrhoeae-2014. MMWR Recomm Rep 2014;63(RR-02):1-19.
8. Reed JL, Zaidi MA, Woods TD, et al. Impact of post-visit contact on emergency department utilization for adolescent women with a sexually transmitted infection. J Pediatr Adolesc Gynecol 2015;28(3):144-8.
9. Workowski KA, Bolan GA, Centers for Disease Control and Prevention. Sexually transmitted diseases treatment guidelines, 2015. MMWR Recomm Rep 2015; 64(RR-03):1-137.
10. Schechter-Perkins EM, Jenkins D, White LF, et al. Treatment of cases of neisseria gonorrhoeae and chlamydia trachomatis in emergency department patients. Sex Transm Dis 2015;42(7):353-7.
11. Lolar SA, Sherwin RL, Robinson DM, et al. Effectiveness of an urban emergency department call-back system in the successful linkage to treatment of sexually transmitted infections. South Med J 2015;108(5):268-73.
12. de Voux A, Kent JB, Macomber K, et al. Notes from the field: cluster of lymphogranuloma venereum cases among men who have sex with men - Michigan, August 2015-April 2016. MMWR Morb Mortal Wkly Rep 2016;65(34):920-1.
13. Taylor MM, Reilley B, Yellowman M, et al. Use of expedited partner therapy among chlamydia cases diagnosed at an urban Indian health centre, Arizona. Int J STD AIDS 2013;24(5):371-4.
14. Fifer H, Cole M, Hughes G, et al. Sustained transmission of high-level azithromycin-resistant Neisseria gonorrhoeae in England: an observational study. Lancet Infect Dis 2018;18(5):573-81.

15. Allen VG, Mitterni L, Seah C, et al. Neisseria gonorrhoeae treatment failure and susceptibility to cefixime in Toronto, Canada. JAMA 2013;309(2):163–70.
16. Goyal M, Hayes K, Mollen C. Sexually transmitted infection prevalence in symptomatic adolescent emergency department patients. Pediatr Emerg Care 2012; 28(12):1277–80.
17. Woolston SL, Dhanireddy S, Marrazzo J. Ocular syphilis: a clinical review. Curr Infect Dis Rep 2016;18(11):36.
18. Woolston S, Cohen SE, Fanfair RN, et al. A cluster of ocular syphilis cases - Seattle, Washington, and San Francisco, California, 2014-2015. MMWR Morb Mortal Wkly Rep 2015;64(40):1150–1.
19. Carmine L, Castillo M, Fisher M. Testing and treatment for sexually transmitted infections in adolescents–what's new? J Pediatr Adolesc Gynecol 2014;27(2): 50–60.
20. Krivochenitser R, Jones JS, Whalen D, et al. Underrecognition of cervical Neisseria gonorrhoeae and Chlamydia trachomatis infections in pregnant patients in the ED. Am J Emerg Med 2013;31(4):661–3.
21. Samuels EA, Tape C, Garber N, et al. "Sometimes you feel like the freak show": a qualitative assessment of emergency care experiences among transgender and gender-nonconforming patients. Ann Emerg Med 2018;71(2):170–82.e1.
22. Rodriguez A, Agardh A, Asamoah BO. Self-reported discrimination in health-care settings based on recognizability as transgender: a cross-sectional study among transgender U.S. citizens. Arch Sex Behav 2018;47(4):973–85.
23. Maragh-Bass AC, Torain M, Adler R, et al. Risks, benefits, and importance of collecting sexual orientation and gender identity data in healthcare settings: a multimethod analysis of patient and provider perspectives. LGBT Health 2017;4(2): 141–52.
24. Sexton ME, Baker JJ, Nakagawa K, et al. How reliable is self-testing for gonorrhea and chlamydia among men who have sex with men? J Fam Pract 2013;62(2): 70–8.

Management of Human Immunodeficiency Virus in the Emergency Department

Mercedes Torres, MD*, Siamak Moayedi, MD

KEYWORDS

- HIV • AIDS • Emergency medicine • Management • Emergency department

KEY POINTS

- In the United States, the highest proportion of new human immunodeficiency virus (HIV) infections occurs in injection drug users, men who have sex with men, sex workers, transgendered people, and prisoners.
- Diagnosis of acute HIV in the emergency department leads to improved health for the patient and decreased transmission within the community.
- The emergency department is the ideal location for universal HIV screening.
- Hepatotoxicity can occur as a side effect of every class of antiretroviral therapy.
- Emergency providers can provide postexposure prophylaxis for all types of HIV exposures.

Before the development of effective antiretroviral therapy (ART), the epidemiology of the human immunodeficiency virus (HIV) was characterized by high rates of new infections in young adults and children. Life expectancy was less than 2 years at acquired immunodeficiency syndrome (AIDS) diagnosis and there were few treatment options.[1] Presently, the worldwide availability of ART has created a different milieu. The global incidence of HIV has declined from 3.3 million in 2002 to 1.8 million in 2016.[2] The global mortality from AIDS peaked in 2005 at 2.3 million, declining to 1.1 million in 2016, with 36.7 million people living with HIV worldwide. These epidemiologic trends reflect an increasing prevalence, with declining incidence of disease. Global efforts toward eliminating mother-to-child transmissions, optimizing viremic control to prevent transmissions, offering postexposure prophylaxis (PEP), and initiating preexposure prophylaxis (PrEP) have all contributed to this decline in incidence. HIV-infected

Disclosure Statement: Nothing to disclose.
Department of Emergency Medicine, University of Maryland School of Medicine, 110 South Paca Street, Sixth Floor, Suite 200, Baltimore, MD 21201, USA
* Corresponding author. Department of Emergency Medicine, University of Maryland School of Medicine, 110 South Paca Street, Sixth Floor, Suite 200, Baltimore, MD 21201, USA
E-mail address: mtorres@som.umaryland.edu

Emerg Med Clin N Am 36 (2018) 777–794
https://doi.org/10.1016/j.emc.2018.06.008   emed.theclinics.com

patients on ART are now primarily middle-aged and their life expectancy is approaching that of their uninfected counterparts.[1]

Advances in ART have created regimens that are less toxic and more effective with a lower pill burden, therefore improving adherence. Current first-line ART regimens typically consist of 2 nucleoside reverse transcriptase inhibitors (NRTIs) coupled with 1 non-NRTI (NNRTI), protease inhibitor (PI), or integrase strand transfer inhibitor.[3] Because opportunistic infections (OIs) are less frequent, more chronic complications related to prolonged ART use and HIV-associated inflammation have emerged. Chronic inflammation has been linked to an increased incidence of cardiovascular, liver, renal, oncologic, and neurobehavioral disorders among HIV-infected patients.[1,3]

Although progress has been made in the global HIV epidemic, specific populations have not benefited from these efforts. In areas of high HIV prevalence, young women are significantly affected by infection. For low-prevalence settings, including the United States, the highest proportion of new HIV infections is occurring in injection drug users, men who have sex with men (MSM), sex workers, transgendered people, and prisoners. Globally, MSM accounted for 12% of new HIV infections in 2015.[2]

ACUTE HUMAN IMMUNODEFICIENCY VIRUS

The clinical presentation of acute HIV infection is variable and nonspecific, mirroring other more benign viral illnesses such as influenza or Epstein-Barr virus. Fever, rash, retrobulbar headache, fatigue, sore throat, diarrhea, myalgias, and arthralgias are common. It can be challenging to distinguish these symptoms from other disease processes. Symptoms of acute HIV manifest 1 to 2 weeks after exposure and typically last for 2 weeks.[4,5] Although some patients remain asymptomatic, approximately 40% to 90% develop some symptomatology.[4] It often takes multiple health care visits until acute HIV is diagnosed because 83% of cases are missed on initial presentation to a health care provider.[5]

There are some distinctive features of this nonspecific presentation that may increase a provider's suspicion for acute HIV. The characteristic rash is described as an erythematous maculopapular eruption typically involving the face, upper thorax, limbs, palms, and soles.[5] In addition, patients with acute HIV can have sharply demarcated, shallow mucocutaneous ulcerations at sites of sexual contact, including the genitals, mouth, esophagus, or anus.[5] Other diagnoses to consider include herpes simplex virus (HSV), syphilis, and chancroid. Gastrointestinal (GI) symptoms such as nausea, vomiting, anorexia, and diarrhea are common due to infiltration of the GI lymphoreticular system within a few days of developing a detectable viral load.[6]

More severe clinical presentations of acute HIV are less common. It is estimated that 25% of patients with acute HIV present with aseptic meningitis. Cerebrospinal fluid (CSF) analysis demonstrates an elevated protein, normal glucose, and lymphocytic predominance. More than 50% of patients with acute HIV, especially those with higher viral loads, report 1 or more neurologic symptoms. These include problems with concentration or memory, gait disturbances, Parkinsonian movements, and neuropathies.[7] For most patients, neurologic findings are no longer present a month after initiation of ART.[7] Myocarditis, pancreatitis, hepatitis, encephalitis, and rhabdomyolysis without a clear cause have all been attributed to acute HIV as well. Rarely, patients may present with OIs during acute HIV. This has been documented for *Pneumocystis jiroveci*, histoplasmosis, cryptococcal meningitis, cytomegalovirus (CMV) infection, toxoplasmosis, and candidal esophagitis.[5]

Acute HIV is characterized by a rapid increase in viral load and viremia. The degree of symptoms has been correlated with the severity of the cytokine reaction to early viremia. As viremia decreases, the viral load set point is reached and symptoms abate.[5] The extent of the inflammatory response to early infection is associated with increased long-term morbidity and mortality among HIV-infected patients.[4,8] Patients with acute HIV are frequently unaware of their infectivity and transmit disease more easily. More than 50% of new HIV infections are acquired from someone with acute HIV. For every 10-fold increase in viral load, the risk of transmission increases by a factor of 2.5.[4,6,9]

Early diagnosis and treatment of acute HIV has become a public health goal, which translates to emergency department (ED) practice. The benefits of treatment during acute HIV have proven significant. Viral reservoirs are decreased, the inflammatory cascade is curbed, disease progression is slowed, and OIs are less common.[4,5] The result is not only improved health for the HIV-infected individual but also decreased transmissions within the community. With the advent of fourth-generation antigen-antibody serum tests, acute HIV can now be detected within 10 to 21 days after exposure.[10] Point-of-care tests are not as reliable, therefore the US Centers for Disease Control (CDC) recommends laboratory-based testing.[11] A positive antigen-antibody test result, followed by a negative antibody-only test and a positive nucleic acid test is expected in cases of acute HIV (**Fig. 1** shows the testing algorithm).[9,12,13] RT-PCR results greater than 1000 copies/mL indicate likely true positives as the viral load in patients with acute HIV should be several orders of magnitude greater. RT-PCR can detect acute HIV 5 days sooner than the best performing fourth-generation test. However, there is still a window period of 1 to 2 weeks when patients with very early infection may test negative. In cases highly suspicious for acute HIV with negative testing, repeat testing in 1 to 2 weeks is recommended. The greatest benefits are experienced if treatment is started as early as possible.[9]

Pilot programs of ED-based testing and initiation of treatment of acute HIV have shown promising results.[10] Patients with acute HIV require serum evaluation of liver and renal function, HIV viral load, CD4 count, and viral genotyping before initiating ART. Therefore, consultation with an infectious disease (ID) specialist is recommended to determine the medication regimen. Regimens including integrase strand transfer inhibitors show the most rapid decline in viral load, which is a key characteristic of

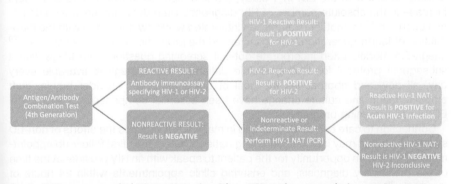

Fig. 1. CDC-recommended HIV testing algorithm. PCR, polymerase chain reaction; NAT, nucleic acid test. (*Data from* CDC. 2018 Quick reference guide: Recommended laboratory HIV testing algorithm for serum or plasma specimens. 2018. Available at: https://stacks.cdc.gov/view/cdc/50872. Accessed February 2, 2018; and CDC and Association of Public Health Laboratories. Laboratory Testing for the Diagnosis of HIV Infection: Updated Recommendations. 2014. Available at: https://doi.org/10.15620/cdc.23447. Accessed February 2, 2018.)

any medication combination for acute HIV. Finally, an essential component of these efforts is robust, reliable follow-up.[9,10]

HUMAN IMMUNODEFICIENCY VIRUS SCREENING

In 2006, the CDC published guidelines recommending universal HIV screening in most outpatient and acute care settings, including EDs.[14] In theory, the ED is the ideal location for this type of universal screening. It is the primary point-of-care for numerous patients without access to health care, including those at highest risk for contracting HIV. When a traditional sexually transmitted infection (STI) clinic HIV screening program was compared with an ED-based HIV screening program, the ED program showed a measureable advantage in that 30% more new infections were detected. This was accomplished with only a fraction of the number of tests performed in the STI clinic (10%) and fewer dedicated staff.[15]

The HIV testing algorithm currently advocated by the CDC is outlined in **Fig. 1**. For EDs that use point-of-care tests, all positive results should be confirmed using a serum-based fourth-generation laboratory test and subsequent tests as indicated on the algorithm.[11,16,17]

One of the largest obstacles to implementing HIV testing in an ED is ensuring that pretest and posttest counseling are available for all patients. Although extensive counseling is clearly beneficial to many patients by dispelling myths about HIV, teaching important prevention strategies, and addressing their concerns, it has proven burdensome to ED staff who are already operating in a setting of inadequate staffing and overcrowding. In recognition of this barrier, CDC recommendations note that prevention counseling should not be required as part of a screening program but rather as a community outreach activity aside from screening. Oral or written information should be provided to all patients screened regarding the meaning of positive and negative test results.[14]

Although it has been more than a decade since the CDC's recommendation for universal HIV screening was released, the question of how to best accomplish the goal of universal HIV screening remains. Parallel staffing models using a separate team of HIV testers have proven beneficial in some circumstances.[18] Inadequate staffing and preexisting time constraints on ED team members are 2 of the primary arguments in favor of this model. Another option is integrating screening into the existing workflow of the ED. In 1 study, a 5-fold increase in HIV testing and 3-fold increase in the absolute number of HIV diagnoses were documented when integration occurred.[19] In another example, an integrated workflow combined with the introduction of fourth-generation testing increased the proportion of patients screened.[20] Integrated models often incorporate opt-out screening questions into triage with a subsequent protocol for testing eligible patients. This strategy is available every day, all day, and approaches the goal of being universal. Provider buy-in, staff empowerment, and culture change have been essential components of successful ED-based screening programs.[19,21]

Connection to care can be difficult and in many cases requires the efforts of non-ED staff.[22–25] Tactics may include contacting patients before their first follow-up appointment, providing an opportunity for the patient to speak with an HIV provider at the time of the preliminary diagnosis, and ensuring clinic appointments within 24 hours of diagnosis.[26]

INFECTIOUS COMPLICATIONS OF HUMAN IMMUNODEFICIENCY VIRUS

Table 1 outlines common infectious complications of HIV, with details regarding their symptomatology, clinical evaluation, and ED management. Although some of these

Table 1
Common opportunistic infections associated with the human immunodeficiency virus

Opportunistic Infection	Cause	CD4 Cells/mm³	EM Presentation	EM Diagnosis	EM Treatment	Special Consideration
Pneumocystis pneumonia	Pneumocystis jiroveci (fungus)	<200	Dyspnea, fever, nonproductive cough, tachypnea	Clinical suspicion Hypoxemia, lactate dehydrogenase >500 mg/dL Chest radiograph: diffuse bilateral interstitial infiltrates Inpatient: bronchoalveolar lavage or PCR	TMP-SMX Methylprednisolone (if Po_2 <70 mm Hg) Oxygen	Chest radiograph may appear normal in early disease Normal computed tomography (CT) has high negative predictive value Spontaneous pneumothorax can occur
Toxoplasma encephalitis	Toxoplasma gondii (protozoan)	<50	Headache, confusion, fever, focal deficits	CT of brain plus contrast	Admit for inpatient pyrimethamine plus sulfadiazine plus leucovorin	Sources: cat feces, undercooked meat, raw shellfish Not transmitted person to person
Cryptosporidiosis	Cryptosporidium (protozoan)	<100	Subacute watery diarrhea and cramping	Stool oocyst evaluation	Fluid and electrolyte repletion Nitazoxanide Refer for ART	Severity can range from asymptomatic to cholera-like
Tuberculosis	Mycobacterium tuberculosis	<200	Cough, fever, night sweats, weight loss, anemia Extrapulmonary: central nervous system (CNS), pericarditis, lymphadenitis, osteomyelitis	Chest radiograph: upper lobe infiltrate plus or minus cavitation (with low CD4 counts cavitation is uncommon and no predilection for upper lobes) Sputum or fluid (pleural, pericardial, CSF, or ascites) analysis for AFB and nucleic-acid amplification testing	Admit Respiratory isolation Inpatient initiation of direct observed 4-drug therapy	Leading cause of death from ID globally Extrapulmonary presentations increase with degree of immunodeficiency

(continued on next page)

Table 1
(continued)

Opportunistic Infection	Cause	CD4 Cells/mm³	EM Presentation	EM Diagnosis	EM Treatment	Special Consideration
MAC disease	*Mycobacterium avium*	<50	Fever, night sweats, weight loss, diarrhea, and abdominal pain	Anemia, elevated alkaline phosphatase, hepatomegaly, splenomegaly, lymphadenopathy (paratracheal, retroperitoneal) CT imaging and cultures	Likely admit for inpatient workup, including biopsy Macrolide plus ethambutol	ART will lead to IRIS, which is clinically indistinguishable from active MAC infection
Candidiasis	*Candida albicans* (yeast)	<200	Thrush, odynophagia, retrosternal pain	Clinical definitive diagnosis of esophageal candidiasis requires endoscopy	Admission depends on severity Fluconazole	In contrast to hairy leukoplakia, white plaques of thrush can be scraped off
Cryptococcal meningitis	*Cryptococcus neoformans* (encapsulated yeast)	<100	Subacute meningitis with fever and headache	Lumbar puncture with high opening pressure CSF analysis for antigen	Admit for amphotericin therapy	Meningeal symptoms, such as neck stiffness and photophobia, occur in only 25% of patients
HSV	HSV types 1 and 2	<100	Orolabial and anogenital lesions	If clinical diagnosis is unclear: HSV DNA PCR or viral culture	Acyclovir or valacyclovir Admit for intravenous acyclovir in severe cases	Consider HSV encephalitis and keratitis
CMV retinitis	CMV	<50	Peripheral: floaters Central: decrease visual acuity and central field defects	Ophthalmoscopy: full-thickness necrotizing retinitis with fluffy white lesions plus or minus retinal hemorrhage	Urgent ophthalmology consultation Ganciclovir	Delay ART initiation until CMV therapy is complete to avoid immune reconstitution uveitis
Varicella-zoster virus (VZV) diseases	VZV	<200	Cutaneous eruption of small vesicles in dermatomal distribution preceded by painful prodrome	If clinical diagnosis is unclear: VZV PCR	Admit for disseminated disease (CNS, pulmonary, optic neuritis, cranial nerve palsies) Treat severe or complicated cases with intravenous acyclovir	In patients with CD4 <100, consider progressive outer retinal necrosis associated with a high rate of vision loss

Abbreviations: AFB, Acid Fast Bacilli; EM, Emergency Medicine; SMX, Sulfamethoxazole; TMP, Trimethoprim.
Data from Panel on opportunistic infections in HIV-infected adults and adolescents. Guidelines for the prevention and treatment of opportunistic infections in HIV-infected adults and adolescents: recommendations from the Centers for Disease Control and Prevention, the National Institutes of Health, and the HIV Medicine As-

infections have become less common with widespread ART availability, none have been eradicated completely. Most of these complications are rare when not linked to HIV infection and, therefore, may clue the diagnostician to the presence of HIV infection. Finally, many of these infections may also present as part of immune reconstitution inflammatory syndrome (IRIS) after ART is initiated.

IMMUNE RECONSTITUTION INFLAMMATORY SYNDROME

IRIS describes a phenomenon of immune activation resulting in new or worsening symptoms of OIs occurring within several months of initiation of ART. It affects approximately 20% of HIV-infected patients.[16] There are 2 types of IRIS, paradoxic and unmasking. In the paradoxic form, patients experience worsening of a previously diagnosed OI that was initially responding to treatment. Paradoxic IRIS is a diagnosis of exclusion. Providers must rule out worsening of the OI due to antimicrobial resistance, nonadherence, or an adverse drug reaction before the making this diagnosis. In unmasking IRIS, patients develop symptoms of a previously undiagnosed OI. In these cases, it is important to rule out worsening of the underlying HIV infection (declining CD4 count, increasing viral load) that can occur with treatment failure before attributing the symptoms to IRIS.[27,28]

HIV-infected patients presenting with worsening or new OI symptoms are more likely to ultimately be diagnosed with IRIS if certain clinical or historical features are present. Historically, patients who were recently started on ART for the first time are at greater risk of IRIS. Clinically, patients presenting with manifestations of disseminated opportunistic disease should increase suspicion for IRIS. Patients with lower baseline CD4 counts and higher baseline viral loads before the initiation of ART are at greater risk. In addition, a higher incidence of IRIS has been documented in patients who experience a rapid decline in HIV viral load after ART initiation.[28]

Mycobacterium tuberculosis infection (TB) is commonly implicated in IRIS, with an estimated frequency of 15.7% worldwide.[29] The presentation is typically paradoxic, rather than unmasking. Clinical features include fever, enlarged lymph nodes, worsening radiographic infiltrates, and enlarging effusions. Intraabdominal manifestations can occur in up to 40% of cases.[28] TB-IRIS is more likely in patients presenting with extrapulmonary or disseminated disease. In patients with TB meningitis, a positive CSF culture for TB is more likely in IRIS cases.[27,28] Although starting ART early in disease portends significantly decreased rates of all-cause mortality, this practice has shown an increased rate of TB-IRIS and mortality from TB-IRIS specifically. Steroids and other immune-modulating medications have been used to treat TB-IRIS.[29]

Other OIs that cause IRIS include *Mycobacterium avium* complex (MAC), *Cryptococcus neoformans*, CMV, *P jiroveci* pneumonia, and progressive multifocal leukoencephalopathy (PML). In each of these disease processes, certain characteristics are helpful for distinguishing IRIS from primary active disease (**Table 2**).

MAC-IRIS presents clinically as painful lymphadenitis and fever, similar to the presentation of active MAC. Inflammatory changes are more focal, involving peripheral, pulmonary or thoracic, or intraabdominal lymph nodes. The presence of hypercalcemia and well-organized granulomas on biopsy are 2 clues used to distinguish IRIS from active disease.[27,28]

Although most IRIS events occur within the first 8 weeks of ART initiation, the onset of cryptococcal infection can be delayed. It is characterized by a relapsing aseptic meningitis, increased intracranial pressure with leukocytosis on lumbar puncture, and new focal neurologic deficits on examination.[30,31] Cryptococcal IRIS develops in 30% of patients with a past history of cryptococcal disease and mortality is high,

Table 2
Distinguishing features of selected immune reconstitution inflammatory syndrome pathogens

Pathogen	IRIS-Specific Characteristics
MAC	Localized lymphadenitis Organized granulomas Hypercalcemia
Cryptococcus neoformans	Higher CSF white blood cell count and opening pressure (compared with active disease) Negative CSF fungal culture
CMV	Retinitis in area of preexisting retinal lesion Presence of vitritis or uveitis
Pneumocystis jiroveci	Organizing pneumonia after tapering steroids
PML	Contrast enhancement of lesions on MRI (active disease shows lack of contrast enhancement)

Adapted from Beatty GW. Immune reconstitution inflammatory syndrome. Emerg Med Clin North Am 2010;28(2):410; with permission.

approaching 70%. For ART-naive patients with active cryptococcal disease, survival rates improve when ART is started after the first 5 weeks of antifungal treatment.[16,30] Other treatments include steroids and serial lumbar punctures to decrease increased intracranial pressure.[27]

Viral OIs that manifest as IRIS include CMV, HSV, varicella-zoster virus (VZV), and PML. Patients with CMV-IRIS present with painless loss of visual acuity or the development of floaters. Symptoms can develop anywhere from a few weeks to a few years after the initiation of ART. CMV-IRIS is associated with vitritis, papillitis, or uveitis with a proliferation of inflammatory cells within the eye.[27,28] HSV and VZV can present as IRIS and are often clinically indistinguishable from active disease.[27] PML, caused by the John Cunningham virus, presents with a wide range of findings, including new motor deficits, visual disturbances, and cognitive impairment. Patients with a paradoxic PML-IRIS suffer more severe disease and have a less favorable prognosis when compared with unmasking PML-IRIS. The only distinguishing feature of PML-IRIS is the presence of contrast enhancement of lesions on MRI when compared with the nonenhancing lesions of active disease. The benefits of steroids for treatment are not clear and prognosis can be poor in severe cases.[28,32]

SERIOUS ANTIRETROVIRAL THERAPY SIDE EFFECTS

The advent of ART has created a large population of patients worldwide who are now experiencing the diagnosis of HIV as a chronic, manageable illness. Although early ART regimens focused on highly toxic drugs with serious side effects, recently developed regimens demonstrate excellent disease control with less toxicity. Life-threatening side effects, such as hypersensitivity and lactic acidosis, are less common in resource-rich settings but may still occur in patients living in areas with fewer resources.

Table 3 outlines some of the most notable acute side effects of ART. Acute symptomatic lactic acidosis due to mitochondrial toxicity, although rare, may occur at any time while taking an NRTI. It begins with nonspecific symptoms but can accelerate into a severe, life-threatening complication. Most patients on NRTIs have an asymptomatic, chronic mild elevation in lactate, which requires no intervention. However, patients with moderate or severe symptoms of lactic acidosis require discontinuation

Table 3
Antiretroviral therapy side effects seen in the emergency department

Side Effect	ART Involved	Clinical Manifestations	EM Diagnosis	EM Management
Lactic acidosis or hepatic steatosis	NRTIs Highest risk • Didanosine • Stavudine	Nonspecific findings • Fatigue • Malaise • Dyspnea • Nausea or vomiting • Abdominal pain • Hepatomegaly • Peripheral edema • Ascites Severe symptoms • Cardiomyopathy • Encephalopathy • Pancreatitis • Pancytopenia • Hepatic failure • Cardiopulmonary shock	Venous pH <7.3 (and) bicarbonate <20 mEq/L (and) Lactate 2–5: mild Lactate 5–10: moderate Lactate >10: severe Elevated LFTs, CPK, lipase possible	Moderate–severe Discontinue NRTI Treat end-organ dysfunction Supportive care: Bicarbonate infusions Hemodialysis Mechanical ventilation
Hepatotoxicity (hepatitis)	High risk: • Nevirapine (early) • Ritonavir plus or minus saquinavir Can occur to some degree with all classes of ART	• Fatigue • Nausea or vomiting • RUQ pain • Fulminant liver failure	AST or ALT>3–5 times normal or patient baseline before ART	Rule out viral hepatitis, IRIS, toxic ingestion Supportive care Consult with ID provider to consider discontinuation of medication if nevirapine or severe symptoms
Hyperbilirubinemia	PIs highest risk: • Atazanavir • Indinavir	• Jaundice • No other signs of hepatic failure	Hyperbilirubinemia without increased transaminase levels	Consult with ID provider regarding ART continuation
Pancreatitis	NRTIs (especially didanosine)	Within first 5 mo: • Nausea or vomiting • Abdominal pain • Fever	Lipase level 2–3 times > normal range	Discontinuation of offending medication Supportive care: IVF, bowel rest, analgesia

(continued on next page)

Table 3
(continued)

Side Effect	ART Involved	Clinical Manifestations	EM Diagnosis	EM Management
Hypersensitivity	Abacavir can occur with all classes to some degree	Within first 8 wk: • Fever • Rash • Nausea or vomiting • Myalgias • Headache • Diarrhea • Pruritus • Lymphadenopathy • Hypotension • Cough • Dyspnea • Pharyngitis (worsens with each dose)	Clinical diagnosis (unlikely for abacavir hypersensitivity to occur given genetic screen for HLA-B*5701 done before starting this medication)	Discontinue abacavir (resolves 48–72 h)
Skin rash	NNRTIs (most): nevirapine (often) NRTIs: abacavir (see hypersensitivity) PIs: amprenavir-sulfa allergy link	Within first few wk: • Mild-moderate rash (most) • Stevens-Johnson syndrome • Toxic epidermal necrolysis • Drug rash with eosinophilia and systemic symptoms	Clinical diagnosis	Discontinue NNRTI (especially nevirapine) in consultation with ID specialist Prophylactic steroids or antihistamines not recommended
Hyperglycemia	PIs (especially indinavir)	Within first 11 wk: • Polyuria • Polydipsia • Polyphagia	Serum glucose, pH, bicarbonate, anion gap	Initiate standard treatment with IVF, oral medications, and insulin, if needed
Avascular necrosis (AVN) and osteopenia or osteoporosis	PIs tenofovir	Hip pain Spine pain	• CT or MRI for AVN • Radiograph or CT for fracture	AVN: conservative or surgical management Discuss initiation of bisphosphonates, raloxifene or calcitonin with ID specialist

Abbreviations: CPK, Creatine Phosphokinase; IVF, Intravenous Fluid; LFT, Liver Function Test.
Data from Refs.[34–39]

of the offending NRTI and supportive care. Women and pregnant patients have an increased risk of this toxicity. Interestingly, pancreatitis has also been linked to mitochondrial toxicity of NRTIs. Stavudine and didanosine have historically been implicated most in cases of symptomatic lactic acidosis and pancreatitis.[33–35]

Emergent hepatobiliary side effects of ART include hepatitis and hyperbilirubinemia. Hepatotoxicity has been documented as a side effect of every class of ART, although the NNRTI nevirapine and the PI ritonavir are common offenders.[34–36] Even newer classes, such as the integrase strand transfer inhibitors, can cause hepatotoxicity, although less commonly. Importantly, when a patient on ART presents with hepatotoxicity, the differential diagnosis must include acute infectious hepatitis, IRIS, and acetaminophen toxicity, as well as this ART-related side effect. Differentiation between these etiologic factors is complicated and may require the intervention of an ID specialist to decide if discontinuation of the possible offending ART is prudent. Conversely, hyperbilirubinemia without evidence of hepatic injury can be fairly benign, is reversible, and may not require discontinuation of the likely culprit if the patient is otherwise asymptomatic.[34–37]

Although all classes of ART can cause a hypersensitivity reaction, abacavir, an NRTI, is notorious for its potential to cause life-threatening hypersensitivity, presenting with fever, rash, and other nonspecific findings. Identification of a genetic test for HLA-B*5701, the gene linked to this toxicity, has dramatically decreased the frequency of this emergent presentation. Other dermatologic presentations of ART toxicities can range from a nonspecific drug rash to Stevens-Johnson syndrome and toxic epidermal necrolysis. Skin rashes commonly occur within a few weeks of initiation of an NNRTI, especially nevirapine. Consultation with an ID specialist is recommended to decide if other offending ART agents should be discontinued.[34]

Alterations in glucose metabolism are commonly experienced by patients on PIs. Although most of the clinical consequences are nonemergent, new-onset insulin resistance or worsening of baseline glucose management can progress to severe hyperglycemia or diabetic ketoacidosis. These metabolic changes typically occur within the first 3 months of therapy with a PI and can be managed with standard therapy. PIs are not typically discontinued when these toxicities occur because therapy for insulin resistance can be provided concurrently.[34,35,38]

Other emergent presentations that may be due to ART toxicities include hip or spine pain related to avascular necrosis (AVN) or osteoporosis with fracture. PI use has been linked to bone demineralization, as has HIV infection itself.[34,39,40] Although radiographs are useful for screening for these complications in symptomatic patients, computed tomography or MRI is recommended in cases of possible AVN and surgical intervention may be required.

POSTEXPOSURE PROPHYLAXIS

Over the past 30 years, emergency physicians have been tasked with prescribing PEP for HIV exposures in the occupational setting. Only 1 case of occupational transmission despite PEP has been confirmed since 1999, demonstrating the success of interventions in this regard.[41] In the past decade, emergency providers have expanded their practice to also provide postexposure counseling and ART to patients with high-risk nonoccupational HIV exposures. These include situations of sexual assault, unprotected high-risk consensual sex, and injection drug use. Current nonoccupational PEP (nPEP) and occupational PEP (oPEP) management strategies are based on shared knowledge about the transmissibility of HIV and prevention efforts over the history of this disease.

Although there are no randomized controlled trials demonstrating the efficacy of HIV PEP, 1 case-controlled study published in 1997 along with observational data collected by the CDC has formed the basis for current recommendations regarding the prescription of PEP. In this study, the authors documented an 81% reduction in the odds of HIV transmission between providers experiencing a percutaneous exposure promptly treated with zidovudine compared with those not receiving any ARTs.[42,43] Given the ethical dilemmas of further human research on PEP, the research community has focused on laboratory-based primate studies of simian immunodeficiency virus in macaques to demonstrate the benefits of PEP and define current guidelines for exposed humans.[44] In 1 review of 25 primate-based studies of PEP regimens, the seroconversion rate was 89% lower among animals that received PEP. Through the years, these studies have shown improved efficacy, lower side effects, and an increasing potency with current PEP regimens.[44]

The CDC-based guidelines for oPEP and nPEP are summarized in **Box 1**.[43] Emergency providers must attempt to make a prompt determination of the HIV status of the exposed person, as well as the source. The efficacy of PEP is demonstrated as soon as possible after the exposure, up to 72 hours. When rapid HIV testing results are not available for the source (more commonly) or the exposed person, providers should assume that the source is HIV-infected and that the exposed person is not HIV-infected. Patients with high-risk exposures should be treated with PEP based on this assumption, given that PEP can be discontinued at a later date if considered inappropriate. When available, the source should have HIV testing performed and be interviewed regarding the history of their HIV infection, previous or current treatment with ART, and recent laboratory results, including viral load.[43]

Determination of the risk involved in any particular exposure is complicated given the variety of exposure routes. Each case requires a detailed history regarding the specific events of the exposure to decide if PEP is recommended. Specific rates of HIV transmission per act are detailed in **Table 4**. Furthermore, the level of risk depends on the body fluid involved (**Table 5**). The highest risk activities include anal receptive sex, intravenous needle-sharing, and percutaneous blood exposures in the occupational setting. Body fluids that may transmit HIV include blood; semen; CSF; and synovial, peritoneal, pleural, amniotic, pericardial, or visibly bloody body fluids of any type.[45]

Exposure involving biting, spitting, or throwing body fluids is considered a negligible risk and PEP is not recommended.[43] Additional scenarios for which PEP is not

---

Box 1
Centers for Disease Control guidelines for antiretroviral postexposure prophylaxis

- HIV exposure must have occurred within 72 hours of PEP initiation
- Substantial risk of HIV transmission
- Baseline HIV status of exposed person is negative
- 28-day course of HIV PEP prescribed
- 3-drug regimen prescribed
- Evaluation for other possible infectious exposures (eg, STI, hepatitis B or C)
- Evaluate for possible pregnancy in exposed person

Data from Announcement: updated guidelines for antiretroviral postexposure prophylaxis after sexual, injection-drug use, or other nonoccupational exposure to HIV - United States, 2016. MMWR Morb Mortal Wkly Rep 2016;65(17):458.

Table 4
Risk of human immunodeficiency virus transmission based on type of exposure

Blood-Based Exposure Risk Per Act (%)	
Percutaneous (occupational)	0.3
Percutaneous (needle-sharing)	0.63
Mucous membrane	0.09
Nonintact skin	<0.09
Sexual Exposure Risk (per act)	
Anal sex (receptive)	1.38
Anal sex (insertive)	0.11
Vaginal sex (receptive)	0.08
Vaginal sex (insertive)	0.04
Oral sex Oral-anal sex Sharing sex toys	Lower than above but precise risk unknown

Data from Kuhar DT, Henderson DK, Struble KA, et al. Updated US Public Health Service guidelines for the management of occupational exposures to human immunodeficiency virus and recommendations for postexposure prophylaxis. Infect Control Hosp Epidemiol 2013;34(9):875–92; and Tan DHS, Hull MW, Yoong D, et al. Canadian guideline on HIV pre-exposure prophylaxis and nonoccupational postexposure prophylaxis. CMAJ 2017;189(47):E1448–58.

recommended include contact of intact skin with potentially infectious blood or body fluids, and contact with saliva (nondental), urine, vomit, or feces that is not visibly contaminated with blood.[41] Another low-risk scenario is a percutaneous injury from a needle discarded in a public setting. To date, there have been no HIV transmissions ever documented via this exposure.[43] Any patient who is on PrEP and is taking it as prescribed should not be prescribed a PEP regimen. If a patient has not taken any PrEP in the week preceding the exposure or is sporadically compliant, PEP can be considered.[43,46]

Laboratory evaluation of patients with substantial risk exposures includes testing for HIV, hepatitis B (surface antigen, surface antibody, and core antigen), hepatitis C, and pregnancy. When a prescription for PEP is possible, evaluation of liver and renal function is necessary to facilitate appropriate ART choice and future monitoring for side effects.[43]

Table 5
Risk of human immunodeficiency virus transmission based on body fluid

Body Fluids Potentially Infectious	Body Fluids Not Infectious Unless Visibly Bloody
Blood	Feces
CSF	Nasal and respiratory secretions
Synovial fluid	Sputum and saliva
Peritoneal fluid	Sweat
Pleural fluid	Tears
Pericardial fluid	Urine
Amniotic fluid	Vomit

Data from Kuhar DT, Henderson DK, Struble KA, et al. Updated US Public Health Service guidelines for the management of occupational exposures to human immunodeficiency virus and recommendations for postexposure prophylaxis. Infect Control Hosp Epidemiol 2013;34(9):875–92.

When the provider and patient agree that PEP is indicated, medications are most effective if initiated promptly and taken for a full 28-day course. In the 2016 CDC guidelines for nPEP, first-line PEP is a 3-drug regimen, consisting of tenofovir disoproxil fumarate (TDF) 300 mg and emtricitabine (FTC) 200 mg once daily, with raltegravir (RAL) 400 mg twice daily or dolutegravir (DTG) 50 mg once daily. Specific changes to the aforementioned regimen are provided in the CDC guidelines for children, pregnant women, and people with decreased renal function. Consultation with an ID expert is recommended for any case in which regimens other than first-line are considered. Medications that should never be given as part of a PEP regimen include nevirapine (risk of liver failure and Stevens-Johnson reaction), abacavir (risk of hypersensitivity without time for genetic testing), and efavirenz (risk of central nervous system toxicity and rapid viral resistance).[43]

Common side effects reported with the TDF-FTC–based regimens include nausea, vomiting, diarrhea, fatigue, and skin discoloration. Serious problems, including renal failure and worsening of underlying hepatitis B infection on withdrawal of the medication, can occur. Severe skin and hypersensitivity reactions can occur when using RAL. In addition, caution is advised if combining RAL or DTG with antacids, laxatives, or any polyvalent cation–containing (magnesium, aluminum, iron, calcium, zinc) medications due to their ability to decreased GI absorption of RAL or DTG.[43]

In recent years, by minimizing side effects and decreasing the pill burden of PEP, adherence rates have been improving.[47] In a cohort study of patients on PEP after sexual exposure to HIV, 70% reported adherence to their regimen. Eighty-three percent of the cohort was MSM and 72% were on PEP after a high-risk episode of anal sex. Patients were found to be more likely to adhere to their regimens if they were prescribed a TDF-FTC backbone.[48] MSM are increasingly at risk of HIV infection; 63% of new HIV infections in 2010 were in this category of risk.[49] The incidence of HIV in young, urban, black MSM is 43% versus 13% among their white counterparts.[49] Research demonstrates that PEP is most cost-effective in this demographic.

Another group of high-risk patients with historically low PEP adherence are victims of sexual assault. In a study of victims of sexual assault in Ontario, Canada, only 24% of subjects with high-risk exposures completed a 28-day course of PEP. Common reasons for nonadherence include adverse drug effects and an inability to incorporate the medication into daily routines. Additional barriers include lack of access to medications, lack of funds to pay for PEP, lack of follow-up services, concern for insurance coverage of PEP, stigma, and posttraumatic stress.[43]

One tactic to increase adherence among vulnerable populations is to provide antiretroviral pills for patients to take with them on ED discharge. A starter pack (consisting of 4–7 days of medication) plus a prescription for the rest, or a complete pill pack of the entire 28-day regimen are provided in some EDs at the initial ED visit. In a study of these 2 options, provision of a 28-day course of PEP at the time of PEP initiation resulted in fewer refusals of PEP (11.4% vs 22%) and higher completion rates (70% vs 53%) when compared with provision of a starter pack and prescription.[50] In this comparison, out of all subjects who successfully completed the full 28-day course of PEP, 71% were given the full regimen on initiation, and 29% were provided a starter pack with a prescription for the rest.[50] These results argue strongly in favor of providing a full 28-day course of PEP to vulnerable populations with concerns for barriers to adherence.

Pill burden is often cited as a barrier to adherence with medication regimens of all types, including PEP. To address this concern, research has recently focused on a single, once-daily pill.[47] Adherence to this 28-day regimen was 71% compared with the CDC's current first-line PEP regimen (TDF-FTC plus RAL) at 57%. The number of missed doses and subjects lost to follow-up declined with the single-pill regimen.[47]

PREEXPOSURE PROPHYLAXIS FOR HUMAN IMMUNODEFICIENCY VIRUS

PrEP has proven effective for prevention of HIV transmission among patients with repeated high-risk exposures, resulting in a 44% reduction in HIV incidence.[51] Examples of scenarios in which PrEP has shown promise include MSM or transgendered women, HIV-discordant couples, commercial sex workers, people with a high number of sexual partners and recent incidence of STI, and people who use injection drugs in a high-risk manner.[4] Recent research supports the practice of PrEP prescription for individuals with ongoing high-risk behaviors, especially in MSM and transgendered women who have sex with men.[46,49,52] This population accounted for 82% of all newly diagnosed HIV infections in 2015.[52] PrEP clinical trials in MSM have demonstrated a decreased seroconversion incidence ranging from 85% to 92% when drug levels are detectable (at least 4 pills taken per week). PrEP use among injection drug users has been shown to decrease the incidence of HIV approximately 70%.[4]

Given that PrEP is a longer term prescription, it is most appropriately prescribed and monitored by primary care or ID specialists. However, emergency providers are in a unique position to identify high-risk patients and initiate PrEP in underresourced communities.[4] Recent estimates are that 25% of HIV-negative MSM in the United States have indications for PrEP prescription.[52] Reaching these patients and initiating this preventive strategy is a current public health challenge. It is postulated that if PrEP uptake in the MSM population increased to more than 40%, the incidence of HIV would decrease by one-third or more than 10 years.[49,52] Given the public health benefits of this intervention, the role of emergency providers in identification, referral, and initiation of PrEP in appropriate patients is arguably significant.[49]

Initiation of PrEP from the ED requires several baseline laboratory tests and a clear follow-up plan. All patients starting a PrEP regimen should have a documented negative HIV antigen-antibody test within the past 3 days, given that the 2-drug regimen of PrEP (tenofovir and emtricitabine) would be insufficient for the treatment of HIV infection. Signs or symptoms of acute HIV should be absent. If there are any concerns about the possibility of acute HIV, an HIV viral load should be sent. In addition, patients should have baseline testing of kidney and liver function. Patients with a history of hepatitis B should be referred to an ID specialist for PrEP prescription given the medication's activity against this virus and concern for rebound effects on medication withdrawal. Women of childbearing age should have a negative pregnancy test documented and, if pregnant, they should be referred to a specialist for decision regarding the initiation of PrEP. Finally, it is recommended that patients eligible for PrEP be tested and treated for any STI given that their presence can greatly increase the risk of HIV transmission. Prescribing physicians should emphasize the importance of compliance with daily dosing of PrEP to ensure its efficacy, arrange a firm plan for close follow-up as an outpatient, and only prescribe a maximum of a 1-month supply initially from the ED.[4]

SUMMARY

As the incidence of HIV continues to decline, a paradigm shift to a chronic care disease model is occurring. Research focusing on management of HIV as a chronic inflammatory state shows promise for new types of therapies and interventions to control the virus. Optimized therapy provides hope for a functional cure in the future. Given the expansion of HIV transmission prevention efforts and successes in treatment worldwide, the future management of HIV will focus primarily on geriatric populations.[1] These changes represent great progress in HIV care. Emergency providers continue to play a key role in the management of acute infection, primary diagnosis, complications, ART toxicities, and HIV exposures during this shifting epidemiology.

REFERENCES

1. Deeks SG, Lewin SR, Havlir DV. The end of AIDS: HIV infection as a chronic disease. Lancet 2013;382(9903):1525–33.
2. UNAIDS. UNAIDS Data 2017. 2017. Available at: http://www.aidsdatahub.org/sites/default/files/publication/UNAIDS_Global_AIDS_Update_2017_Data_book_2017_en.pdf. Accessed February, 2018.
3. Maartens G, Celum C, Lewin SR. HIV infection: epidemiology, pathogenesis, treatment, and prevention. Lancet 2014;384(9939):258–71.
4. Stanley K, Lora M, Merjavy S, et al. HIV prevention and treatment: the evolving role of the emergency department. Ann Emerg Med 2017;70(4):562–72.e3.
5. Richey LE, Halperin J. Acute human immunodeficiency virus infection. Am J Med Sci 2013;345(2):136–42.
6. Cohen MS, Shaw GM, McMichael AJ, et al. Acute HIV-1 Infection. N Engl J Med 2011;364(20):1943–54.
7. Hellmuth J, Fletcher JL, Valcour V, et al. Neurologic signs and symptoms frequently manifest in acute HIV infection. Neurology 2016;87(2):148–54.
8. Sereti I, Krebs SJ, Phanuphak N, et al. Persistent, albeit reduced, chronic inflammation in persons starting antiretroviral therapy in acute HIV infection. Clin Infect Dis 2017;64(2):124–31.
9. Rutstein SE, Ananworanich J, Fidler S, et al. Clinical and public health implications of acute and early HIV detection and treatment: a scoping review. J Int AIDS Soc 2017;20(1):21579.
10. Jacobson KR, Arora S, Walsh KB, et al. High feasibility of empiric HIV treatment for patients with suspected acute HIV in an emergency department. J Acquir Immune Defic Syndr 2016;72(3):242–5.
11. CDC. 2018 quick reference guide: recommended laboratory HIV testing algorithm for serum or plasma specimens. 2018. Available at: https://stacks.cdc.gov/view/cdc/50872. Accessed February 2, 2018.
12. Fitzgerald N, Cross M, O'Shea S, et al. Diagnosing acute HIV infection at point of care: a retrospective analysis of the sensitivity and specificity of a fourth-generation point-of-care test for detection of HIV core protein p24. Sex Transm Infect 2017;93(2):100–1.
13. Lewis JM, Macpherson P, Adams ER, et al. Field accuracy of fourth-generation rapid diagnostic tests for acute HIV-1: a systematic review. AIDS 2015;29(18):2465–71.
14. Branson BM, Handsfield HH, Lampe MA, et al. Revised recommendations for HIV testing of adults, adolescents, and pregnant women in health-care settings. MMWR Recomm Rep 2006;55(RR-14):1–17 [quiz: CE1–4].
15. Lyss SB, Branson BM, Kroc KA, et al. Detecting unsuspected HIV infection with a rapid whole-blood HIV test in an urban emergency department. J Acquir Immune Defic Syndr 2007;44(4):435–42.
16. Boulougoura A, Sereti I. HIV infection and immune activation: the role of coinfections. Curr Opin HIV AIDS 2016;11(2):191–200.
17. CDC. Laboratory testing for the diagnosis of HIV infection: updated recommendations. 2014. Available at: https://doi.org/10.15620/cdc.23447. Accessed February 2, 2018.
18. Walensky RP, Reichmann WM, Arbelaez C, et al. Counselor- versus provider-based HIV screening in the emergency department: results from the universal screening for HIV infection in the emergency room (USHER) randomized controlled trial. Ann Emerg Med 2011;58(1 Suppl 1):S126–32, e1–4.

19. Hankin A, Freiman H, Copeland B, et al. A comparison of parallel and integrated models for implementation of routine HIV screening in a large, urban emergency department. Public Health Rep 2016;131(Suppl 1):90–5.

20. Signer D, Peterson S, Hsieh YH, et al. Scaling up HIV testing in an academic emergency department: an integrated testing model with rapid fourth-generation and point-of-care testing. Public Health Rep 2016;131(Suppl 1):82–9.

21. Isaac JK, Sanchez TH, Brown EH, et al. How compliance measures, behavior modification, and continuous quality improvement led to routine HIV screening in an emergency department in Brooklyn, New York. Public Health Rep 2016; 131(Suppl 1):63–70.

22. White DA, Scribner AN, Schulden JD, et al. Results of a rapid HIV screening and diagnostic testing program in an urban emergency department. Ann Emerg Med 2009;54(1):56–64.

23. Centers for Disease Control and Prevention (CDC). Rapid HIV testing in emergency departments–three U.S. sites, January 2005-March 2006. MMWR Morb Mortal Wkly Rep 2007;56(24):597–601.

24. Brown J, Shesser R, Simon G. Establishing an ED HIV screening program: lessons from the front lines. Acad Emerg Med 2007;14(7):658–61.

25. Gift TL, Hogben M. Emergency department sexually transmitted disease and human immunodeficiency virus screening: findings from a national survey. Acad Emerg Med 2006;13(9):993–6.

26. Brown J, Shesser R, Simon G, et al. Routine HIV screening in the emergency department using the new US Centers for Disease Control and Prevention Guidelines: results from a high-prevalence area. J Acquir Immune Defic Syndr 2007; 46(4):395–401.

27. Dhasmana DJ, Dheda K, Ravn P, et al. Immune reconstitution inflammatory syndrome in HIV-infected patients receiving antiretroviral therapy: pathogenesis, clinical manifestations and management. Drugs 2008;68(2):191–208.

28. Beatty GW. Immune reconstitution inflammatory syndrome. Emerg Med Clin North Am 2010;28(2):393–407.

29. Bell LC, Breen R, Miller RF, et al. Paradoxical reactions and immune reconstitution inflammatory syndrome in tuberculosis. Int J Infect Dis 2015;32:39–45.

30. Meya DB, Manabe YC, Boulware DR, et al. The immunopathogenesis of cryptococcal immune reconstitution inflammatory syndrome: understanding a conundrum. Curr Opin Infect Dis 2016;29(1):10–22.

31. Boulware DR, Bonham SC, Meya DB, et al. Paucity of initial cerebrospinal fluid inflammation in cryptococcal meningitis is associated with subsequent immune reconstitution inflammatory syndrome. J Infect Dis 2010;202(6):962–70.

32. Shahani L, Shah M, Tavakoli-Tabasi S. Immune reconstitution inflammatory syndrome in a patient with progressive multifocal leukoencephalopathy. BMJ Case Rep 2015;2015:1–3.

33. John M, Moore CB, James IR, et al. Chronic hyperlactatemia in HIV-infected patients taking antiretroviral therapy. AIDS 2001;15(6):717–23.

34. Dybul M, Fauci AS, Bartlett JG, et al. Panel on clinical practices for the treatment of HIV. Guidelines for using antiretroviral agents among HIV-infected adults and adolescents. Recommendations of the panel on clinical practices for treatment of HIV. MMWR Recomm Rep 2002;51(RR-7):1–55.

35. Lugassy DM, Farmer BM, Nelson LS. Metabolic and hepatobiliary side effects of antiretroviral therapy (ART). Emerg Med Clin North Am 2010;28(2):409–19.

36. Gunthard HF, Saag MS, Benson CA, et al. Antiretroviral drugs for treatment and prevention of HIV infection in adults: 2016 Recommendations of the International Antiviral Society-USA Panel. JAMA 2016;316(2):191–210.

37. Nunez M, Lana R, Mendoza JL, et al. Risk factors for severe hepatic injury after introduction of highly active antiretroviral therapy. J Acquir Immune Defic Syndr 2001;27(5):426–31.

38. Tsiodras S, Mantzoros C, Hammer S, et al. Effects of protease inhibitors on hyperglycemia, hyperlipidemia, and lipodystrophy: a 5-year cohort study. Arch Intern Med 2000;160(13):2050–6.

39. Tebas P, Powderly WG, Claxton S, et al. Accelerated bone mineral loss in HIV-infected patients receiving potent antiretroviral therapy. AIDS 2000;14(4):F63–7.

40. Hileman CO, Overton ET, McComsey GA. Vitamin D and bone loss in HIV. Curr Opin HIV AIDS 2016;11(3):277–84.

41. Weber DJ, Rutala WA. Occupational health update: focus on preventing the acquisition of infections with pre-exposure prophylaxis and postexposure prophylaxis. Infect Dis Clin North Am 2016;30(3):729–57.

42. Kaplan JE, Dominguez K, Jobarteh K, et al. Postexposure prophylaxis against human immunodeficiency virus (HIV): new guidelines from the WHO: a perspective. Clin Infect Dis 2015;60(Suppl 3):S196–9.

43. Announcement: updated guidelines for antiretroviral postexposure prophylaxis after sexual, injection-drug use, or other nonoccupational exposure to HIV - United States, 2016. MMWR Morb Mortal Wkly Rep 2016;65(17):458.

44. Irvine C, Egan KJ, Shubber Z, et al. Efficacy of HIV postexposure prophylaxis: systematic review and meta-analysis of nonhuman primate studies. Clin Infect Dis 2015;60(Suppl 3):S165–9.

45. Kuhar DT, Henderson DK, Struble KA, et al. Updated US Public Health Service guidelines for the management of occupational exposures to human immunodeficiency virus and recommendations for postexposure prophylaxis. Infect Control Hosp Epidemiol 2013;34(9):875–92.

46. Tan DHS, Hull MW, Yoong D, et al. Canadian guideline on HIV pre-exposure prophylaxis and nonoccupational postexposure prophylaxis. CMAJ 2017;189(47): E1448–58.

47. Mayer KH, Jones D, Oldenburg C, et al. Optimal HIV postexposure prophylaxis regimen completion with single tablet daily elvitegravir/cobicistat/tenofovir disoproxil fumarate/emtricitabine compared with more frequent dosing regimens. J Acquir Immune Defic Syndr 2017;75(5):535–9.

48. Thomas R, Galanakis C, Vezina S, et al. Adherence to post-exposure prophylaxis (PEP) and incidence of HIV seroconversion in a major North American cohort. PLoS One 2015;10(11):e0142534.

49. Kelley CF, Kahle E, Siegler A, et al. Applying a PrEP continuum of care for men who have sex with men in Atlanta, Georgia. Clin Infect Dis 2015;61(10):1590–7.

50. Ford N, Venter F, Irvine C, et al. Starter packs versus full prescription of antiretroviral drugs for postexposure prophylaxis: a systematic review. Clin Infect Dis 2015;60(Suppl 3):S182–6.

51. Grant RM, Lama JR, Anderson PL, et al. Preexposure chemoprophylaxis for HIV prevention in men who have sex with men. N Engl J Med 2010;363(27):2587–99.

52. LeVasseur MT, Goldstein ND, Tabb LP, et al. The effect of PrEP on HIV incidence among men who have sex with men in the context of condom use, treatment as prevention, and seroadaptive practices. J Acquir Immune Defic Syndr 2018; 77(1):31–40.

Infectious Disease Emergencies in Oncology Patients

Lauren Cantwell, MD, Jack Perkins, MD*

KEYWORDS

- Oncology • Infection • Neutropenic fever • Neutropenia • Pneumonia
- Catheter-related infections • Fungal infections

KEY POINTS

- Recognition of neutropenia in oncology patients is paramount in the evaluation and management of infectious disease pathology.
- Oncology patients, particularly neutropenic oncology patients, often present with subtle signs and symptoms of infectious pathology.
- Atypical infectious processes must be considered in the evaluation.
- It is always optimal to discuss the evaluation, management, and disposition with patients' oncologist.

INTRODUCTION

Patients with cancer represent a unique and vulnerable patient population seen in the emergency department (ED). Malignancies can impact oncology patients' immune defenses in numerous ways. For example, skin cancers resulting in epithelial breakdown provide access for the development of cellulitis. Mass lesions may cause obstruction of the airways, urinary system, or other organs, thus, interfering with normal emptying, a natural host defense.[1] Many leukemia's, T-cell lymphoma, and Hodgkin disease result in deficits of humoral immunity, cellular immunity, phagocytosis, or splenic clearance of microorganisms. Patients with certain hematologic malignancies may have had a splenectomy as part of their treatment, which increases susceptibility to encapsulated organisms and some protozoa (**Fig. 1**).[1]

However, by far the most significant threat to oncology patients is the development of neutropenia and the consequent increased risk from several infectious pathogens. Although many oncology patients develop neutropenia as a consequence of chemotherapy, some patients develop neutropenia as a consequence of their primary

Department of Emergency Medicine, Virginia Tech Carilion School of Medicine, 1 Riverside Circle, 4th Floor, Roanoke, VA 24014, USA
* Corresponding author.
E-mail address: Jcperkins@carilionclinic.org

Emerg Med Clin N Am 36 (2018) 795–810
https://doi.org/10.1016/j.emc.2018.06.009
0733-8627/18/© 2018 Elsevier Inc. All rights reserved.

emed.theclinics.com

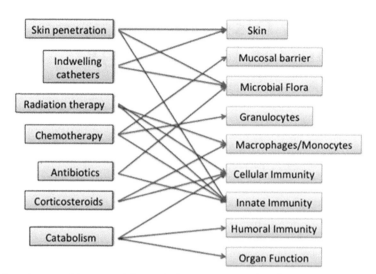

Fig. 1. Impairment of immune defense during treatment of malignancy.

malignancy (eg, leukemia). Patients with hematologic malignancies are more likely to be neutropenic than those with solid tumor malignancies.[2,3] As a result, patients with hematologic malignancies are often more susceptible to infections; thus, it is not unexpected that more than half of all deaths in hematologic malignancies are attributable to infectious disease complications.[4,5] As chemotherapy treatments become more intensive and more common, it should be expected that the incidence of neutropenia will also increase with a corresponding increase in the incidence of neutropenic fever. Therefore, neutropenic fever remains a condition that must be well understood by emergency providers (EPs), in addition to other infectious disease emergencies that may manifest in oncology patients.

NEUTROPENIC FEVER

Unfortunately, fever may be the only sign of infection in neutropenic patients because of a reduced ability to mount an inflammatory response. Consequently, it is common for the EP to be underwhelmed when evaluating patients with a neutropenic fever, as they often present well before they are septic. It is important to remember that any patient undergoing chemotherapy will have an oncologist who has given the patient detailed instructions on the dangers of fever during the course of chemotherapy. Thus, patients will take their temperatures at home often and will routinely present to the oncology clinic or the ED well before other systemic symptoms are evident. The danger lies in being falsely reassured by well-appearing patients with a neutropenic fever who has minimal host defenses to prevent the development of sepsis and associated morbidity and mortality. Fever in neutropenic patients is a medical emergency that needs to be quickly recognized, evaluated, and treated.[6] Broad-spectrum antibiotics covering both gram-positive and gram-negative pathogens are recommended within 1 hour of the identification of neutropenic fever.[7] If not treated promptly, oncology patients with a neutropenic fever can have mortality rates from 5% to 20% depending on coexisting infections and comorbidities. The mortality rate approaches 50% if neutropenic patients present in septic shock.[6]

Febrile neutropenia is defined by the Infectious Disease Society of America (IDSA) as the following[7]:

- A single oral temperature measurement higher than 38.3°C (101°F) or a temperature of 38°C (100.4°F) or higher for longer than 1 hour
- Neutropenia: absolute neutrophil count (ANC) less than 500 or less than 1000/μL with a predicted rapid decline to fewer than 500/μL

The possibility of neutropenia should be considered immediately in febrile patients with hematologic malignancies. In one study of patients with acute myeloid leukemia, 91% of febrile episodes during induction chemotherapy were neutropenic.[8]

The remaining sections of this article focus on numerous infectious disease complications that can occur both in neutropenic and non-neutropenic oncology patients. Although evaluation and management are similar in many conditions, specific considerations may be necessary in neutropenic patients and are mentioned in detail in these specific situations.

Infectious Disease Pathology (Both Neutropenic and Non-neutropenic Oncology Patients)

Skin and soft tissue infections

Skin lesions and cellulitis are common in oncology patients. Non-neutropenic patients are more likely to present classically with areas of pain, warmth, erythema, and possible induration or fluctuance. Group A Streptococcus and Staphylococcus aureus remain the most common pathogens and should be treated per the IDSA's guidelines.[7] Risk factors for methicillin-resistant S aureus should be assessed as with nononcology patients. Neutropenic patients may present with minimal physical signs or symptoms, which is why a detailed head-to-toe physical examination is so important in these patients. Neutropenic patients may also develop pathology from unusual pathogens with atypical presentations, such as Pseudomonas aeruginosa (eg, ecthyma gangrenosum), Candida species (eg, maculopapular rash), Escherichia coli, or herpes simplex virus (HSV) (eg, erythema multiforme).[1] One final consideration is to make sure a deep skin and soft tissue infection is considered in any septic patient who has a suspected skin or soft tissue source. Aggressive imaging and surgical consultation is recommended in this patient cohort, as surgical management may be required.

Oral infections

Chemotherapy toxicity can cause breakdown in the oral mucosa and increased susceptibility to pathogens. Mucositis is the clinical manifestation of mucosal barrier injury. It can affect all mucosal surfaces but will be most readily visible on examination if it is present in the oropharynx. Other mucosal surfaces may require endoscopy or other invasive imaging to evaluate. Common signs and symptoms of oral mucositis are edema, erythema, pain, ulceration, pseudomembranes, and xerostomia.[9] It is also common for patients to have fever with mucositis; thus, this clinical entity should be in the differential diagnosis of causes of neutropenic fever.[10,11] The National Cancer Institute has developed criteria to categorize the severity of mucositis among other adverse effects of therapy (**Table 1**).[12]

Although not always infectious, breakdown in the mucosal barrier predisposes to infection. Oral ulcerations caused by cytotoxic chemotherapy have been associated with Streptococcus viridians bacteremia.[13] Severe mucositis can be caused by HSV or other viruses (eg, cytomegalovirus [CMV]).[9] Oral candidiasis or thrush is also common but may be simply a visible clue to more severe infections, such as candida esophagitis.

Table 1 National Cancer Institute oral mucositis grading				
Grade 1	**Grade 2**	**Grade 3**	**Grade 4**	**Grade 5**
Asymptomatic or mild symptoms; intervention not indicated	Moderate pain, not interfering with oral intake; modified diet indicated	Severe pain, interfering with oral intake	Life-threatening consequences; urgent intervention indicated	Death

Data from Common terminology criteria for adverse events, US Dept of Health and Human Services. CTCAE Version 5.0. 2017. Available at: https://ctep.cancer.gov/protocolDevelopment/electronic_applications/ctc.htm. Accessed March 20, 2018.

Pulmonary infections

Neutropenic oncology patients with pneumonia can have a mortality approaching 55%.[14] Non-neutropenic oncology patients are susceptible to types of pneumonia that mimic those most commonly occurring in the general population. Despite this, these patients may be more frequently hospitalized and, thus, susceptible to infection with hospital-acquired pathogens. In neutropenic patients, it is important to consider more unusual pathogens. Some consideration should be given to *Aspergillus fumigatus, Mycoplasma pneumoniae, Chlamydia pneumoniae, Legionella pneumophila,* and *Nocardia asteroides* especially if the patient has had such pathology previously.[15] *Pneumocystis jiroveci* pneumonia (PCP) is a consideration in patients with acute lymphocytic leukemia or lymphoma due to T-cell dysfunction.[16] Viral pneumonia will be difficult to differentiate from bacterial pathology, however, special consideration should be given to the potential for influenza, respiratory syncytial virus (RSV), and parainfluenza.[16] CMV pneumonia is an additional consideration in hematopoietic stem cell transplant (HSCT) recipients.[17] When evaluating neutropenic patients with suspected pulmonary infectious pathology, it is important to recognize the limitations of plain chest radiography in detecting infiltrates. The lack of neutrophils makes it less likely an infiltrate will develop; thus, stronger consideration should be given to computed tomography (CT) to further evaluate suspicions of pneumonia.[18]

Cardiovascular infections

Endocarditis should be considered in oncology patients with a new murmur or febrile patients with an indwelling central venous catheter (CVC). Many oncology patients receiving chemotherapy will have a port. Although the physical examination should always be comprehensive in febrile oncology patients, those with CVCs should receive special inspection for evidence of embolic disease (eg, Janeway lesions, Osler nodes). Blood cultures are extremely important in suspected endocarditis patients, as positive cultures factor prominently in establishing the diagnosis per modified Duke Criteria.[19]

GASTROINTESTINAL INFECTIONS

Common abdominal infectious pathologies, such as appendicitis, cholecystitis, diverticulitis, hepatitis, and colitis, among others, should be considered in the differential of oncology patients who present with abdominal pain or other signs or symptoms suggesting a gastrointestinal (GI) cause. Patients who have solid tumors are at a higher risk for mechanical complications due to obstruction. Certain diagnoses warrant special consideration in oncology patients and specifically those patients who are neutropenic. Even without the use of antibiotics, patients receiving chemotherapy are predisposed to developing *Clostridium difficile* diarrhea.[20] *C difficile* should be considered in any oncology patient who presents with new-onset diarrhea regardless of whether they have received recent antibiotics. Other causes of diarrhea must be considered in neutropenic patients and include but are not limited to bacterial colitis (eg, *Shigella, Salmonella*), CMV colitis, parasitic infections (eg, *Entamoeba histolytica*), mucositis, ischemic colitis, and typhlitis.[21]

Typhlitis

Typhlitis (neutropenic enterocolitis) should be considered in neutropenic patients with fever and right-lower quadrant pain or cramping. It is associated with diarrhea (often bloody) and most often occurs after cytotoxic chemotherapy with multiple medications implicated.[22,23] Chemotherapy results in damage to the mucosal surfaces of the intestinal wall and then bacterial invasion of that wall. Untreated, it can quickly lead to bacteremia, sepsis, and death.[24]

Abdominal CT with contrast is the diagnostic modality of choice, although ultrasound can sometimes identify bowel wall thickening.[23] Gorschlüter and colleagues[25] determined that the combination of fever, abdominal pain, and any bowel wall thickening less than 4 mm in the transverse plane on CT or ultrasound indicates typhlitis. In one study of 53 patients with typhlitis, the most common radiographic findings were bowel wall thickening (100%), mesenteric stranding (51%), intestinal dilatation (38%), mucosal enhancement (28%), and pneumatosis intestinalis (21%).[26] Pneumatosis intestinalis in particular is specific to typhlitis in neutropenic patients.[26] As the infection progresses, it can extend to involve the ascending colon and the terminal ileum.

Most cases of typhlitis can be treated conservatively with broad-spectrum antibiotics to cover gram-negative bacilli and anaerobes found in the GI tract (**Box 1**). Peritonitis, perforation, or significant GI bleeding are all possible consequences of typhlitis. Consequently, early surgical consultation is imperative for these patients while in the ED to make sure surgical intervention can be achieved in a timely manner if necessary.[23,24]

Central Nervous System Infections

History and physical should include consideration of evidence that would suggest potential central nervous system (CNS) infection. Headaches, neck pain and/or stiffness, fevers, focal neurologic deficits, and altered mental status should be carefully assessed with the understanding that immunocompromised patients may not manifest classic symptoms.

Meningitis, encephalitis, and mass lesions are all infectious considerations.[1]

Patients with lymphoma or chronic lymphocytic leukemia who are undergoing chemotherapy, patients who have received HSCT, and those patients with prolonged neutropenia or deficiencies in cellular immunity (eg, chronic corticosteroids) are at risk

---

Box 1
Antibiotic treatment of neutropenic colitis

1. Piperacillin (semisynthetic penicillin)/tazobactam (β lactamase inhibitor) 4.5 g IV Q6h

2. Cefepime 2.0 g IV Q8h or ceftazidime 1.0 g IV Q8–12 h (third-generation cephalosporins) plus metronidazole 1.0 g IV Q6h

3. Imipenem/cilastatin (antipseudomonal penicillins) 500.0 mg IV Q6h or 1.0 g IV Q6–8 h

Abbreviation: IV, intravenous.

Data from Freifeld AG, Bow EJ, Sepkowitz KA, et al. Clinical practice guideline for the use of antimicrobial agents in neutropenic patients with cancer: 2010 update by the Infectious Diseases Society of America. Clin Infect Dis 2011;52(4):e56–93; and Cloutier RL. Neutropenic enterocolitis. Emerg Med Clin North Am 2009;27(3):415–22.

for *Cryptococcus neoformans* and *Listeria monocytogenes* infections.[27,28] Splenectomy patients or antibody-deficient patients (eg, chronic lymphocytic leukemia, multiple myeloma, monoclonal antibody therapy) are at risk for infection with encapsulated bacteria, such as *Streptococcus pneumonia, Haemophilus influenzae, and Neisseria meningitidis.*[29] Additionally, patients with chronic lymphocytic leukemia may not mount an adequate immune response to vaccination.[29]

Encephalitis is most frequently caused by viral infections. Deficiency in T-cell function or T-cell number whether by disease or by chemotherapy increases the risk for viral encephalitis. Varicella-zoster virus, CMV, HSV, and JC virus are the most common opportunistic pathogens.[27]

Infectious mass lesions (eg, abscess) can be viral, bacterial, parasitic, or fungal. *N asteroides, Cryptococus neoformans, A fumigatus, Toxoplasma gondii* (parasite), and Epstein-Barr virus lymphoproliferative disease can all present as mass lesions.[27] Consequently, when obtaining brain imaging in oncologic patients with suspected CNS infectious pathology, it is recommended to consider intravenous contrast, which will increase sensitivity for mass lesions.

Genitourinary Infections

Urinary tract infections (UTIs) are common sources of infection in oncology patients. Historical features, such as suprapubic pain, dysuria, frequency, retention, and new incontinence, should increase suspicion for a UTI.[30] An indwelling catheter increases the risk of UTI; however, caution is advised, as this also increases the risk of colonization and the likelihood of an abnormal urinalysis and urine microscopy.[31] Although a urinalysis is a fairly standard piece of the evaluation in patients with an unknown source of infectious pathology, those patients without any localizing symptoms (eg, suprapubic pain, dysuria, frequency) may be erroneously diagnosed with a UTI because of a contaminated urine specimen or colonization.

The likelihood of ascending UTI (eg, pyelonephritis) increases in those patients at risk of obstructive pathology (eg, bladder, ovarian, renal, lower GI malignancy).[1] Bedside ultrasound may be used to rapidly assess for hydronephrosis, which is suggestive of ureteral occlusion.

Vulvovaginal candidiasis should be considered in patients with a history of pruritis, vaginal discharge, vaginal soreness, or dyspareunia. Recent antibiotic use is a known risk factor.[32] Oncology patients often take prophylactic antibiotics, which can make them more prone to developing mucosal candidiasis. Uncomplicated infections can be treated with either topical antifungals or a one-time dose of fluconazole.[33]

Catheter-related bloodstream infections

Indwelling CVCs are common in oncology patients and are an additional source of potential infection in this patient population. Fifteen million CVCs are inserted yearly in the United States with 200,000 catheter-related bloodstream infections (CRBSIs) reported per year.[34] Risk factors that increase the risk of developing a CRBSI include prolonged hospitalization before catheter placement, duration of catheterization, neutropenia, total parenteral nutrition, and heavy microbial colonization of the catheter insertion site or hub.[35] Subcutaneous ports are associated with a lower risk of infection.[35]

Despite the presence of a CVC, the catheter should remain the last consideration on the list of likely sources of systemic infection. The urinary tract, anorectal area, and upper respiratory tract are all more likely sources of infectious pathology than the CVC.[36] The most common pathogens responsible for CRBSIs are coagulase-negative staphylococci, Escherichia Coli species, *Candida* species, and *S aureus*. CVCs are also associated with a higher incidence of candidemia.[37]

Catheter infections can present as exit site infections, tunnel infections, or pocket infections. Exit site infections have erythema, induration, and/or tenderness within 2 cm of the exit site. Tunnel infections are defined by the same symptoms but greater than 2 cm from the exit site and along the subcutaneous track of a tunneled catheter.[35] Fully implanted devices may develop pocket infections with similar symptoms around the site of the implant. Phlebitis may mimic infection. If there is any exudate from an exit site or draining area that is suspicious for infection, it should be collected and sent for culture.[35] Rare but serious catheter-related septic central venous thrombosis can occur. It does not have unique clinical features but should be suspected in the context of continued bacteremia despite catheter removal.[38]

When there is concern for bloodstream infection, at least one blood culture should be drawn through venipuncture (eg, peripheral site), as higher rates of false-positive cultures are associated with cultures obtained through a catheter.[35,39] A second culture from the furthest distal port on the indwelling line should also be obtained.[35]

In the ED it is important for staff who need to access indwelling CVCs to take precautions to help prevent catheter-related infections. Catheter hubs, injection ports, and connectors should be disinfected with alcohol-chlorhexidine preparation or 70% alcohol before use.[35] Topical antibiotic ointment or creams can promote fungal infection and antimicrobial resistance and should not be used around insertion sites.[35,40] Mupirocin ointment can also damage the polyurethane catheter.[35]

Fungal infections

The most common fungal pathogens are *A fumigatus* and Candida spp species.[41] In most circumstances, fungal blood cultures in the ED are not indicated. However, empirical (ie, treating before documented infection) antifungal treatment may be appropriate in certain circumstances; in this case fungal blood cultures would be necessary. Previous history of fungal infections increases the risk of subsequent fungal infections and warrants discussion of empirical antifungal treatment with the patients' oncologist and/or infectious disease consultant.[42] A review of the patients' past medical history is of tremendous value, especially in those patients who have neutropenic fever. Sepsis due to fungemia is clinically indistinguishable from bacterial sepsis, so knowing which patients are at a higher risk (eg, previous fungemia) is valuable.[43]

Prevention of fungal infections is crucial for certain high-risk patients, particularly those with an allogenic HSCT and patients receiving induction or reinduction regimes for acute leukemia. These patients should be isolated from mold and fungi as much as possible. Precautions should include private rooms without plants or cut flowers and no connection to construction sites.[44]

Viral infections

Patients with either hematologic malignancies or who have HSCT are very susceptible to severe respiratory viral illnesses. The most common viruses seen are RSV, influenza virus, and parainfluenza virus (PIV). RSV and influenza classically occur more frequently during the winter months, with PIV more prevalent during the summer. Patients can present predominately with upper respiratory tract infection (URTI) symptoms (eg, cough, rhinorrhea, nasal congestion, sinusitis, sore throat) or lower respiratory symptoms. In viral lower respiratory tract infections (LRTI), the URTI symptoms progress to include dyspnea, hypoxemia, and new or changing pulmonary infiltrates on chest radiography.[45] Progression to LRTI increases the likelihood of mortality in immunosuppressed patients. Older age, smoking history, neutropenia, lymphocytopenia, graft-vs-host disease, and allogenic HSCT are risk factors for progression to LRTI.

Polymerase chain reaction (PCR) testing for influenza, RSV, and PIV is available in some hospitals, although the utility can be hampered by lengthy turnaround times. Although the mainstay of therapy for most viral illnesses is supportive care, in select cases (eg, influenza) antiviral therapy may be beneficial.[46]

- *RSV*: Ribavirin is a broad-spectrum nucleoside analogue with activity against DNA and RNA viruses. It has been shown to be effective in preventing progression from URTI to LRTI as well as decreasing mortality in adult allogeneic HSCT recipients.[47]
- *Influenza*: The influenza virus changes rapidly from year to year, which alters efficacy of vaccination and also of treatment options. Vaccination has been shown to lower mortality in patients with cancer.[48] Currently, early initiation of neuraminidase inhibitor therapy is important in preventing progression to LRTI and the associated increased mortality.[45] There are few prospective randomized control studies looking at antivirals to treat influenza in higher risk populations; however, antivirals, such as neuraminidase inhibitors, are widely used.[49] One retrospective case-control study showed that oseltamivir was well tolerated in a population of HSCT patients.[50] Lung transplant patients are at particularly high risk of death due to influenza.[49] Early initiation of antiviral treatment of influenza in both HSCT recipients and recipients of solid organ transplants has been shown to decrease intensive care unit admission and reduce mortality.[51,52]

Initial Workup

The initial step in evaluating oncologic patients with suspected infectious pathology is to determine if those patients are neutropenic. A complete blood count (CBC) with a differential is required for this purpose. Neutropenia is the most common complication associated with chemotherapy and can vastly alter the amount of workup required. Additional tests for most patients should include a complete metabolic panel, a chest radiograph (ideally 2 views if possible), and strong consideration of blood cultures obtained from 2 separate sites. Blood cultures can be associated with false-positive results because of skin contamination; therefore, multiple sets of blood cultures help inform their interpretation and appropriate clinical decision-making. If patients are neutropenic and is febrile, blood cultures are mandatory. If a CVC is present, one set of blood cultures should be collected simultaneously from the CVC and a separate peripheral site.[7,35] Additional tests, such as sputum gram stain and culture, urinalysis, and lumbar puncture, should be considered based on the individual patient and suspected pathology. A broad differential exists for new-onset diarrhea; consideration of stool culture, ova and parasite, and *C difficile* toxin or PCR in certain patients is appropriate.

Chest radiography is an important screening tool, and patterns of infiltrates may aid in establishing a differential (**Table 2**). False-negative and false-positive chest films are

Table 2
Characteristic patterns of pulmonary infiltrate in immunocompromised patients

Infiltrate	Infectious	Noninfectious
Localized	Bacterial pneumonia	Tumor, local hemorrhage or infarction
Nodular	Fungal pneumonia (*Aspergillus fumigatus, Nocardia asteroides, Mucormycosis*)	Tumor
Diffuse	Viral pneumonia Atypical bacterial pneumonia (*Chlamydia pneumoniae, PCP, Toxoplasma gondii*)	Radiation pneumonitis Drug-induced lung injury Diffuse alveolar hemorrhage Congestive heart failure

a risk in this patient population. Providers should consider chest CT for better characterization of suspected pulmonary infections or identification of pulmonary embolus. **Table 2** outlines potential findings on chest films and considerations based on those findings in immunocompromised patients.

Chemotherapy medications can also cause pulmonary pathology that can easily be mistaken for infectious causes.[53,54] Bleomycin is the most common cause; however, multiple other chemotherapy drugs can have similar effects. Radiation treatment can also cause radiation pneumonitis.

Other markers of inflammation such as procalcitonin, C-reactive protein, and interleukin-6 (IL-6) may be considered; however, these markers must be used cautiously in this patient population. Febrile neutropenic patients are at a high risk for bacterial pathology; thus, inflammatory markers should not influence the decision to start antibiotic therapy.[55]

Procalcitonin is a prohormone of calcitonin produced after stimulation with proinflammatory cytokines or endotoxin.[55] Values less than 1.0 ng/mL are less likely to be associated with bacteremia; however, a localized infection may still be present.[56] Patients with pneumonia, but not bacteremia, had average procalcitonin values of 0.22 ng/mL. In comparison, bacteremic patients had a median procalcitonin of 1.8 ng/mL. The same study also showed markedly higher IL-6 levels in patients with bacteremia compared with patients without bacteremia, although IL-6 levels are likely of limited use in the ED setting.[55] Additionally, in neutropenic patients, there is evidence that the increase in procalcitonin can be slower, especially in fungal or viral infections. Very high values of procalcitonin greater than 2.0 mg/mL may help raise suspicion of bacteremia and poor prognosis in the ED; however, the positive predictive value varies widely in studies. Procalcitonin is likely of more value in the inpatient setting to guide or de-escalate antibiotic therapy.[56]

Bacterial pathogens and antibiotic treatment

The predominant bacterial pathogens in febrile neutropenic patients have shifted over the past few decades. Since the 1980s, gram-positive organisms have replaced gram-negative organisms as the most frequently isolated bacterial pathogens overall and continue to increase in prevalence.[2,57] In one study, gram-positive organisms accounted for 62% of all nosocomial bloodstream infections in 1995 and increased to 76% in 2000. In the same years, gram-negative organisms accounted for 22% and 14% of nosocomial bloodstream infections, respectively.[58]

Part of the shift in pathogen prevalence may be related to the increased use of empirical antibiotics.[37,59] Low-risk patients who have received little or no prophylaxis continue to show most gram-negative organisms (eg, *Escherichia coli, Klebsiella pneumoniae, Pseudomonas aeruginosa*). Higher-risk patients who receive antibacterial prophylaxis are showing an increased prevalence of gram-positive organisms (*S aureus, Streptococcus* species).[60] The increase in gram-positive organisms may also be related to the increased use of indwelling catheters providing an entry point for skin flora.[57] *P aeruginosa* is also showing increasing resistance to current therapies.

Most studies have focused on the neutropenic population, but several studies have started to emerge that examine the epidemiology of bacteremia among non-neutropenic oncology patients.[2,3] Differences have been found in the frequency of bacterial pathogens isolated from the bloodstream in oncology patients who are not neutropenic. A 2004 study of patients with solid tumors (neutropenia is less common in these patients than in hematologic malignancies) showed that 82% of febrile episodes occurred in non-neutropenic patients. Of the pathogens isolated, 47% were gram-negative bacteria, 34% gram-positive bacteria, 3% anaerobes, 2% fungi, and 14% polymicrobial.[3]

Initial antibiotic therapy for high-risk patients requiring hospitalization for intravenous antibiotics should be monotherapy with either an antipseudomonal β-lactam agent, such as cefepime, a carbapenem, or piperacillin-tazobactam. For patients with hypotension, pneumonia, or suspected/proven antimicrobial resistance, an aminoglycoside, fluoroquinolone, and/or vancomycin may be added. Antibiotics active against aerobic gram-positive cocci should be added for suspected catheter-related or skin/soft tissue infection (**Table 3**).[7]

Risk stratification of neutropenic patients

The first step in risk stratifying patients presenting in the ED is a calculation of their ANC, which requires a CBC with a differential.[7,57] The ANC is calculated using the following equation: total white blood cell count × (percentage of neutrophils + percentage of bands). The ANC is then classified into mild, moderate, or severe neutropenia (**Table 4**). Severe neutropenia is defined as an ANC less than 500 cells per microliter or an ANC that is expected to drop to less than 500 cells per microliter in the next 48 hours. The ANC nadir is often 12 to 14 days after the first dose of chemotherapy.[61]

Additional high-risk features are patients who are expected to have prolonged neutropenia lasting greater than 7 days or those with profound neutropenia less than 100 cells per microliter.

The Multinational Association for Supportive Care in Cancer (MASCC) risk index is a well-validated tool that EPs should be aware of as a method to help identify low-risk patients. The tool incorporates multiple objective criteria, such as blood pressure, active chronic obstructive pulmonary disease (COPD), tumor type, prior fungal infections, age, presence of dehydration requiring intravenous fluids, and outpatient status. Burden of illness is scored depending on the severity of symptoms (**Table 5**). The points for burden of illness are not cumulative. A maximum total score is 26. Low-risk characteristics are defined by a MASCC score of 21 or greater, whereas high risk is defined as an MASCC score less than 21. In the initial study, 551 patients were considered low risk using the threshold of 21. Of these, 32 (6%) developed a serious medical complication, including 6 deaths (1%). By comparison, in the group identified as high risk for complications, 39% of patients experienced a serious medical complication, whereas 14% died.[7,62]

Another tool has recently emerged to help assess the risk of febrile neutropenia in patients with solid tumors. The Clinical Index of Stable Febrile Neutropenia (CISNE) (**Table 6**) provides a score from 0 to 8 to classify patients as low risk (0 points), intermediate risk (1–2 points), or high risk (≥3 points). The variables considered are as follows: Eastern Cooperative Oncology Group performance status ≥2 or greater (2 points), COPD (1 point), chronic cardiovascular disease (1 point), mucositis of grade 2 or greater (1 point; as determined by the National Cancer Institute Common Toxicity

Table 3 Empirical antibiotics therapy for neutropenic fever	
First-line therapy	Cefepime
	Carbapenem (meropenem or imipenem-cilastatin)
	Piperacillin-tazobactam
Suspected antimicrobial resistance OR complications: hypotension, pneumonia	Aminoglycosides
	Fluoroquinolones
	Vancomycin
Suspected catheter-related infection, skin/soft tissue infection, pneumonia, OR hemodynamic instability	Vancomycin
	Linezolid
	Daptomycin

Table 4 Classification of neutropenia	
	ANC (Cells per Microliter)
Mild	1000–1500
Moderate	500–999
Severe	100–500
Profound	<100

Data from Freifeld AG, Bow EJ, Sepkowitz KA, et al, Infectious Diseases Society of America. Clinical practice guideline for the use of antimicrobial agents in neutropenic patients with cancer: 2010 update by the Infectious Diseases Society of America. Clin Infect Dis 2011;52(4):e56–93; and Flowers CR, Seidenfeld J, Bow EJ, et al. Antimicrobial prophylaxis and outpatient management of fever and neutropenia in adults treated for malignancy: American Society of Clinical Oncology clinical practice guideline. J Clin Oncol 2013;31(6):794–810.

Criteria), monocytes 200/μL (1 point), and stress-induced hyperglycemia (2 points). Stress-induced hyperglycemia was defined as a glucose of 121 mg/dL or greater or 250 mg/dL or greater if patients have a history of diabetes mellitus or if patients are receiving corticosteroids. National Cancer Institute grade 2 mucositis was defined as at least the presence of patchy ulcerations or pseudomembranes or moderate pain with a modified diet indicated.[63] Early monocytopenia has been shown to correlate with neutropenia after chemotherapy and was shown among the most predictive independent variables in the creation of CISNE.[64,65]

A recent study compared the CISNE score with the MASCC score in febrile neutropenic patients presenting to the ED and found the CISNE to be more specific in the identification of low-risk patients compared with MASCC.[66] This new scoring system shows promise; however, this study included both hematologic as well as solid malignancies and the CISNE tool was validated specifically in patients with a solid malignancy.[63,66] More studies are needed to further assess this tool's applicability.

DISPOSITION OF NEUTROPENIC PATIENTS WITH FEVER

All dispositions of febrile neutropenic patients must be done in collaboration with the patients' oncologist. However, it is valuable to calculate the MASCC score so this may

Table 5 Multinational Association for Supportive Care in Cancer risk index	
Patient Characteristics	**Points**
No hypotension (systolic BP <90 mm Hg)	5
Burden of illness; no or mild symptoms[a]	5
Solid tumor or no previous invasive fungal disease	4
No chronic obstructive pulmonary disease	4
No dehydration	3
Burden of illness; moderate symptoms[a]	3
Outpatient	3
Age <60 y	2

Abbreviation: BP, blood pressure.
[a] Not cumulative
Data from Klastersky J, Paesmans M, Rubenstein EB, et al. The multinational association for supportive care in cancer risk index: a multinational scoring system for identifying low-risk febrile neutropenic cancer patients. J Clin Oncol 2000;18(16):3038–51.

Table 6
Clinical Index of Stable Febrile Neutropenia score

Patient Characteristics	Points
ECOG performance status $\geq$2	2
Stress-induced hyperglycemia[a]	2
Chronic cardiovascular disease	1
Chronic obstructive pulmonary disease	1
NCI mucositis $\geq$2	1
Monocytes	1

Abbreviations: ECOG, Eastern Cooperative Oncology Group; NCI, National Cancer Institute.

[a] Stress-induced hyperglycemia: 121 mg/dL or greater or 250 mg/dL or greater if patients have history of diabetes mellitus or if patients are receiving steroids.

From Carmona-Bayonas A, Gómez J, González-Billalabeitia E, et al. Prognostic evaluation of febrile neutropenia in apparently stable adult cancer patients. Br J Cancer 2011;105(5):612–7.

be used in the discussion. Although patients with a low-risk MASCC score of 21 or greater may be managed in the outpatient setting with oral antibiotics, the final disposition and treatment decisions should be made in consultation with the patients' oncologist.[7] Any ill-appearing (eg, septic) patient should be admitted; using the MASCC score in these patients is inappropriate. Keep in mind that the oncologist is often relying on your clinical impression of their patients, as they may only be available through phone consultation.[7] Although the new CISNE score can be considered by the EP and discussed with the patients' oncologist, studies are needed to determine the full applicability of this tool in the final ED disposition.

SUMMARY

Oncology patients are a unique population in the ED. Their disease and treatments often put them at an increased risk for infection, which needs to be rapidly assessed on presentation. Neutropenic patients in particular can demonstrate minimal symptoms even in the setting of severe infection or develop more atypical infections. The following points are important to remember in all oncology patients presenting to the ED.

- A thorough history and physical examination should assess for subtle signs or symptoms of infection.
- A detailed review of the patients' chart can be of tremendous value, especially if patients are presenting with neutropenic fever.
- Early identification of neutropenia will help risk stratify patients.
- Consideration of both common and unusual infectious disease pathologies is necessary depending on the malignancy, treatment, and whether neutropenia is present.
- Rapid initiation of appropriate antibiotics in patients with neutropenic fever is strongly recommended.
- Discussion with patients' oncologist before discharge helps ensure agreement with the plan and facilitate close follow-up.

REFERENCES

1. Finberg R. Infections in patients with cancer. [Chapter: 86]. In: Longo D, Fauci AS, Kasper DL, et al, editors. Harrison's principles of internal medicine. 18th edition. New York: McGraw Hill Companies Inc; 2012. p. 712–22.

2. Kang CI, Song JH, Chung DR, et al, Korean Network for Study on Infectious Diseases (KONSID). Bloodstream infections in adult patients with cancer: Clinical features and pathogenic significance of staphylococcus aureus bacteremia. Support Care Cancer 2012;20(10):2371–8.
3. Anatoliotaki M, Valatas V, Mantadakis E, et al. Bloodstream infections in patients with solid tumors: associated factors, microbial spectrum and outcome. Infection 2004;32(2):65–71.
4. Nosari A, Barberis M, Landonio G, et al. Infections in haematologic neoplasms: autopsy findings. Haematologica 1991;76(2):135–40.
5. Hersh EM, Bodey GP, Nies BA, et al. Causes of death in acute leukemia: a ten-year study of 414 patients from 1954-1963. JAMA 1965;193:105–9.
6. Lyman GH, Rolston KV. How we treat febrile neutropenia in patients receiving cancer chemotherapy. J Oncol Pract 2010;6(3):149–52.
7. Freifeld AG, Bow EJ, Sepkowitz KA, et al, Infectious Diseases Society of America. Clinical practice guideline for the use of antimicrobial agents in neutropenic patients with cancer: 2010 update by the infectious diseases society of America. Clin Infect Dis 2011;52(4):e56–93.
8. Gupta A, Singh M, Singh H, et al. Infections in acute myeloid leukemia: An analysis of 382 febrile episodes. Med Oncol 2010;27(4):1037–45.
9. Epstein JB. Mucositis in the cancer patient and immunosuppressed host. Infect Dis Clin North Am 2007;21(2):503–22, vii.
10. van der Velden WJ, Herbers AH, Netea MG, et al. Mucosal barrier injury, fever and infection in neutropenic patients with cancer: Introducing the paradigm febrile mucositis. Br J Haematol 2014;167(4):441–52.
11. Blijlevens NA, Logan RM, Netea MG. Mucositis: from febrile neutropenia to febrile mucositis. J Antimicrob Chemother 2009;63(suppl_1):i36–40. Available at:https://doi.org/10.1093/jac/dkp081.
12. Common terminology criteria for adverse events, US Dept of Health and Human Services. CTCAE Version 5.0. 2017. Available at: https://ctep.cancer.gov/protocolDevelopment/electronic_applications/ctc.htm. Accessed March 20, 2018.
13. Bochud PY, Eggiman P, Calandra T, et al. Bacteremia due to viridans streptococcus in neutropenic patients with cancer: clinical spectrum and risk factors. Clin Infect Dis 1994;18(1):25–31.
14. Sampsonas F, Kontoyiannis DP, Dickey BF, et al. Performance of a standardized bronchoalveolar lavage protocol in a comprehensive cancer center: a prospective 2-year study. Cancer 2011;117(15):3424–33.
15. Aoun M, Klastersky J. Respiratory infections in the immunocompromised patient. Int J Antimicrob Agents 1993;3(Suppl 1):S99–108.
16. Heussel CP, Kauczor HU, Ullmann AJ. Pneumonia in neutropenic patients. Eur Radiol 2004;14(2):256–71.
17. Travi G, Pergam SA. Cytomegalovirus pneumonia in hematopoietic stem cell recipients. J Intensive Care Med 2014;29(4):200–12.
18. Upchurch CP, Grijalva CG, Wunderink RG, et al. Community-acquired pneumonia visualized on CT scans but not chest radiographs: pathogens, severity, and clinical outcomes. Chest 2018;153(3):601–10.
19. Baddour LM, Wilson WR, Bayer AS, et al. Infective endocarditis in adults: diagnosis, antimicrobial therapy, and management of complications. Circulation 2015;132:1435–86.
20. Dupont HL. Diagnosis and management of clostridium difficile infection. Clin Gastroenterol Hepatol 2013;11(10):1216–23 [quiz: e73].

21. Krones E, Hgenauer C. Diarrhea in the immunocompromised patient. Gatroen-terol Clin North Am 2012;41(3):677–701.
22. Shahani L. Typhlitis: a neutropenic complication. BMJ Case Rep 2012;2012. https://doi.org/10.1136/bcr.02.2012.5815.
23. Nesher L, Rolston KV. Neutropenic enterocolitis, a growing concern in the era of widespread use of aggressive chemotherapy. Clin Infect Dis 2013;56(5):711–7.
24. Bayramoglu A, Saritemur M, Citirik F, et al. A rare cause of acute abdomen for which broad-spectrum antibiotics should be initiated in emergency service: ty-phlitis. Am J Emerg Med 2015;33(5):738.e1-3.
25. Gorschlüter M, Mey U, Strehl J, et al. Neutropenic enterocolitis in adults: system-atic analysis of evidence quality. Eur J Haematol 2005;75(1):1–13.
26. Kirkpatrick ID, Greenberg HM. Gastrointestinal complications in the neutropenic patient: characterization and differentiation with abdominal CT. Radiology 2003; 226(3):668–74.
27. Pruitt AA. Nervous system infections in patients with cancer. Neurol Clin 2003; 21(1):193–219.
28. Schuchat A, Swaminathan B, Broome CV. Epidemiology of human listeriosis. Clin Microbiol Rev 1991;4(2):169–83.
29. Srivastava S, Wood P. Secondary antibody deficiency - causes and approach to diagnosis. Clin Med (Lond) 2016;16(6):571–6.
30. Askew K. Urinary tract infections and hematuria. In: Tintinalli JE, Stapczynski J, Ma O, et al, editors. Tintinalli's emergency medicine: a comprehensive study guide. 8th edi-tion. New York: McGraw-Hill; 2016. Available at: http://accessemergencymedicine. mhmedical.com/content.aspx?bookid=1658&sectionid=109433563. Accessed July 26, 2018.
31. Schulz L, Hoffman RJ, Pothof J, et al. Top ten myths regarding the diagnosis and treatment of urinary tract infections. J Emerg Med 2016;51(1):25–30.
32. Grigoriou O, Baka S, Makrakis E, et al. Prevalence of clinical vaginal candidiasis in a university hospital and possible risk factors. Eur J Obstet Gynecol Reprod Biol 2006;126(1):121–5.
33. Pappas PG, Kauffman CA, Andes DR, et al. Clinical practice guideline for the management of candidiasis: 2016 update by the infectious diseases society of America. Clin Infect Dis 2016;62(4):e1–50.
34. Chee L, Brown M, Sasadeusz J, et al. Gram-negative organisms predominate in Hickman line-related infections in non-neutropenic patients with hematological malignancies. J Infect 2008;56(4):227–33.
35. Weber DJ, Rutala WA. Central line-associated bloodstream infections: prevention and management. Infect Dis Clin North Am 2011;25(1):77–102.
36. Aufderheide TP. Peripheral arteriovascular disease. In: Marx JA, Hockberger RS, Walls RM, et al, editors. Rosen's emergency medicine: concepts and clinical practice. 8th edition. Philadelphia (PA): Elsevier/Saunders; 2014. p. 1138–56.
37. Velasco E, Byington R, Martins CS, et al. Bloodstream infection surveillance in a cancer centre: a prospective look at clinical microbiology aspects. Clin Microbiol Infect 2004;10(6):542–9.
38. Ghanem G, Adachi J, Han XY, et al. Central venous catheter-related strep-tomyces septic thrombosis. Infect Control Hosp Epidemiol 2007;28(5): 599–601.
39. Mermel LA, Allon M, Bouza E, et al. Clinical practice guidelines for the diagnosis and management of intravascular catheter-related infection: 2009 update by the Infectious Diseases Society of America. Clin Infect Dis 2009;49(1):1–45.

40. Zakrzewska-Bode A, Muytjens HL, Liem KD, et al. Mupirocin resistance in coagulase-negative staphylococci, after topical prophylaxis for the reduction of colonization of central venous catheters. J Hosp Infect 1995;31(3):189–93.

41. Marr KA. Fungal infections in oncology patients: update on epidemiology, prevention, and treatment. Curr Opin Oncol 2010;22(2):138–42.

42. Cornely OA, Gachot B, Akan H, et al. Epidemiology and outcome of fungemia in a cancer cohort of the Infectious Diseases Group (IDG) of the European Organization for Research and Treatment of Cancer (EORTC 65031). Clin Infect Dis 2015; 61(3):324–31.

43. Rolston KV. Neutropenic fever and sepsis: evaluation and management. Cancer Treat Res 2014;161:181–202.

44. Patterson TF, Thompson GR, Denning DW, et al. Executive summary: practice guidelines for the diagnosis and management of aspergillosis: 2016 update by the infectious diseases society of America. Clin Infect Dis 2016;63(4):433–42.

45. Chemaly RF, Shah DP, Boeckh MJ. Management of respiratory viral infections in hematopoietic cell transplant recipients and patients with hematologic malignancies. Clin Infect Dis 2014;59(Suppl 5):S344–51.

46. Takhar SS, Moran GJ. Serious viral infections. In: Tintinalli JE, Stapczynski J, Ma O, et al, editors. Tintinalli's emergency medicine: a comprehensive study guide. 8th edition. New York: McGraw-Hill; 2016. Available at: http://accessemergencymedicine. mhmedical.com/content.aspx?bookid=1658&sectionid=109412038. Accessed July 26, 2018.

47. Shah DP, Ghantoji SS, Shah JN, et al. Impact of aerosolized ribavirin on mortality in 280 allogeneic haematopoietic stem cell transplant recipients with respiratory syncytial virus infections. J Antimicrob Chemother 2013;68:1872–80.

48. Vinograd I, Eliakim-Raz N, Farbman L, et al. Clinical effectiveness of seasonal influenza vaccine among adult cancer patients. Cancer 2013;119(22):4028–35.

49. Ison MG. Clinical use of approved influenza antivirals: therapy and prophylaxis. Influenza Other Respir Viruses 2013;7(Suppl 1):7–13.

50. Vu D, Peck AJ, Nichols WG, et al. Safety and tolerability of oseltamivir prophylaxis in hematopoietic stem cell transplant recipients: a retrospective case-control study. Clin Infect Dis 2007;45(2):187–93.

51. Kumar D, Michaels MG, Morris MI, et al, American Society of Transplantation H1N1 Collaborative Study Group. Outcomes from pandemic influenza A H1N1 infection in recipients of solid-organ transplants: a multicentre cohort study. Lancet Infect Dis 2010;10(8):521–6.

52. Ljungman P, de la Camara R, Perez-Bercoff L, et al, Infectious Complications Subcommittee, Spanish Group of Haematopoietic Stem-cell Transplantation. Outcome of pandemic H1N1 infections in hematopoietic stem cell transplant recipients. Haematologica 2011;96(8):1231–5.

53. Bommart S, Bourdin A, Makinson A, et al. Infectious chest complications in haematological malignancies. Diagn Interv Imaging 2013;94(2):193–201.

54. Anderson EJ. Respiratory infections. In: Stosor V, Zembower T, editors. Infectious complications in cancer patients. Cancer treatment and research, vol. 161. Cham (Switzerland): Springer; 2014. p. 203–36.

55. von Lilienfeld-Toal M, Dietrich MP, Glasmacher A, et al. Markers of bacteremia in febrile neutropenic patients with hematological malignancies: Procalcitonin and IL-6 are more reliable than c-reactive protein. Eur J Clin Microbiol Infect Dis 2004;23(7):539–44.

56. Sakr Y, Sponholz C, Tuche F, et al. The role of procalcitonin in febrile neutropenic patients: Review of the literature. Infection 2008;36(5):396–407.

57. White L, Ybarra M. Neutropenic fever. In: Perkins J.C., Davis J.E. hematology/oncology emergencies. Hematol Oncol Clin North Am 2017;31(6).

58. Wisplinghoff H, Seifert H, Wenzel RP, et al. Current trends in the epidemiology of nosocomial bloodstream infections in patients with hematological malignancies and solid neoplasms in hospitals in the united states. Clin Infect Dis 2003; 36(9):1103–10.

59. Jagarlamudi R, Kumar L, Kochupillai V, et al. Infections in acute leukemia: an analysis of 240 febrile episodes. Med Oncol 2000;17(2):111–6.

60. Ramphal R. Changes in the etiology of bacteremia in febrile neutropenic patients and the susceptibilities of the currently isolated pathogens. Clin Infect Dis 2004; 39(Suppl 1):S25–31.

61. Bow E. Treatment and prevention of neutropaenic fever syndromes in adult cancer patients at low risk for complications. In: Marr KA, editor. Waltham (MA): Online resource (UpToDate); 2018. Available at: www.uptodate.com. Accessed March 20, 2018.

62. Klastersky J, Paesmans M, Rubenstein EB, et al. The multinational association for supportive care in cancer risk index: a multinational scoring system for identifying low-risk febrile neutropenic cancer patients. J Clin Oncol 2000;18(16):3038–51.

63. Carmona-Bayonas A, Jiménez-Fonseca P, Virizuela Echaburu J, et al. Prediction of serious complications in patients with seemingly stable febrile neutropenia: validation of the clinical index of stable febrile neutropenia in a prospective cohort of patients from the FINITE study. J Clin Oncol 2015;33(5):465–71.

64. Carmona-Bayonas A, Gómez J, González-Billalabeitia E, et al. Prognostic evaluation of febrile neutropenia in apparently stable adult cancer patients. Br J Cancer 2011;105(5):612–7.

65. Oguz A, Karadeniz C, Ckitak EC, et al. Which one is a risk factor for chemotherapy-induced febrile neutropenia in childhood solid tumors: early lymphopenia or monocytopenia? Pediatr Hematol Oncol 2006;23(2):143–51.

66. Coyne CJ, Le V, Brennan JJ, et al. Application of the MASCC and CISNE risk-stratification scores to identify low-risk febrile neutropenic patients in the emergency department. Ann Emerg Med 2017;69(6):755–64.

Approach to Transplant Infectious Diseases in the Emergency Department

Diana Zhong, MD[a], Stephen Y. Liang, MD, MPHS[b,c,*]

KEYWORDS

- Solid organ transplantation • Hematopoietic cell transplantation
- Infectious diseases • Emergency department

KEY POINTS

- Patients who have undergone solid organ transplantation or hematopoietic cell transplantation are medically complex and at high risk of infection.
- Transplant patients can present with subtle or atypical presentations of infection; therefore, emergency physicians must maintain a high index of suspicion for infection.
- The infectious differential for posttransplant patients is broad but can be guided by a timeline of immunosuppression.
- Patients who are critically ill or have potentially life-threatening infections should be managed and resuscitated appropriately and in a timely manner, through targeted laboratory testing and imaging, broad-spectrum antimicrobials, resuscitation, specialty consultation, and hospital admission.

INTRODUCTION

Modern advances in solid organ transplantation (SOT) and hematopoietic cell transplantation (HCT), including breakthroughs in surgical technique and immunosuppression, have significantly improved survival and long-term clinical outcomes. As the multidisciplinary field of transplantation medicine continues to evolve and innovate,

Disclosure Statement: S.Y. Liang reports no conflicts of interest in this work. S.Y. Liang is the recipient of a KM1 Comparative Effectiveness Research Career Development Award (KM1CA156708-01) and received support through the Clinical and Translational Science Award (CTSA) program (UL1RR024992) of the National Center for Advancing Translational Sciences as well as the Barnes-Jewish Patient Safety & Quality Career Development Program, which is funded by the Foundation for Barnes-Jewish Hospital.

[a] Department of Medicine, University of Washington, 1959 Northeast Pacific Street, Box 356429, Seattle, WA 98195, USA; [b] Division of Emergency Medicine, Washington University School of Medicine, 4523 Clayton Avenue, Campus Box 8072, St Louis, MO 63110, USA; [c] Division of Infectious Diseases, Washington University School of Medicine, 4523 Clayton Avenue, Campus Box 8051, St Louis, MO 63110, USA
* Corresponding author. 4523 Clayton Avenue, Campus Box 8051, St Louis, MO 63110.
E-mail address: syliang@wustl.edu

Emerg Med Clin N Am 36 (2018) 811–822
https://doi.org/10.1016/j.emc.2018.06.010
0733-8627/18/© 2018 Elsevier Inc. All rights reserved.

those who have undergone a transplant will continue to be some of the most medically complex and severely immunocompromised patients an emergency physician will care for in the emergency department (ED).

SOT is the surgical placement or replacement of a donated organ to address end-stage organ failure. In 2017, 34,770 SOTs were performed in the United States alone, a number that has continued to increase annually.[1,2] Although kidneys remain the most frequently transplanted organ to date, heart, liver, pancreas, lung, and intestinal transplantation have also become increasingly common over the past decade.[2,3]

HCT encompasses the introduction of hematopoietic progenitor cells to restore function to failing bone marrow or immune systems. It is performed for a wide range of indications, including leukemia, lymphoma, multiple myeloma, and certain nonmalignant diseases (eg, sickle cell disease, immunodeficiency diseases). In 2016, the most common indications for HCT in the United States were multiple myeloma and lymphoma, comprising 63% of all HCTs.[4] HCT is categorized by donor type (allogeneic vs autologous) and source of progenitor cells (bone marrow, peripheral blood, or umbilical cord blood). In allogeneic transplantation, hematopoietic cells are derived from a relative or unrelated donor. In autologous transplants, cells are harvested from a patient's own body. In 2015, 12,570 autologous HCTs, 3804 related donor allogeneic HCTs, and 4918 unrelated donor allogeneic HCTs were performed in the United States.[5]

EDs play a critical role in post-transplantation care.[6] At one high-volume transplant center, nearly 40% of abdominal organ transplant recipients sought ED care within 1 year after transplantation, with three-quarters of visits resulting in hospital admission.[7] In California, Florida, and New York, 57% of patients who underwent kidney transplantation visited an ED within the first 2 years after implant; almost half of these ED visits resulted in hospitalization.[8] Although ED utilization by HCT patients has not been well quantified, it is likely to be significant. Many similarities exist between SOT and HCT patients when it comes to the need for long-term immunosuppression, rendering both populations distinctly vulnerable to infectious diseases. Conversely, certain aspects also set these two populations apart. In this review, the authors provide emergency physicians with an approach to assessing transplant patients' underlying risk for infection, creating a broad differential of infectious diseases suited to that risk, and managing their initial infectious disease care in the ED.

GENERAL PRINCIPLES

Infections are common in patients who have undergone SOT and HCT. Infections after SOT are often from surgical complications and later from chronic immunosuppression to prevent graft rejection. Infections after HCT relate to chemotherapy and sometimes the radiation used to eliminate the underlying malignancy and ensuing immunosuppression to prevent donor graft rejection. Depending on the depth of immunosuppression required, both SOT and HCT patients may be vulnerable to opportunistic pathogens, including viruses and fungi. Should SOT patients experience graft rejection or HCT patients develop graft-versus-host disease (GVHD), additional immunosuppression may be necessary, further increasing their susceptibility to infection. In GVHD, T cells present in the donor graft are activated, recognize the recipient (host) as foreign, and mount an immune reaction against host tissues (eg, skin, liver, gastrointestinal tract). Significant health care exposure at the time of and after transplantation also increases their risk of infection due to nosocomial pathogens.

Generally speaking, the risk of infection after SOT or HCT is greatest immediately after the procedure. Incidence of infection ranges anywhere from 25% to 80% during the critical first year following SOT.[9] Infection accounts for 20% of all deaths occurring within the first 100 days after HCT among those who have undergone HLA-matched sibling or unrelated donor allogeneic transplantation.[4] In a study that followed HCT patients for 30 months after the procedure, 93% experienced infections, with more than half involving the bloodstream.[10] Infections after SOT or HCT can be severe and even life-threatening. The incidence of sepsis is 20% to 60% among SOT recipients, with in-hospital mortality ranging from 5% to 40%.[11] Infections significantly influence long-term transplant outcomes, endangering graft survival and contributing to chronic rejection.[12] A significant proportion of post-transplantation ED visits are due to infectious complications; almost half result in hospital admission.[6–8,13–15]

Four basic principles can help guide the emergency physician's approach to infectious disease emergencies in post-transplantation patients:

1. *Beware of atypical clinical presentations and findings of infection.*
2. *Establish the timeline since transplantation, and use this as a guide for building a differential of potential infectious diseases along the continuum of immunosuppression.*
3. *Although infections are common and wide ranging after transplantation, maintain a broad differential that includes noninfectious causes of fever in this population.*
4. *Recognize critical infection, initiate timely antimicrobial therapy and resuscitation when indicated, and understand that a full infectious disease evaluation often requires inpatient admission.*

ATYPICAL CLINICAL PRESENTATIONS OF INFECTION AFTER TRANSPLANTATION

Recognizing the signs and symptoms of infection in SOT and HCT patients can be challenging. Immunosuppressive therapy can impair the inflammatory response; thus, a transplant patient may not exhibit a classic physiologic response to infection. Up to 40% of infections in this population will present without a fever.[9,16] Subtle symptoms, such as a mild cough or scant diarrhea, can mask a serious underlying infection. In SOT patients, altered anatomy after surgery further mutes the usual physical manifestations of infection. In lung transplant recipients, airway defense mechanisms are compromised by surgical denervation, decreased mucociliary clearance, and blunted cough reflex. As a result, patients with pneumonia of their transplanted lungs may not develop a significant cough.[17] Renal transplants are often heterotopic, meaning the graft is implanted in a different location, usually the iliac fossa. Pyelonephritis involving the transplanted kidney will, therefore, present with pain localized to that site rather than costovertebral angle tenderness associated with infection of a native kidney. Laboratory and other diagnostic testing in SOT and HCT patients with infection may also be less revealing than that of immunocompetent patients because of impaired inflammatory responses.[18,19] Leukocytosis is often absent. On chest radiography, infiltrates may be absent or minimal in the setting of pneumonia.[20] Pyuria can be absent despite a urinary tract infection (UTI). A paucity of classic findings indicating infection should not dissuade an emergency physician from further clinical investigation if the index of suspicion for infection is high based on a patient's level of immunosuppression.

TRANSPLANTATION TIMELINES AND CREATING THE INFECTIOUS DISEASE DIFFERENTIAL

Unique temporal frameworks help characterize the phases of immunosuppression following SOT and HCT. Each phase carries its own inherent risk for certain infections, although exceptions to the rule frequently exist. Both timelines start with the initial transplant and proceed along a continuum of immunosuppression to prevent graft rejection, tailored to each patient's unique clinical situation.

"Net state of immunosuppression" is determined by their immunosuppressive regimen, underlying disease process, medical comorbidities, use of antimicrobial prophylaxis, and other risk factors (eg, chronic urinary catheter, vascular access device).[9,21] Most patients receive antimicrobial prophylaxis against *Pneumocystis jiroveci* pneumonia (PJP) (eg, trimethoprim/sulfamethoxazole, dapsone, or inhaled pentamidine) and cytomegalovirus (CMV) (eg, valganciclovir).[22] Antifungal prophylaxis can vary. Fluconazole is used primarily for *Candida* prophylaxis and voriconazole and itraconazole for broader coverage against *Candida, Aspergillus,* and most molds; posaconazole has the widest spectrum of coverage, including *Candida, Aspergillus*, and mucormycosis.[23] The risk of an opportunistic infection (OI) increases as immunosuppression increases, usually within a month after transplantation.

Most transplant patients with an uncomplicated clinical course will see their immunosuppression decreased over time. As a result, their risk for infection will return closer to normal as they transition to maintenance immunosuppression.[21] However, those with complications, including graft rejection or GVHD, often require continuation or intensification of their immunosuppression, prolonging their vulnerability to infection.

INFECTIONS AFTER SOLID ORGAN TRANSPLANTATION

The timeline for infection after SOT can be broken down into 3 phases: early (<1 month after transplantation), intermediate (1–6 months after transplantation), and late (>6 months after transplantation).

Early (<1 Month After Transplantation)

Many infections occurring immediately after SOT are related to surgery and hospitalization. During the postoperative period, it is important to consider surgical site infections and anastomotic stenosis or leaks. In one study, 15% of renal transplant patients developed a surgical site infection.[24] Bile leaks occur in up to 20% of liver transplant patients, often at the anastomotic site, and typically present early on, whereas other surgical complications (eg, biliary strictures) arise later.[25] In kidney transplantation patients, UTIs are the most common bacterial infection requiring hospitalization. Patients may be further predisposed to UTIs if they have complications, such as ureteral stricture or obstruction.[12,26] Health care–associated infections due to medical devices, including central line–associated bloodstream infection and catheter-associated UTI, are also possible. Infections due to antibiotic-resistant organisms are common, including methicillin-resistant *Staphylococcus aureus* (MRSA), vancomycin-resistant *Enterococcus* (VRE), as well as health care–associated organisms, such as *Clostridium difficile*, and resistant *Candida* species, particularly in the setting of prolonged hospitalization and antibiotic exposure. *C difficile* infection affects up to 30% of SOT patients, often with severe disease. Depending on the season, respiratory viruses, including respiratory syncytial virus (RSV) and influenza, can be nosocomially acquired.[22,27]

Donor-derived infections are another important consideration during the early posttransplantation period. The serologic status of the donor and recipient to various organisms (eg, CMV, Epstein-Barr virus [EBV], *Toxoplasma gondii*) can aid the assessment of infection risk, although this information may not be readily available in the ED. Donor allografts can become contaminated or colonized with fungi (eg, *Aspergillus*) or bacteria (eg, MRSA). Less commonly, grafts may harbor viruses (eg, West Nile virus, hepatitis B virus [HBV], hepatitis C virus [HCV], human immunodeficiency virus [HIV]),

Mycobacterium tuberculosis, or endemic fungi, such as *Histoplasma*.[22,27] Toxoplasmosis is the most common protozoal infection in SOT patients.[28] Patients with toxoplasmosis may be asymptomatic or present with nonspecific symptoms, such as fever and lymphadenopathy. Central nervous system (CNS) toxoplasmosis usually presents as encephalitis. Toxoplasmosis can also manifest as myocarditis, interstitial pneumonitis, or chorioretinitis. Transmission of *Toxoplasma* infection from a seropositive donor to a seronegative recipient is greatest in heart transplant patients, with up to 75% developing toxoplasmosis in the absence of prophylaxis.[29] *Strongyloides* infection can often be innocuous initially but carries a mortality rate of 50% to 80% in the setting of hyperinfection syndrome or rapid acceleration of infection due to immunosuppression. Hyperinfection syndrome presents as rash, abdominal pain, and pneumonitis but may also masquerade with a bacterial superinfection in the form of gram-negative meningitis and bacteremia.[28,30] Chagas disease, an infection due to *Trypanosoma cruzi*, can present with myocarditis, encephalitis, or cutaneous manifestations (eg, panniculitis).[28]

Intermediate (1–6 Months After Transplantation)

Opportunistic infections abound during the intermediate phase because of prolonged immunosuppression. SOT patients are at an increased risk for viral infections, including primary infection and reactivation of latent infections. CMV syndrome can present with fever, weakness, myalgia, arthralgia, and myelosuppression with viremia. Tissue-invasive CMV disease can affect any organ, most commonly causing pneumonitis, as well as enteritis, hepatitis, meningoencephalitis, and retinitis. Disseminated CMV infection can be fatal. Finally, CMV infection can lead to early or late rejection of renal transplants, cardiac vasculopathy in heart transplants, and bronchiolitis obliterans in lung transplants.[22,27]

EBV is another important viral infection and may present initially with fever, malaise, fatigue, weight loss, and lymphadenopathy. EBV infection can be complicated by posttransplant lymphoproliferative disorder (PTLD), a disease with varied presentations ranging from benign polyclonal B-cell proliferation to malignant B-cell lymphoma. Suspect PTLD in patients who present with constitutional symptoms and extranodal masses. The risk of PTLD is greatest in EBV-negative recipients who develop a primary infection.[31]

Other viral infections can include herpes simplex virus (HSV), HBV, HCV, human T-lymphotropic virus, and polyomaviruses. BK virus is a notable polyomavirus in renal transplant patients that can cause nephropathy or hemorrhagic cystitis. Patients with polyomavirus-associated nephropathy will typically present with renal dysfunction, sometimes with ureteral obstruction from stenosis or stricture.[26] JC virus, another polyomavirus, is the etiologic agent for progressive multifocal leukoencephalopathy (PML), a severe demyelinating disease of the CNS. Symptoms of PML can include visual disturbances, hemiparesis, and behavioral changes.[22,27,32]

Opportunistic fungal infections during the intermediate period include pneumocystis pneumonia, *Nocardia*, *Cryptococcus*, *Aspergillus*, mucormycosis, *Candida*, and endemic fungi. *Aspergillus* is the most common cause of respiratory fungal infection but may present as disseminated disease.[33] Mucormycosis, due to *Rhizopus, Mucor, or Rhizomucor* spp, classically manifests as rhino-orbital-cerebral disease with symptoms of acute sinusitis, fever, nasal ulceration and necrosis, periorbital or facial swelling, decreased vision, ophthalmoplegia, and headache, with the potential for cerebral extension. Isolated pulmonary mucormycosis presents as fever and hemoptysis. Candidemia can be associated with septic shock, which carries a high mortality. *Candida* can also cause intra-abdominal infections, including peritonitis and abdominal abscesses.[34] Endemic fungi, including *Histoplasma*, *Blastomyces*, and *Coccidioides*, should be considered depending on donor and recipient geographic risk factors and exposure history.

Bacterial and mycobacterial infections, including those due to *Listeria monocytogenes* and *M tuberculosis*, are also possible during the intermediate phase.[11,12] SOT patients have an increased risk of bacterial meningitis, most commonly caused by *Streptococcus pneumoniae* and *L monocytogenes*.[35] In one study, SOT patients had a 110-fold increased risk of *Listeria* infection compared with the general population.[36] The frequency of tuberculosis in SOT patients is 20 to 70 times greater than that of the general population. Most cases of tuberculosis in SOT patients result from reactivation of latent infection after initiation of immunosuppression.[37]

Late (≥6 Months After Transplantation)

As immunosuppression is tapered to maintenance doses, the types of infection encountered in SOT patients begin to resemble those encountered in community dwellers. Nevertheless, SOT patients still bear a comparatively higher risk of infection due to community-acquired and opportunistic pathogens. Community-acquired pathogens include common respiratory viruses, such as influenza and RSV,[38] as well as bacteria, including *S pneumoniae*, *Mycoplasma*, *Legionella*, and *Listeria*.[22] UTIs are also common, particularly among renal transplant patients.[39,40]

Cryptococcal infections frequently present after the first year, manifesting as a CNS infection, pulmonary infection, or disseminated infection. CNS cryptococcal infections vary in presentation in HIV-negative patients, ranging from months of subacute symptoms to acute illness within days. Most commonly, patients will present with a subacute meningoencephalitis with fever, headache, lethargy, personality changes, and memory loss. Pulmonary infection can present as pneumonia or with severe illness, including acute respiratory distress syndrome.[33]

INFECTIONS AFTER HEMATOPOIETIC CELL TRANSPLANTATION

In many ways, the timeline of infection after HCT mirrors that of SOT patients. After transplantation, immune constitution typically occurs several months after autologous HCT but often a year or longer following allogeneic HCT. In patients who develop chronic GVHD, immune reconstitution may be dramatically delayed or never occur.[41] Donor source and degree of donor-recipient HLA compatibility also impede immune reconstitution.[42] As with SOT patients, the timeline after HCT can be divided into 3 phases: pre-engraftment (transplant to neutrophil recovery or about <15–45 days after HCT), early postengraftment (day 30 to day 100), and late postengraftment (after day 100).[43]

Pre-engraftment (Transplant to Neutrophil Recovery, <15–45 Days After Hematopoietic Cell Transplantation)

This period is marked by significant neutropenia as well as mucocutaneous damage (eg, mucositis). Patients are at an increased risk for bacteremia, particularly due to gram-negative organisms, as a consequence of mucosal translocation.[43] Neutropenic fever in HCT patients can be an indication of a life-threatening infection and is considered a medical emergency.[44] HCT patients are also at an increased risk for reactivation of HSV as well as fungal infections, including *Candida* and *Aspergillus*.[41] Diarrhea should raise a concern for *C difficile* infection, which frequently occurs before engraftment in the setting of neutropenia and antimicrobial use.[10] Oftentimes, patients may still have indwelling central venous catheters during this period, predisposing them to bloodstream infection.[41] In one study of HCT patients diagnosed with bacteremia, 56% were due to gram-positive and 21% were due to gram-negative bacteria, with *Pseudomonas aeruginosa* being the predominant organism in the latter group. Mortality is significantly higher in HCT patients who develop gram-negative bacteremia.[10]

Early Postengraftment (Day ~30 to Day 100 After Hematopoietic Cell Transplantation)

Impaired cell-mediated immunity dominates during this phase as immunosuppression sets in. A diagnosis of acute GVHD may require escalation of immunosuppressive therapy, further increasing the depth of immunosuppression. Viral infections are common, including herpesviruses, such as CMV and EBV, as well as the BK virus. In one study, CMV was the most common viral infection diagnosed in HCT patients.[10] Fungal infections, such as PJP and *Aspergillus*, are likewise frequent.[41,43] Some HCT patients may have residual mucocutaneous damage with persistent neutropenia, rendering them prone to the types of infections encountered during the pre-engraftment period.

Late Postengraftment (Day ~30 to Day 100 After Hematopoietic Cell Transplantation)

Patients with chronic GVHD requiring prolonged and increased immunosuppression remain at highest risk for infection, particularly involving CMV and EBV, similar to the early postengraftment phase, as well as VZV. They are also vulnerable to infection with encapsulated bacteria, (eg *S pneumoniae*), [43] PJP, and *Aspergillus*.[41]

The frequency of tuberculosis in HCT patients is 10 to 40 times higher than that of the general population. Risk factors include allogeneic transplantation from an unrelated donor, chronic GVHD (and resultant immunosuppressive treatment with corticosteroids), unrelated or mismatched allograft, and use of certain conditioning regimens; the type and severity of the patients' underlying primary hematologic disorder also influences their risk for tuberculosis.[37]

NONINFECTIOUS CAUSES OF FEVER IN TRANSPLANT PATIENTS

Although infectious diseases are a common cause of fever in SOT and HCT patients, it is important to maintain a broad differential diagnosis that also encompasses noninfectious causes. Graft rejection, thrombosis, adverse medication effects, and malignancy are all potential causes of fever in this high-risk patient population.[45] In HCT, symptoms, such as diarrhea or rash, may represent GVHD rather than infection; however, infection must be ruled out first as a cause of these symptoms.[42]

INITIAL MANAGEMENT IN THE EMERGENCY DEPARTMENT

Initial ED evaluation and management of infectious disease in SOT or HCT patients should focus on 3 priorities: recognizing the severity of the infection, identifying its source, and initiating appropriate antimicrobial therapy and resuscitation in a timely manner.

Sepsis and neutropenic fever are imminently life-threatening infectious disease emergencies in post-transplantation patients. Both are time-sensitive diagnoses that require expedited collection of microbiologic cultures and early administration of empirical antibiotics. To this effect, initial ED assessment of SOT or HCT patients must focus on recognizing these two conditions quickly. Clinical criteria for sepsis and septic shock in SOT and HCT patients are no different than that of the general population codified in current international guidelines.[46,47] Tools such as the quick Sequential Organ Failure Assessment (qSOFA) may assist in identifying critically ill patients but remain under active investigation in settings outside of the intensive care unit and have not been widely studied in SOT or HCT populations.[48,49] Neutropenic fever is defined by an absolute neutrophil count of less than 500 cells per cubic millimeter or less than 1000 cells per cubic millimeter with an anticipated decline to less than 500 cells per cubic millimeter over the next 48 hours in the presence of a single oral temperature measurement of 38.3°C (101°F) or greater or a temperature of 38.0°C (100.4°F) or greater sustained over a 1-hour period.[44] Some patients may have functional neutropenia, a condition in which malignancy or medical therapy causes qualitative neutrophil defects that increase patients' risk of infection despite a normal neutrophil count.

ED evaluation of SOT or HCT patients should begin with a complete blood cell count with differential, comprehensive chemistry panel, urinalysis, and chest radiograph at a minimum. If sepsis or a bloodstream infection is suspected, at least 2 sets of blood cultures should be obtained from different sites immediately and before the administration of antibiotics, whenever possible.[47] If patients have a central venous catheter, blood cultures should be drawn from each catheter lumen and from a peripheral site.[50] Fungal blood cultures should be considered in patients who are neutropenic or otherwise at high risk for developing an invasive fungal infection.[44]

A thorough physical examination is necessary to identify and investigate potential sources of infection. Microbiologic cultures should be obtained from appropriate sites (eg, sputum, urine, wound/abscess) in the presence of localizing signs and symptoms of infection. In patients with concern for respiratory infection, respiratory virus testing (including influenza and RSV) should be performed. Based on patient presentation, risk factors, and laboratory assay availability, urinary antigen testing for *S pneumoniae*, *Legionella*, and *Histoplasma* can aid the diagnosis. In patients presenting with diarrhea and a recent history of antibiotic exposure, stool testing for *C difficile* infection should be pursued. Serum biomarkers for *Aspergillus* and other fungal infections, including galactomannan antigen or beta-D-glucan, disease-specific serologies, and specialized polymerase chain reaction assays, can help expand the ED workup but are best ordered in consultation with an infectious disease specialist.[18]

Computed tomography (CT) of the brain and lumbar puncture should be considered in SOT and HCT patients with suspected CNS infection. MRI is appropriate when looking for signs of opportunistic CNS infections, including PML. In patients with pulmonary complaints and an increased risk for invasive pulmonary aspergillosis or other OIs, emergency physicians should have a low threshold for obtaining a CT of the chest.[33] In neutropenic patients with fever, abdominal pain, and diarrhea, a CT of the abdomen and pelvis should be performed to evaluate for neutropenic enterocolitis, also known as typhlitis.[51,52] Neutropenic enterocolitis is a life-threatening infection of the cecum, ileum, and sometimes the ascending and transverse colon.

Empirical antimicrobial therapy in the ED for sepsis, neutropenic fever, and other serious undifferentiated infection should broadly cover gram-positive and gram-negative bacteria using an antipseudomonal agent (eg, cefepime, meropenem, or piperacillin-tazobactam). If there is a concern for infection due to methicillin-resistant *Staphylococcus aureus* (eg, central line-associated bloodstream infection, skin and soft tissue infection, pneumonia, critical illness, hemodynamic instability), additional gram-positive coverage should be added (eg, vancomycin). If patients have risk factors for infection or have had a history of colonization or infection due to antibiotic-resistant bacteria (eg, MRSA, VRE, resistant gram-negative bacteria), empirical coverage directed against these organisms may be considered.[44] When available, hospital antibiograms can provide invaluable guidance in selecting empirical antibiotics with low observed resistance rates for specific organisms (eg,

P aeruginosa). Likewise, review of patients' medical record and prior microbiologic data can also help direct empirical therapy.

Antifungal therapy with empirical liposomal amphotericin B should be initiated if a rapidly progressive acute pulmonary process or disseminated fungal infection is suspected.[33] For less critically ill patients with suspicion for fungal infections, other less toxic antifungal agents can be considered. First-line therapy for invasive aspergillosis is voriconazole, although isavuconazole and posaconazole are options as well. Echinocandins are sometimes added for synergistic effect.[17,33] If *Candida* infection is suspected, the empirical therapy of choice is an echinocandin, such as micafungin or caspofungin. Azoles (eg, fluconazole) should be avoided as first-line empirical therapy because of increasing resistance.[47,53] In patients with concern for mucormycosis, empirical therapy with liposomal amphotericin B is appropriate.

In patients with sepsis and those with neutropenic fever, broad-spectrum antimicrobial therapy should be administered as soon as possible, preferably within 1 hour of recognition.[46] Source control (eg, abscess drainage, removal of an infected central venous catheter or urinary catheter, surgical debridement for rhino-orbital-cerebral mucormycosis) should likewise ensue quickly. Volume resuscitation (30 mL/kg intravenous crystalloid solution within the first 3 hours) and vasopressor therapy should be initiated in the face of sepsis and septic shock adhering to current guidelines and best practices.[46,47]

Critically ill SOT and HCT patients should be admitted to the hospital for further resuscitation, antibiotic therapy, and diagnostic evaluation. The decision to admit clinically stable patients can be more nuanced; patient dispositions are best made in consultation with specialists in infectious diseases, transplantation medicine, and/or hematology/oncology as appropriate. Scoring systems for certain infectious diseases can help inform admission decisions. For example, in the case of pneumonia, the CURB-65 [Confusion, Uremia (blood urea nitrogen >7 mmol/L or 19mg/dL), Respiratory rate (≥30 breaths/minute), Blood pressure (systolic <90 mmHg or diastolic ≤60 mmHg), age ≥65 years] and Pneumonia Severity Index can be used to identify high-risk patients requiring hospitalization. However, it is important to understand that neither scoring system takes into account immunosuppression or transplantation as a risk factor for severe disease. Consequently, emergency physicians must rely on clinical judgment and a global risk assessment to safely and appropriately manage these complex patients.[18] Serious infections in SOT and HCT patients can present with subtle symptoms that have the potential to progress rapidly. Therefore, emergency physicians should have a lower threshold to admit these patients for more specialized inpatient evaluation (eg, bronchoscopy, fluid aspiration, tissue biopsy) and management, including adjustment of immunosuppression.

SUMMARY

The approach to transplant-related infectious diseases can be daunting and challenging, given the broad range of infections possible along a complex spectrum of immunosuppression. This circumstance is compounded by the fact that infections in SOT and HCT patients often present differently than in the immunocompetent host. Opportunistic infections are common. A temporal framework of transplantation and ensuing immunosuppression helps emergency physicians assess post-transplantation patients' overall risk for different types of infection over time. Timely evaluation, management, and disposition from the ED should hinge on a thorough history and physical examination, laboratory testing, imaging, and specialty consultation, along with empirical antimicrobial therapy and resuscitation when clinically appropriate.

REFERENCES

1. National Data. Secondary National Data March 29, 2018. 2018. Available at: https://optn.transplant.hrsa.gov/data/view-data-reports/national-data/. Accessed March 29, 2018.
2. National Data: Transplants By Organ Type January 1, 1988-February 28, 2018. Based on OPTN data as of March 29, 2018. Secondary National Data: Transplants By Organ Type January 1, 1988-February 28, 2018. Based on OPTN data as of March 29, 2018 March 29, 2018. 2018. Available at: https://unos.org/data/. Accessed March 29, 2018.
3. OPTN/SRTR 2016 annual data report: introduction. Am J Transplant 2018; 18(Suppl 1):10–7.
4. D'Souza A, FC. Current Uses and Outcomes of Hematopoietic Cell Transplantation (HCT): CIBMTR Summary Slides. Secondary Current Uses and Outcomes of Hematopoietic Cell Transplantation (HCT): CIBMTR Summary Slides. 2017. Available at: http://www.cibmtr.org/. Accessed March 29, 2018.
5. Transplant Activity Report. Secondary Transplant Activity Report April 15, 2017. 2017. Available at: https://bloodcell.transplant.hrsa.gov/research/transplant_data/transplant_activity_report/index.html. Accessed March 29, 2018.
6. Li AH, Lam NN, Naylor KL, et al. Early hospital readmissions after transplantation: burden, causes, and consequences. Transplantation 2016;100(4):713–8.
7. McElroy LM, Schmidt KA, Richards CT, et al. Early postoperative emergency department care of abdominal transplant recipients. Transplantation 2015; 99(8):1652–7.
8. Schold JD, Elfadawy N, Buccini LD, et al. Emergency department visits after kidney transplantation. Clin J Am Soc Nephrol 2016;11(4):674–83.
9. Long B, Koyfman A. The emergency medicine approach to transplant complications. Am J Emerg Med 2016;34(11):2200–8.
10. Schuster MG, Cleveland AA, Dubberke ER, et al. Infections in hematopoietic cell transplant recipients: results from the organ transplant infection project, a Multicenter, Prospective, Cohort Study. Open Forum Infect Dis 2017;4(2):ofx050.
11. Florescu DF, Sandkovsky U, Kalil AC. Sepsis and challenging infections in the immunosuppressed patient in the intensive care unit. Infect Dis Clin North Am 2017; 31(3):415–34.
12. Arpali E, Al-Qaoud T, Martinez E, et al. Impact of ureteral stricture and treatment choice on long-term graft survival in kidney transplantation. Am J Transplant 2018. https://doi.org/10.1111/ajt.14696.
13. Savitsky EA, Votey SR, Mebust DP, et al. A descriptive analysis of 290 liver transplant patient visits to an emergency department. Acad Emerg Med 2000;7(8): 898–905.
14. Unterman S, Zimmerman M, Tyo C, et al. A descriptive analysis of 1251 solid organ transplant visits to the emergency department. West J Emerg Med 2009; 10(1):48–54.
15. Dalrymple LS, Romano PS. Emergency department visits after kidney transplantation. Clin J Am Soc Nephrol 2016;11(4):555–7.
16. Sawyer RG, Crabtree TD, Gleason TG, et al. Impact of solid organ transplantation and immunosuppression on fever, leukocytosis, and physiologic response during bacterial and fungal infections. Clin Transplant 1999;13(3):260–5.
17. Adegunsoye A, Strek ME, Garrity E, et al. Comprehensive care of the lung transplant Patient. Chest 2017;152(1):150–64.

18. Pagalilauan GL, Limaye AP. Infections in transplant patients. Med Clin North Am 2013;97(4):581–600, x.
19. Pelletier SJ, Crabtree TD, Gleason TG, et al. Characteristics of infectious complications associated with mortality after solid organ transplantation. Clin Transplant 2000;14(4 Pt 2):401–8.
20. Wilmes D, Coche E, Rodriguez-Villalobos H, et al. Bacterial pneumonia in kidney transplant recipients. Respir Med 2018;137:89–94.
21. Fishman JA. Infections in immunocompromised hosts and organ transplant recipients: essentials. Liver Transpl 2011;17(Suppl 3):S34–7.
22. Fishman JA. Infection in solid-organ transplant recipients. N Engl J Med 2007; 357(25):2601–14.
23. Patel TS, Eschenauer GA, Stuckey LJ, et al. Antifungal prophylaxis in lung transplant recipients. Transplantation 2016;100(9):1815–26.
24. Harris AD, Fleming B, Bromberg JS, et al. Surgical site infection after renal transplantation. Infect Control Hosp Epidemiol 2015;36(4):417–23.
25. Senter-Zapata M, Khan AS, Subramanian T, et al. Patient and graft survival: biliary complications after liver transplantation. J Am Coll Surg 2018;226(4):484–94.
26. Karuthu S, Blumberg EA. Common infections in kidney transplant recipients. Clin J Am Soc Nephrol 2012;7(12):2058–70.
27. Green M. Introduction: infections in solid organ transplantation. Am J Transplant 2013;13(Suppl 4):3–8.
28. Franco-Paredes C, Jacob JT, Hidron A, et al. Transplantation and tropical infectious diseases. Int J Infect Dis 2010;14(3):e189–96.
29. Khurana S, Batra N. Toxoplasmosis in organ transplant recipients: evaluation, implication, and prevention. Trop Parasitol 2016;6(2):123–8.
30. Coster LO. Parasitic infections in solid organ transplant recipients. Infect Dis Clin North Am 2013;27(2):395–427.
31. Allen UD, Preiksaitis JK, AST Infectious Diseases Community of Practice. Epstein-Barr virus and posttransplant lymphoproliferative disorder in solid organ transplantation. Am J Transplant 2013;13(Suppl 4):107–20.
32. Cook L. Polyomaviruses. Microbiol Spectr 2016;4(4). https://doi.org/10.1128/microbiolspec.DMIH2-0010-2015.
33. De La Cruz O, Silveira FP. Respiratory fungal infections in solid organ and hematopoietic stem cell transplantation. Clin Chest Med 2017;38(4):727–39.
34. Saxena S, Gee J, Klieger S, et al. Invasive fungal disease in pediatric solid organ transplant recipients. J Pediatric Infect Dis Soc 2017. https://doi.org/10.1093/jpids/pix041.
35. van Veen KE, Brouwer MC, van der Ende A, et al. Bacterial meningitis in solid organ transplant recipients: a population-based prospective study. Transpl Infect Dis 2016;18(5):674–80.
36. Qayyum QJ, Scerpella EG, Moreno JN, et al. Report of 24 cases of Listeria monocytogenes infection at the University of Miami Medical Center. Rev Invest Clin 1997;49(4):265–70.
37. Aguado JM, Silva JT, Samanta P, et al. Tuberculosis and transplantation. Microbiol Spectr 2016;4(6). https://doi.org/10.1128/microbiolspec.TNMI7-0005-2016.
38. Paulsen GC, Danziger-Isakov L. Respiratory viral infections in solid organ and hematopoietic stem cell transplantation. Clin Chest Med 2017;38(4):707–26.
39. Uysal E, Dokur M, Bakir H, et al. The reasons of renal transplant recipients' admission to the emergency department; a case series study. Emerg (Tehran) 2016; 4(4):207–10.

40. Trzeciak S, Sharer R, Piper D, et al. Infections and severe sepsis in solid-organ transplant patients admitted from a university-based ED. Am J Emerg Med 2004;22(7):530–3.

41. Wingard JR, Hsu J, Hiemenz JW. Hematopoietic stem cell transplantation: an overview of infection risks and epidemiology. Infect Dis Clin North Am 2010; 24(2):257–72.

42. Socie G, Ritz J. Current issues in chronic graft-versus-host disease. Blood 2014; 124(3):374–84.

43. Tomblyn M, Chiller T, Einsele H, et al. Guidelines for preventing infectious complications among hematopoietic cell transplantation recipients: a global perspective. Biol Blood Marrow Transplant 2009;15(10):1143–238.

44. Freifeld AG, Bow EJ, Sepkowitz KA, et al. Clinical practice guideline for the use of antimicrobial agents in neutropenic patients with cancer: 2010 update by the Infectious Diseases Society of America. Clin Infect Dis 2011;52(4):e56–93.

45. Venkat KK, Venkat A. Care of the renal transplant recipient in the emergency department. Ann Emerg Med 2004;44(4):330–41.

46. Howell MD, Davis AM. Management of sepsis and septic shock. JAMA 2017; 317(8):847–8.

47. Rhodes A, Evans LE, Alhazzani W, et al. Surviving sepsis campaign: international guidelines for management of sepsis and septic shock: 2016. Crit Care Med 2017;45(3):486–552.

48. Freund Y, Lemachatti N, Krastinova E, et al. Prognostic accuracy of sepsis-3 criteria for in-hospital mortality among patients with suspected infection presenting to the emergency department. JAMA 2017;317(3):301–8.

49. Haydar S, Spanier M, Weems P, et al. Comparison of QSOFA score and SIRS criteria as screening mechanisms for emergency department sepsis. Am J Emerg Med 2017;35(11):1730–3.

50. Mermel LA, Allon M, Bouza E, et al. Clinical practice guidelines for the diagnosis and management of intravascular catheter-related infection: 2009 Update by the Infectious Diseases Society of America. Clin Infect Dis 2009;49(1):1–45.

51. Lebon D, Biard L, Buyse S, et al. Gastrointestinal emergencies in critically ill cancer patients. J Crit Care 2017;40:69–75.

52. Rodrigues FG, Dasilva G, Wexner SD. Neutropenic enterocolitis. World J Gastroenterol 2017;23(1):42–7.

53. Pappas PG, Kauffman CA, Andes DR, et al. Clinical practice guideline for the management of candidiasis: 2016 update by the Infectious Diseases Society of America. Clin Infect Dis 2016;62(4):e1–50.

Biothreat Agents and Emerging Infectious Disease in the Emergency Department

Amesh A. Adalja, MD

KEYWORDS

- Emerging infectious disease • Bioterrorism • Biosecurity • Biothreats
- Health security

KEY POINTS

- An astute emergency medicine clinician can minimize the cascading effects of an infectious disease emergency.
- The use of diagnostic tools to make a specific diagnosis is key.
- Early infectious disease consultation is advised with any uncertainty.

INTRODUCTION

Emergency physicians in every location in the world, in developed and developing countries alike, will undoubtedly be confronted with the possibility of an emerging infectious disease in their career. A subset of these physicians may be faced with a patient who has potentially been exposed to biological weapons. Of the myriad infectious disease emergencies an emergency physician contends with, these 2 possibilities are the gravest and most impactful. In such scenarios, the emergency department (ED) clinician can be the key in recognizing or containing an outbreak.

The challenge inherent with emerging infectious diseases presenting in the ED is that such cases can be camouflaged, lurking amongst innumerable infectious disease clinical syndromes, from common colds to viral rashes. This article provides guidance to emergency physicians as to how to approach this challenging problem as well as familiarizing readers with specific microbial threats of high consequence.

DEVELOPING A GENERAL APPROACH

A key method for detecting the presence of an emerging infectious disease syndrome or a biological weapons exposure in an ED patient is to develop a general approach

No relevant conflicts of interest.
Johns Hopkins Center for Health Security, Bloomberg School of Public Health, Johns Hopkins University, 601 E. Pratt Street, Baltimore, MD 21202, USA
E-mail address: AAdalja1@jhu.edu

Emerg Med Clin N Am 36 (2018) 823–834
https://doi.org/10.1016/j.emc.2018.06.011
0733-8627/18/© 2018 Elsevier Inc. All rights reserved.

that seeks out key historical and physical examination clues. This approach is not different from what is included in a full history and physical examination but requires meticulous attention to certain aspects of the history.

Travel History and Situational Awareness

Travel history becomes a key focus of the history because many infectious diseases, especially of the emerging variety, have delimited borders in which they are prevalent. The travel history must be coupled, however, with situational awareness as to what infections are known to be present in specific parts of the world. Such a task is daunting for most physicians and, therefore, it is important that they know where such resources can be found. Both the Centers for Disease Control and Prevention (CDC) (www.cdc.gov/travel) and ProMED (Program for Monitoring Emerging Diseases) (www.promedmail.org) are 2 such resources that are easy to access and continually updated. Using these resources, a busy provider can quickly assess which specific infection risks any given country might confer.

An important component of the travel history is understanding the dates of travel and how they relate to the incubation period of specific infections. Travel must be contextualized and integrated with incubation period, because domestic infections acquired before or after travel might be mistaken for a travel-related infection.

Additionally, EDs in a given geographic locale (eg, metropolitan area, county, or state) should develop a mechanism to have insight into changes in ED volume, chief complaint mix, and unusual diagnoses at other EDs in the region. Much of this can be accomplished through leveraging emergency health care coalitions and local or state health departments to develop tools to enhance insight into the vicissitudes of a given region's ED-relevant infectious disease problems through syndromic surveillance programs.

Exposure History

An important component of an individual's risk for particular infections is related to exposures. Attention must be paid to animal exposures (domestic and wild), eating habits, occupation, and hobbies. Additionally, it is essential to determine if a person has had any sick contacts or has attended a mass gathering, because an ED physician might be seeing one of the first formal presentations of a wider outbreak.

SPECIFIC AGENTS

Of the specific biological agents, the category A agents (anthrax, plague, tularemia, and botulism), and certain viral hemorrhagic fevers (VHFs) (eg, Ebola, Marburg, Machupo, and Lassa fever) are of the highest priority. **Table 1** provides salient points regarding the treatment of the category A biothreat agents.

In all cases of uncertainty, prompt consultation with an infectious disease physician is recommended.

Anthrax

Anthrax is caused by the gram-positive bacillus, *Bacillus anthracis*. It is a ubiquitous spore-forming gram-positive bacterium that is found naturally in the soil worldwide. It is a disease of herbivores. Humans can contract 1 of 4 forms of the infection: cutaneous, inhalational, injectional, and gastrointestinal.[1,2] Of these forms, cutaneous is by far the most common and represents a majority of cases.[3] An intentional release of anthrax is expected to result in primarily inhalational cases.[1] Anthrax is not contagious from person to person and no special precautions are required.[4]

Table 1
Treatment and prophylaxis of category A agents

Agent	Typical Incubation Period	Treatment	Prophylaxis
Anthrax (meningitis not excluded)	1–7 d	Ciprofloxacin, 500 mg IV q12h; linezolid, 6000 mg IV q12h; and meropenem, 1 g IV q24h, plus antitoxin therapy	Vaccine + ciprofloxacin, 500 mg PO BID, or doxycycline, 100 mg PO BID
Tularemia	3–5 d	Gentamicin, 5 mg/kg IV q24h	Ciprofloxacin, 500 mg PO BID, or doxycycline, 100 mg PO BID
Plague	1–3 d	Gentamicin, 5 mg/kg IV q24h	Ciprofloxacin, 500 mg PO BID, or doxycycline, 100 mg PO BID
Botulism	12–72 h	Heptavalent antitoxin	
Smallpox	12–14 d	Vaccine	Vaccine

Cutaneous anthrax is characterized by a painless black ulceration (**Fig. 1**) that occurs on the site of exposure. Infection is more common in those exposed to animal products contaminated with spores, such as meat, drum skins, or wool. After an incubation period of approximately 7 days, the lesion characteristically begins as a papule and progresses to a black eschar. Diagnosis is often clinical, although culture, biopsy, polymerase chain reaction (PCR), and serology confirm the diagnosis. Mortality is low if the disease is recognized and treated with appropriate antimicrobials. Treatment regimens include oral ciprofloxacin or doxycycline (although penicillin may be used if susceptibility is known) for 7 days. If exposure was through a biological attack, treatment duration is extended to 60 days to cover incubating spores that may have been inhaled. Injectional anthrax has been exclusively linked to use of contaminated illicit drugs whereas gastrointestinal anthrax is due to ingestion of contaminated food.[3,4]

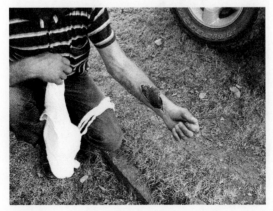

Fig. 1. Painless black eschar of cutaneous anthrax. (*Courtesy of* Archil Navdarashvili, Centers for Disease Control and Prevention. Available at: https://phil.cdc.gov/Details.aspx?pid=19826.)

Inhalational anthrax is the deadliest form of anthrax and occurs on inhalation of as little as 1 spore. Anthrax was historically known as *wool sorter's disease* because of its linkage with the occupation of wool sorting, in which spores on sheep's wool became aerosolized. The disease is characterized not by pneumonia but by mediastinal widening (**Fig. 2**) that can progress rapidly to shock. Toxin-laden pleural effusions may be present. The disease begins after a week-long incubation period and is typically biphasic with flulike symptoms (with the notable exception of rhinorrhea) occurring before a terminal phase. When anthrax of any form progresses, the grave complication of hemorrhagic meningitis can occur.[3]

The treatment of systemic anthrax syndromes (inhalational, gastrointestinal, and injectional) involves first ruling out the presence or absence of meningitis via a lumbar puncture. If meningitis is confirmed or cannot be ruled out, the treatment regimen should include 3 central nervous system penetrating drugs, 1 of which should be a protein synthesis inhibitor (eg, linezolid) and 1 of which should be bactericidal (eg, meropenem). The third drug could be ciprofloxacin. If meningitis has been ruled out, ciprofloxacin and clindamycin or linezolid could be used for treatment (with de-escalation of ciprofloxacin to penicillin once drug susceptibility is known). Treatment is for 2 weeks to 3 weeks.[5] Adjunctive antibody therapies, available from the CDC, such as anthrax immune globulin, raxibacumab, and obiltoxaximab, also should be given.[5] Additionally, if present, pleural effusions, pericardial effusions, and ascites should be drained, a factor that has likely improved survival rates from inhalational anthrax in the modern era.[6]

Postexposure prophylaxis, for those exposed to anthrax spores, includes both an abbreviated 3-dose regimen of the vaccine coupled with 60 days of oral ciprofloxacin or doxycycline (antibody therapies can be used in this manner when no other prophylaxis method can be used).[3]

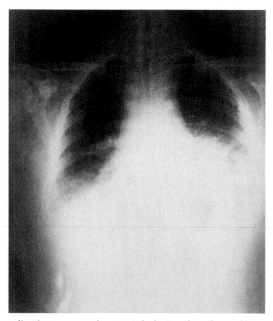

Fig. 2. Widened mediastinum secondary to inhalational anthrax. (*Courtesy of* Dr Philip S. Brachman, Centers for Disease Control and Prevention. Available at: https://phil.cdc.gov/Details.aspx?pid=1118.)

In a mass event the post-exposure prophylaxis regimen for adults can be shortened to 42 days after the first vaccine dose or 2 weeks after the last vaccine dose, which ever comes later.

Plague

Plague is caused by the gram-negative bacillus *Yesinia pestis* and is endemic in many parts of the world, including the Western United States. This zoonotic infection is naturally spread from rodents, such as prairie dogs, to humans via the bite of a flea. There are 3 forms of plague: bubonic (the most common), pneumonic, and septicemic. If used as a bioweapon, plague is expected to present in its pneumonic form.[7]

Bubonic plague is characterized by marked painful lymphadenopathy (**Fig. 3**) that develops after a 2-day to 6-day incubation period whereas pneumonic plague (**Fig. 4**) may be indistinguishable from ordinary community-acquired pneumonia but has a mortality rate that can reach 50%. Pneumonic plague has a 1-day to 3-day incubation period. Pneumonic plague is transmissible from person to person through respiratory droplets and requires patients be placed in droplet isolation.[3,7]

Diagnosis of pneumonic plague in an intentional attack requires a high index of suspicion and can be made through PCR, serology, and/or culture.[3,7]

The treatment of plague is with aminoglycoside antibiotics, such as gentamicin or streptomycin, for 7 days to 10 days, whereas postexposure prophylaxis of those exposed to an aerosol in a bioweapon attack consists of oral ciprofloxacin or doxycycline.[3,7]

Tularemia

Tularemia is caused by the gram-negative bacillus *Francisella tularenesis* and is naturally a zoonotic infection that is common in many parts of the United States. Naturally, tularemia may occur through tick, fly, and mosquito bites or through contact with reservoir animals (eg, rabbits). Contaminated uncooked food or water can also be a vehicle for spread. The most common presentation of tularemia is the ulceroglandular cutaneous form whereas a biologic attack likely results in pneumonic tularemia. Tularemia is not contagious between humans.[8]

Tularemia is notable for its low infectious dose in which inhalation of just a small number of bacilli can result in disease. Because of this, it is important to notify laboratory personnel about the possibility of tularemia, so they are able to don appropriate personal protective equipment when working with clinical specimens.[3,8]

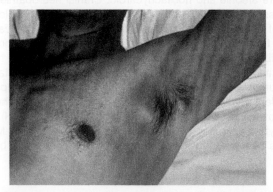

Fig. 3. Axillary bubo associated with plague. (*Courtesy of* Margaret Parsons and Dr Karl F. Meyer, Centers for Disease Control and Prevention. Available at: https://phil.cdc.gov/Details.aspx?pid=2061.)

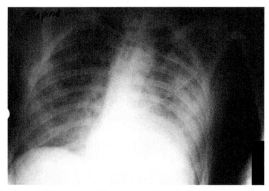

Fig. 4. Pneumonic plague. (*Courtesy of* Dr Jack Poland, Centers for Disease Control and Prevention. Available at: https://phil.cdc.gov/Details.aspx?pid=4079.)

Pneumonic tularemia occurs after a 3-day to 5-day incubation period and is essentially indistinguishable from community-acquired pneumonia. Even physicians who live in endemic areas often miss the diagnosis of tularemia in its various form, highlighting the need for tularemia to be in the differential diagnosis of compatible syndromes in endemic areas.[9] Temperature-pulse disassociation may be present and can serve as a clue to diagnosis.[8]

The treatment of tularemia is aminoglycoside antibiotics, such as gentamicin or streptomycin, for 7 days to 10 days. Postexposure prophylaxis, to those exposed to an aerosol in a biological weapons attack, is with oral doxycycline or ciprofloxacin.[3,8]

Botulism

Botulism is caused by the acetylcholine release-blocking neurotoxin released by *Clostridium botulinum*, a ubiquitous spore-forming gram-positive rod. There are several forms of naturally occurring botulism: infant, wound, and gastrointestinal. These forms result from exposure to spores of the bacteria, which then germinate and elaborate toxin. In a biological attack, inhalational botulism is expected, and it manifests similar to gastrointestinal botulism. Botulism is not contagious.[3,10]

After 12 hours to 36 hours postexposure to spores, clinical botulism occurs. It is characterized by a symmetric, flaccid, descending paralysis without sensory symptoms. Patients are afebrile and not tachycardic. Cranial neuropathies are common. Paralysis progresses to involve respiratory muscles and can be prolonged, requiring long durations of mechanical ventilation. Diagnosis is largely clinical. Confirmatory mouse bioassay testing is used to determine which of the several botulinum toxinotypes is responsible.[3,10]

Heptavalent antitoxin, which neutralizes toxinotypes A to G, is obtainable from the CDC and can neutralize toxin. Antibiotics and BabyBIG (California Department of Public Health, a bivalent botulinum antitoxin used in infant botulism) are not indicated.[3,10] There was controversy over the existence of an eighth toxinotype (H) but it has been shown to be a hybrid toxin and is neutralized by A-type antitoxin.[11] More recently, a toxinotype X has been described and is unable to be neutralized by any available antitoxin.[12]

Smallpox

Smallpox is the only human infectious disease that has been eradicated from the planet. As such, there is little current clinical experience with this disease. Smallpox is a significantly contagious disease that is spread via airborne, respiratory droplet, or direct contact route. Fomites are also known to spread the virus.[3,13]

The clinical presentation of smallpox begins with flulike symptoms after a 14-day incubation period which is followed by the characteristic rash. The rash begins in a papular form and then progresses to umbilicated lesions and finally to pustules that crust and scab. A person with smallpox is contagious only from the appearance of the rash until the rash is scabbed, a key factor that led to its control.[3,13]

The rash of smallpox (**Fig. 5**) must be distinguished from similar rashes that can be seen with varicella. Several points of distinction are important. The rash of smallpox is centrifugal with more lesions on the face and extremities while the varicella rash is centripetal. The lesions of the smallpox rash are all at identical stages with identical appearances whereas the rash of varicella may have lesions of different stages. The case fatality rate of smallpox was historically 25%.[3,13]

A diagnosis of smallpox would be a national security emergency of the highest order because even 1 case represents either a laboratory accident or a biological attack. Because smallpox vaccination is no longer routine, there is a sizable amount of the world population that lacks immunity. Any suspicion of smallpox should prompt infectious disease consultation, airborne isolation procedures, and notification of local, state, and national public health authorities. The CDC has a telephone consultation service in place to discuss potential cases with experts.

A diagnosis of smallpox initially is based on clinical suspicion while confirmatory testing by PCR, viral culture, or electron microscopy is performed under appropriate biosafety conditions.[3,13]

There is no Food and Drug Administration–approved treatment of smallpox currently, although several experimental antiviral compounds are in late stages of clinical development and might be accessible. The smallpox vaccine is effective as postexposure prophylaxis, even during the incubation period, and should be given to all patient contacts, who also will be placed under public health surveillance. The vaccine is contraindicated in the immunosuppressed and pregnant and those with eczema. Experimental attenuated vaccines may be more suitable for these individuals.[14–16] Additionally, the smallpox vaccine carries a risk of myocarditis.[17]

Viral Hemorrhagic Fever

VHFs are caused by a diverse group of viruses, each with its own unique microbiological, epidemiologic, and clinical features. Of this group, which ranges from yellow fever

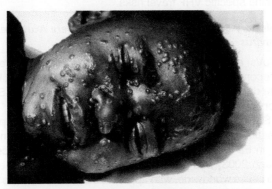

Fig. 5. Smallpox. (*Courtesy of* Centers for Disease Control and Prevention. Available at: https://phil.cdc.gov/Details.aspx?pid=3; with permission.)

to Ebola, certain are more important as potential biological weapons than others. In the biological weapons context, it is the filoviruses (Ebola and Marburg) as well as the arenaviruses (Lassa fever, Machupo, and others) that merit concern.

Despite their differences, this group of viruses is characterized by a clinical presentation that often includes general malaise, fever, rash, prostration, pharyngitis, nausea, vomiting, and diarrhea. Disease can rapidly progress to shock and multiple organ dysfunction syndrome with disseminated intravascular coagulation and hemorrhagic manifestations.[18]

Diagnosis can be made using molecular tests, but a high index of suspicion is needed to differentiate these infections from ordinary septic shock. In the ED patient, travel to endemic areas, exotic animal exposure, or laboratory work with VHFs might be the only clue to the etiology. In a biological attack, a cluster of patients with similar symptoms may present to several EDs in a given region. Any suspicion of a VHF should prompt immediate consultation with an infectious disease physician and state and local health authorities.[18]

Although these viruses are spread via blood and body fluid exposure and do not spread between humans via the airborne route, the experience of the United States during the 2014 West Africa Ebola outbreak has influenced infection control recommendations. The 2 nosocomial infections at a hospital in Texas have led to recommendations for strict airborne and body fluid isolation for patients suspected of having a VHF, with transfer to definitive care at specialized units for confirmed cases.[19]

Treatment is generally supportive and has proved life-saving in the case of Ebola. The recent experience with Ebola highlighted the fact that simple supportive care with fluids and electrolytes brought fatality rates down from 90% to less than 40%.[20] There are several experimental treatments and vaccines (which can be used for postexposure prophylaxis) that are available for filovirus infections and arenavirus infections that would likely be used in any domestic VHF cases caused by these groups of viruses.[21] For Ebola exposures, the experimental vaccine would be indicated for postexposure prophylaxis whereas a combination of experimental antiviral agents (eg, favipiravir) and antibody-based therapies, such as ZMapp, might be indicated after consultation with CDC. Lassa fever can be treated with intravenous ribavirin, which is available via CDC.

The possibility of VHF infection should be considered in those with severe illness and travel to areas in which these infections are endemic, such as parts of Africa (eg, Democratic Republic of Congo, Uganda, and Nigeria) or South America (eg, Brazil and Argentina). Consultation of the CDC travel Web site (www.cdc.gov/travel) is advised to determine specific VHF travel risks.

Middle East Respiratory Syndrome Coronavirus and Severe Acute Respiratory Syndrome Coronavirus

Coronaviruses (CoVs) are major causes of the common cold and rarely cause severe disease in immunocompetent hosts. There are, however, 2 CoVs that have the capacity to cause severe disease: severe acute respiratory syndrome (SARS)-CoV and Middle East respiratory syndrome (MERS)-CoV.

Although both SARS and MERS present to the ED as ordinary upper or lower respiratory tract infections, they have distinct geographic and epidemiologic features that should alert an ED physician to the possibility of their presence. SARS, which emerged in China in 2003, was a worldwide infectious disease emergency that led to more than 8000 cases worldwide, with approximately 10% of cases fatal—including in the United States. The virus was zoonotic in origin and linked to human consumption of palm civet cats. The spread of the virus was abetted by the presence of superspreading events in which certain individuals infected a disproportionate number of others. The epidemic extinguished once infection control measures were instituted in health care settings and the consumption of palm civet cats ceased.[22]

MERS is also a zoonotic respiratory CoV that emerged in the Arabian Peninsula in 2012 and has been linked to contact with both bats and camels. All cases have an epidemiologic link to the Arabian Peninsula, including a multiple-ED superspreading event that occurred in South Korea. Mortality rates are approximately 30%.[22] In the United States, 2 imported mild cases have been diagnosed in travelers returning from the Middle East.[22]

MERS should be suspected in individuals with upper or lower respiratory infection after travel to the Middle East in the prior 2 weeks, and confirmatory molecular testing can be done in conjunction with state and local health authorities. Many respiratory viral panels have the capacity to identify the presence of a CoV and may be helpful in the work-up. Infectious disease consultation and institution of droplet or airborne precautions are advised.

There are no antivirals or vaccines available for any CoV.

Avian Influenza

Influenza is often considered one of the highest pandemic threats. Prior influenza pandemics have killed millions and have caused severe societal disruption. Each modern pandemic (1918, 1957, 1968, and 2009) has been linked to the emergence of a novel influenza A variant of zoonotic (avian, swine, or a combination) origin.

Zoonotic influenza viruses, in their first forays into humans, can cause a range of illness, ranging from ordinary influenza to fulminant disease, including pneumonia and acute respiratory distress syndrome. Poor to limited nonsustained human-to-human transmission characterizes these viruses in the prepandemic stage, with most cases linked directly or indirectly to poultry exposure. It is when sustained human-to-human transmission occurs that a pandemic is eminent.

Because of this threat, monitoring and surveillance efforts exist for avian influenza infections in humans and poultry. Currently, of the myriad zoonotic influenza infections, the H7N9 strain of influenza A has been deemed the highest threat amongst these viruses currently, although others (such as H5N1) are also important to track.[23]

The ED physician should suspect avian influenza in travelers from China and other areas in which avian influenza is known to circulate, who present within approximately 1 week after travel with upper or lower respiratory tract infection. Additionally, domestic agricultural workers or those with agricultural contact with flulike symptoms (eg, children at fairs) also may harbor zoonotic influenza infections.[24]

Diagnosis is similar to ordinary influenza, but a rapid or standard molecular test may or may not be able to detect influenza. Confirmatory testing is via health authorities. Treatment involves supportive care coupled to antiviral therapy with either oral oseltamivir or, if disease severity is high, intravenous peramivir. Infectious disease consultation and institution of droplet precautions is advised.

Emerging Arboviruses

Mosquito-borne arboviruses have increasingly taken on importance in the field of emerging infectious disease with the explosion of cases of West Nile, chikungunya, and Zika in the Western Hemisphere. Additionally, local transmission of dengue fever has occurred in Florida, Texas, Hawaii, and New York.[25,26]

Chikungunya, dengue fever, and Zika are all spread by the Aedes species of mosquitoes, which have habitats both within and outside the United States and cause clinically indistinguishable syndromes. These syndromes all involve fevers, rash, myalgias, and arthralgias. Conjunctivitis has been noted with Zika. Prolonged debilitating arthralgias can occur with chikungunya whereas severe illness, including shock and hemorrhagic manifestations, can occur with dengue fever (especially with repeat infection with disparate strains).[27,28] Zika has been linked to Guillain-Barré syndrome and requires special counseling regarding sexual transmission and pregnancy given its ability to cause a devastating congenital syndrome.[29,30]

Travel history and residence in an endemic area (eg, Key West, Hawaii, and Texas) are important elements of the history. Diagnostic testing is commercially available for each infection.

Consultation with the CDC travel Web site is advised to assess specific risks for individual patients' travel history. No vaccines or antiviral therapies are available for these infections.

EMERGENCY MEDICINE AND SPECIFIC DIAGNOSIS

Emergency physicians play a crucial and unique role in the defense against emerging infectious disease and are most likely to encounter the first cases of any new infectious disease syndrome. The challenge that the emergency physician faces is that these cases do not announce themselves and are hidden among the sea of chief complaints that any ED sees on a given day.

With many clinical scenarios, a busy physician may not be inclined to pursue a specific diagnosis if it "doesn't change treatment," may lengthen ED length of stay, and will not produce a result while a patient is in the ED, creating follow-up logistical problems. Failing to diagnose an epidemiologically important emerging infectious disease or biological attack, however, can have tremendous cascading effects involving all sectors of society (health care, government, and economy) that can be minimized or averted with a proactive approach.

In the current era, there are several molecular multianalyte tests available, some of which are Clinical Laboratory Improvement Amendments (CLIA) waived and available at point of care for specific infectious disease syndromes, such as gastrointestinal infections, meningitis, and respiratory infections, that can be used to increase the rate of microbial specific diagnoses in ED settings. Biodefense cartridges, which probe for select bioagents, are also available. These tests, in the hands of an astute physician, can improve the nation's resiliency to infectious disease emergencies, and negative results in the right clinical context may prompt further investigation for a specific etiology.

SUMMARY

By having a working knowledge of emerging infectious disease and biothreat landscape, an emergency physician becomes a key component of the infectious disease emergency system.

REFERENCES

1. Christian MD. Biowarfare and bioterrorism. Crit Care Clin 2013;29:717–56.
2. Hanczaruk M, Reischl U, Holzmann T, et al. Injectional anthrax in heroin users, Europe, 2000-2012. Emerg Infect Dis 2014;20:322–3.
3. Adalja AA, Toner E, Inglesby TV. Clinical management of potential bioterrorism-related conditions. N Engl J Med 2015;372:954–62.
4. Martin GJ, Friedlander AM. Bacillus anthracis (anthrax). In: Bennett JE, Dolin R, Blaser MJ, editors. Mandell, Douglas, and Bennett's principles and practice of infectious diseases. 8th edition. Philadelphia: Elsevier; 2014.

5. Hendricks KA, Wright ME, Shadomy SV, et al. Centers for Disease Control and Prevention expert panel meetings on prevention and treatment of anthrax in adults. Emerg Infect Dis 2014;20:e130687.

6. Holty JE, Bravata DM, Liu H, et al. Systematic review: a century of inhalational anthrax cases from 1900 to 2005. Ann Intern Med 2006;144:270–80.

7. Mead PS. Yersinia species (including plague). In: Bennett JE, Dolin R, Blaser MJ, editors. Mandell, Douglas, and Bennett's principles and practice of infectious diseases. 8th edition. Philadelphia: Elsevier; 2014.

8. Penn RL. Francisella tularensis (tularemia). In: Bennett JE, Dolin R, Blaser MJ, editors. Mandell, Douglas, and Bennett's principles and practice of infectious diseases. 8th edition. Philadelphia: Elsevier; 2014.

9. Weber IB, Turabelidze G, Patrick S, et al. Clinical recognition and management of tularemia in Missouri: a retrospective records review of 121 cases. Clin Infect Dis 2012;55:1283–90.

10. Hodowanec A, Bleck TP. Botulism (Clostridium botulinum). In: Bennett JE, Dolin R, Blaser MJ, editors. Mandell, Douglas, and Bennett's principles and practice of infectious diseases. 8th edition. Philadelphia: Elsevier; 2014.

11. Maslanka SE, Luquez C, Dykes JK, et al. A novel botulinum neurotoxin, previously reported as serotype H, has a hybrid-like structure with regions of similarity to the structures of serotypes A and F and is neutralized with serotype A antitoxin. J Infect Dis 2016;213:379–85.

12. Zhang S, Masuyer G, Zhang J, et al. Identification and characterization of a novel botulinum neurotoxin. Nat Commun 2017;8:14130.

13. Peterson BW, Damon IK. Orthopoxviruses: vaccinia (smallpox vaccine), variola (smallpox), monkeypox, and cowpox. In: Bennett JE, Dolin R, Blaser MJ, editors. Mandell, Douglas, and Bennett's principles and practice of infectious diseases. 8th edition. Philadelphia: Elsevier; 2014.

14. Nalca A, Zumbrun EE. ACAM2000: the new smallpox vaccine for United States Strategic National Stockpile. Drug Des Devel Ther 2010;4:71–9.

15. Frey SE, Winokur PL, Salata RA, et al. Safety and immunogenicity of IMVAMUNE smallpox vaccine using different strategies for a post event scenario. Vaccine 2013;31:3025–33.

16. Kennedy JS, Gurwith M, Dekker CL, et al. Safety and immunogenicity of LC16m8, an attenuated smallpox vaccine in vaccinia-naive adults. J Infect Dis 2011;204: 1395–402.

17. Food and Drug Administration. ACAM 2000 prescribing information. Available at: http://www.fda.gov/downloads/biologicsbloodvaccines/vaccines/approved products/ucm142572.pdf. Accessed July 30, 2018.

18. Borio LL, Henderson DA, Hynes NA. Bioterrorism: an overview. In: Bennett JE, Dolin R, Blaser MJ, editors. Mandell, Douglas, and Bennett's principles and practice of infectious diseases. 8th edition. Philadelphia: Elsevier; 2014.

19. Koonin LM, Jamieson DJ, Jernigan JA, et al. Systems for rapidly detecting and treating persons with Ebola virus disease – United States. MMWR Morb Mortal Wkly Rep 2015;64:222–5.

20. Lamontagne F, Fowler RA, Adhikari NK, et al. Evidence-based guidelines for supportive care of patients with Ebola virus disease. Lancet 2018;391:700–8.

21. Hayden FG, Friede M, Bausch DG. Experimental therapies for Ebola virus disease: what have we learned? J Infect Dis 2017;215:167–70.

22. McIntosh K, Perlman S. Coronaviruses, including severe acute respiratory syndrome (SARS) and middle east respiratory syndrome (MERS). In: Bennett JE,

Dolin R, Blaser MJ, editors. Mandell, Douglas, and Bennett's principles and practice of infectious diseases. 8th edition. Philadelphia: Elsevier; 2014.

23. CDC. Summary of influenza risk assessment tool (IRAT) results. Available at: https://www.cdc.gov/flu/pandemic-resources/monitoring/irat-virus-summaries.htm. Accessed February 25, 2018.

24. Schicker RS, Rossow J, Eckel S, et al. Outbreak of influenza A (H3N2) variant virus infections among persons attending agricultural fairs housing infected swine – Michigan and Ohio, July-August 2016. MMWR Morb Mortal Wkly Rep 2016;65: 1157–60.

25. Adalja AA, Sell TK, Bouri N, et al. Lessons learned during dengue outbreaks in the United States, 2001-2011. Emerg Infect Dis 2012;18:608–14.

26. Suffolk County Government. Health commissioner reports dengue virus case. Available at: http://www.suffolkcountyny.gov/Home/tabid/59/ctl/details/itemid/ 1939/mid/2638/health-commissioner-reports-dengue-virus-case.aspx. Accessed February 25, 2018.

27. Thomas SJ, Endy TP, Rothman AL, et al. Flaviviruses (dengue, yellow fever, Japanese encephalitis, West Nile encephalitis, St. Louis encephalitis, tick-borne encephalitis, Kyasanur Forest disease, Alkhurma hemorrhagic fever, Zika). In: Bennett JE, Dolin R, Blaser MJ, editors. Mandell, Douglas, and Bennett's principles and practice of infectious diseases. 8th edition. Philadelphia: Elsevier; 2014.

28. Markoff L. Alphaviruses. In: Bennett JE, Dolin R, Blaser MJ, editors. Mandell, Douglas, and Bennett's principles and practice of infectious diseases. 8th edition. Philadelphia: Elsevier; 2014.

29. Parra B, Lizarazo J, Jimenez-Arango JA, et al. Guillain-Barre syndrome associated with Zika virus infection in Columbia. N Engl J Med 2016;375:1513–23.

30. Rasmussen SA, Jamieson DJ, Honein MA, et al. Zika virus and birth defects—reviewing the evidence for causality. N Engl J Med 2016;374:1981–6.

Infectious Diseases After Hydrologic Disasters

Stephen Y. Liang, MD, MPHS[a,b,*], Nicole Messenger, MD[a]

KEYWORDS

- Flood • Hurricane • Tsunami • Infectious diseases • Soft tissue infections
- Respiratory infections • Gastrointestinal infections • Vector-borne diseases

KEY POINTS

- Skin and soft tissue infections following a hydrologic disaster can arise in the setting of traumatic injury and exposure to contaminated water.
- Gastrointestinal and respiratory infections are common among displaced populations, and are shaped by living conditions, access to clean water, and pre-existing endemic diseases.
- Leptospirosis is a zoonotic infection that has been associated with severe floods and population displacement.
- Vector-borne diseases can be influenced by hydrologic disasters; outbreaks are often multifactorial in nature.
- Disaster responders can reduce their risk of illness due to infectious diseases through careful planning, preparation, and preventive measures.

INTRODUCTION

Natural disasters are defined as disturbances in the ecosystem that impede a native community's ability to adapt, often requiring external interventions for survival.[1] They can arise from hydrologic, atmospheric, or geologic events.[2] Hydrologic events include hurricanes, tsunamis, and storm surges, as well as excessive rainfall, floods, and even drought. Recent hydrologic disasters such hurricanes Harvey, Irma, and Maria in the latter half of 2017 are poignant reminders of the power and destruction these events can unleash. When hydrologic disasters occur, concerns about the threat of

Disclosures: S.Y. Liang reports no conflicts of interest in this work. S.Y. Liang is the recipient of a KM1 Comparative Effectiveness Research Career Development Award (KM1CA156708-01) and received support through the Clinical and Translational Science Award (CTSA) program (UL1RR024992) of the National Center for Advancing Translational Sciences as well as the Barnes-Jewish Patient Safety & Quality Career Development Program, which is funded by the Foundation for Barnes-Jewish Hospital.
[a] Division of Emergency Medicine, Washington University School of Medicine, St Louis, MO, USA; [b] Division of Infectious Diseases, Washington University School of Medicine, St Louis, MO, USA
* Corresponding author. 4523 Clayton Avenue, Campus Box 8051, St Louis, MO 63110.
E-mail address: syliang@wustl.edu

Emerg Med Clin N Am 36 (2018) 835–851
https://doi.org/10.1016/j.emc.2018.07.002
0733-8627/18/© 2018 Elsevier Inc. All rights reserved.

infectious diseases associated with human remains often arise.[2,3] However, endemic infectious diseases affecting vulnerable and displaced populations pose the greatest risk to human health, particularly in resource-poor settings.[2–5] This article discusses general principles of infectious diseases following a hydrologic disaster. Next, it focuses on skin and soft tissue infections, gastrointestinal infections, respiratory infections, and zoonotic and vector-borne infectious diseases commonly encountered among survivors. Finally, it provides personal safety guidance for emergency physicians and other disaster responders providing care after a hydrologic disaster.

PRINCIPLES OF INFECTIOUS DISEASE AFTER HYDROLOGIC DISASTERS

The risk for infectious diseases following a hydrologic disaster can be contextualized using the classic epidemiologic triad or triangle, comprised of an external agent (microorganism), a susceptible host, and an environment that brings the host and agent together. In most instances, agents responsible for infections are ones that existed naturally in the affected region prior to the disaster, albeit with varying levels of contribution to human disease.[3] For this reason, it is possible to generate a rational differential diagnosis of microorganisms responsible for specific infectious disease syndromes based on geography and individual exposure history. Hosts, including survivors and responders alike, are susceptible to infection through traumatic injury and exposure to contaminated environments following a hydrologic event. Poor hygiene, poor sanitation, and lack of access to clean water and uncontaminated food further increase host vulnerability to various common communicable infectious diseases.[2,3] A hydrologic event disrupts the environment on multiple levels and can eliminate pre-existing barriers separating hosts and agents. Water sources can become contaminated with microbe-laden sewage, wastewater, and agricultural runoff.[5] Standing water can serve as a breeding site for arthropod vectors (eg, mosquitos). Displaced human populations lacking shelter are likely to encounter contaminated water, animals, and arthropod vectors, while those in temporary shelter may be subject to infections associated with crowded living conditions.

The timeline following a natural disaster is often broken down into an impact (0–4 days), postimpact (4 days to 4 weeks), and recovery phase (after 4 weeks).[3] Infections during the impact phase are likely to be associated with traumatic injuries (eg, lacerations, punctures) sustained while escaping imminent danger or performing initial clean-up and repairs after a hydrologic event. However, most acute infections including those involving wounds or related to population displacement are likely to emerge during the postimpact phase.[6] Vector-borne diseases (eg, dengue, malaria), uncommon infections related to environmental contamination (eg, leptospirosis), and infections with longer incubation or latent periods are more apt to emerge during postimpact and into the recovery phase.[3,6]

SKIN AND SOFT TISSUE INFECTIONS

Skin and soft tissue infections (SSTIs) are common after hydrologic disasters.[7–10] Compromised skin integrity in the setting of environmental water exposure, traumatic wounds, and water-related dermatologic conditions (eg, contact dermatitis, immersion foot) provide skin and waterborne pathogens an avenue for infecting underlying soft tissue. Gram-positive organisms including *Staphylococcus aureus* and *Streptococcus* species are typical bacterial pathogens associated with these infections, which may be exacerbated in crowded living conditions. During Hurricane Katrina in 2005, a cluster of methicillin-resistant *S aureus* (MRSA) SSTIs involving adults and children occurred at an evacuee facility in Dallas, Texas.[11] Empiric antibiotic therapy directed against these common pathogens, paired with incision and drainage of abscesses when appropriate, is no different from standard clinical practice in many cases.[12]

Gram-negative organisms specifically associated with water exposure also play a role in SSTIs after hydrologic events.[13,14] *Vibrio vulnificus* is naturally found in saltwater or brackish water and has been associated with wound infections in southern US states bordering the Gulf of Mexico. Infections begin with cellulitis around the wound and can progress to the formation of hemorrhagic bullae, altered mental status, and septic shock, with a mortality rate of up to 30%.[15] Patients with underlying liver disease (eg, cirrhosis) and immunosuppression are particularly susceptible to infection and poor outcomes. Eighteen cases of wound-associated *V vulnificus* and *V parahaemolyticus* infection were reported after Hurricane Katrina, with 5 cases resulting in death.[16] Wound and blood cultures are necessary to establish the diagnosis. Severe infections should be treated using a combination of a third-generation cephalosporin (eg, ceftazidime, ceftriaxone) and doxycycline; fluoroquinolones may also be considered.[12,14,17] Timely surgical debridement of the wound reduces mortality in severe wound and necrotizing soft tissue infections involving this organism.[18]

Aeromonas species are gram-negative organisms that inhabit fresh and brackish water and have also been implicated in wound infections following hydrologic disasters. *Aeromonas* species was the most common wound isolate recovered from survivors with SSTI transferred to four hospitals in Bangkok, Thailand, following the 2004 Indian Ocean tsunami.[19] Most survivors likely had contaminated freshwater exposure from surrounding reservoirs after flooding from the tsunami wave.[9] High concentrations of *Aeromonas* species were detected in floodwater from Lake Pontchartrain throughout New Orleans weeks after Hurricane Katrina.[20] Onset of infection is typically within 48 hours and may present as a simple cellulitis, with erythema, warmth, and pain to the affected region. Infection can spread deeper, resulting in myonecrosis and necrotizing soft tissue infection. Antibiotic coverage for *Aeromonas* consists of a combination of doxycycline and either ciprofloxacin or ceftriaxone.[12,14] Wound culture with antibiotic susceptibility testing and surgical debridement when indicated are important guides to appropriate care.

Polymicrobial SSTIs including other gram-negative organisms such as *Pseudomonas aeruginosa*, *Klebsiella pneumoniae*, and *Escherichia coli*, some multidrug-resistant, were common among survivors of the 2004 Indian Ocean tsunami.[19,21,22] Similar microbiological trends were observed in SSTIs following floods in Taiwan after Typhoon Morakot in 2009.[23] In general, a history of immersion in contaminated waters with subsequent SSTI should raise a concern for gram-negative or polymicrobial infection. Broad empiric antibiotic coverage of gram-positive and gram-negative organisms is recommended pending wound culture results. Indolent, late-onset skin infections and those that fail to improve with conventional antibiotic regimens increase suspicion for an uncommon organism. Several cases of cutaneous infection due to *Burkholderia pseudomallei*, the causative agent for melioidosis, and nontuberculous mycobacteria have been reported among tsunami survivors.[24-27]

Necrotizing soft tissue infection (NSTI) complicating contaminated traumatic soft tissue injuries is one of the gravest concerns after a hydrologic disaster. Infections can be polymicrobial (type I), involving aerobic and anaerobic bacteria, or monomicrobial (type II), classically due to group A *Streptococcus* (GAS; also known as *S pyogenes*), other β-hemolytic streptococci, or *S aureus*. GAS was identified using rapid whole-genome sequencing in a case of wound-associated NSTI after floodwater exposure during Hurricane Harvey in Houston, Texas, in 2017.[28] Although less common, *V vulnificus* and *Aeromonas* species can also cause NSTI, with *V vulnificus* NSTI reported in a patient with hepatitis C who was evacuated from New Orleans following a boat rescue during Hurricane Katrina.[16] Cutaneous mucormycosis leading to NSTI has also been described in tsunami survivors with contaminated soft tissue injuries.[29,30] Subtle erythema and edema accompanied by pain out of proportion to physical findings can give way to skin bullae, ecchymosis, necrosis, and systemic toxicity. Progression of disease is often rapid, and death can ensue within hours of presentation. Prompt surgical debridement is combined with empiric broad-spectrum antibacterial or antifungal therapy (eg, liposomal amphotericin B), depending on the organism of concern, and fluid resuscitation.[12]

Clostridium tetani is a toxin-producing anaerobe naturally found in soil. An outbreak involving 106 cases of tetanus was reported a month after the 2014 Indian Ocean tsunami in Indonesia, where population tetanus immunization status was suboptimal at baseline.[31] Traumatic puncture wounds from debris inoculate *C tetani* spores into soft tissue. Subsequent germination and production of tetanus toxin lead to clinical symptoms after an incubation period of 3 to 21 days. With generalized tetanus, the most common form of the disease, painful, involuntary muscle spasm and rigidity frequently involve the jaw (trismus), neck, trunk, and extremities. Diagnosis of tetanus is clinical. Definitive treatment requires wound debridement for source control of spores, administration of human tetanus immune globulin (HTIG) to neutralize unbound toxin (passive immunization), active immunization with tetanus toxoid at a site different from that of HTIG, and initiation of antibiotic therapy (eg, metronidazole, penicillin G). As tetanus is a vaccine-preventable disease, appropriate wound care after a traumatic injury with active and passive immunization against tetanus based on US Centers for Disease Control and Prevention (CDC) guidelines is recommended when resources permit.[32]

GASTROINTESTINAL INFECTIONS

Diarrheal illnesses contribute up to 40% of deaths after a natural disaster, particularly in the setting of population displacement.[3] Contaminated food and water, disrupted sewage systems, compromised sanitation, poor hygiene, and crowded living situations can facilitate fecal-oral transmission of several gastrointestinal pathogens leading to outbreaks and even widespread epidemics of infectious diarrhea, particularly in resource-poor settings and developing countries. In the United States, flooding after several hydrologic disasters has also been associated with diarrheal illness.[33–37]

V cholerae remains a widespread cause of bacterial diarrheal illness globally, with significant morbidity and mortality. An estimated 2.9 million cases of cholera occur annually, resulting in 95,000 deaths across 69 endemic countries, with the greatest global burden of disease centered in sub-Saharan Africa and southeast Asia.[38] *V cholerae* was the most common cause of diarrhea during flood-associated diarrheal epidemics in 1988, 1998, 2004, and 2007 in Bangladesh, where the disease is endemic, significantly affecting older patients and those of lower socioeconomic status.[39–41] In contrast, cholera is rare and sporadic in nonendemic countries such as the United States, with no direct flood-associated cases or epidemics identified after Hurricane Katrina in 2004 or Hurricane Rita in 2005 along the Louisiana Gulf Coast.[16,42] Transmitted through contaminated water, *V cholerae* causes a profuse, secretory diarrhea leading to dehydration, muscle cramps, electrolyte derangements, acute renal failure, altered mentation, and hypotension. Abdominal pain and vomiting are common early on. Definitive diagnosis of cholera is established through stool culture; basic laboratory testing can help identify patients with significant hypoglycemia and electrolyte losses. Treatment centers on aggressive fluid resuscitation and supportive care. Although often reserved for severe cases with significant volume depletion, antibiotic therapy reduces duration of illness, total stool volume, stool shedding of V cholerae, and fluid requirements.[43] Doxycycline, azithromycin, ciprofloxacin, and ceftriaxone are appropriate choices to treat V cholerae, depending on local antibiotic resistance patterns.[44]

Enterotoxigenic E coli has been a significant cause of epidemic diarrhea, particularly among children after flooding in Bangladesh.[39,41] Other enteric pathogens associated with diarrhea after floodwater exposure include Salmonella and Shigella species throughout parts of Asia.[40,45,46] In Massachusetts, the risk of Clostridium difficile infection increased in the 2 weeks following a flood.[47] Diarrhea accompanied by fever, bloody or mucoid stool, severe abdominal pain, or signs of sepsis should prompt stool testing for Salmonella, Shigella, Campylobacter, Yersinia, shiga toxin-producing E coli (0157), and C difficile with guideline-directed antibiotic therapy and fluid resuscitation when indicated.[44]

Norovirus is the most common cause of acute viral gastroenteritis worldwide. Low infectious dose, presence of virus in vomitus, and continued viral shedding in stool weeks after patient recovery make norovirus highly contagious.[48] This is further compounded by its stability on environmental surfaces. Following Hurricane Katrina, an outbreak of acute gastroenteritis caused by norovirus affected more than 1000 evacuees and relief workers in temporary shelter at Reliant Park in Houston, Texas, over a period of 11 days.[49,50] A smaller outbreak of what was likely norovirus occurred in an evacuation shelter in New York City after Hurricane Sandy in 2012.[51] Symptoms including nausea, vomiting, abdominal pain, and nonbloody diarrhea, with or without fever, usually develop within 2 to 3 days of infection. Diagnosis of norovirus is usually clinical, but can be confirmed using molecular or immunologic assays of stool specimens. Treatment, as with other acute viral gastroenteritis, is supportive, and infection prevention measures emphasizing hand hygiene, contact isolation, and rigorous environmental disinfection are critical to halting an outbreak.

Rotavirus was responsible for an outbreak of diarrheal illness in a temporary shelter in India following the 2004 Indian Ocean tsunami, and has been a frequent agent of flood-associated diarrhea in Bangladesh.[40,52] In 2014, rotavirus played a prevalent role in a diarrheal outbreak in Honiara following significant flooding and population displacement that subsequently evolved into a nationwide epidemic throughout the Solomon Islands.[53]

Hepatitis A virus (HAV) and hepatitis E virus (HEV) are endemic in many developing countries, with the greatest mortality reported in sub-Saharan Africa and Asia.[54] Both viruses are transmitted through contaminated food and water and thrive in poor sanitary conditions. Flood-associated outbreaks of HAV and HEV have been reported previously in Sudan and India.[55,56] Severe flooding in 2007 in Anhui Province, China, was significantly associated with an increased incidence of HAV infection in affected areas.[57] In Bangladesh, increased incidence of HEV infection after flooding has been attributed to sewage contamination of piped water, with high mortality rates reported among women in the third trimester of pregnancy.[58] Symptoms can include fever, fatigue, nausea, vomiting, abdominal pain, and jaundice. Most infections are self-limited; a small fraction can progress to acute liver failure. Although HAV infection is readily diagnosed by serology, testing options for HEV may vary and are more limited in availability. Treatment is supportive and should focus on fluid resuscitation and avoiding further hepatic insult. HAV infection is preventable through widely available vaccines; in contrast, HEV vaccines may be more challenging to access.

RESPIRATORY INFECTIONS

Acute respiratory infections are common following natural disasters, particularly among displaced populations and young children.[2] Although data are limited, excess morbidity and mortality caused by acute respiratory infections is significant in crisis-affected populations, with case fatality rates as high as 35%.[59] Overcrowding, poor nutrition, and lack of health care are significant risk factors for infection. The incidence of acute respiratory tract infections increased from 295 to 1205 per 100,000 residents in a Nicaraguan municipality immediately after Hurricane Mitch in 1998.[60] Following the 2014 Indian Ocean tsunami, syndromic surveillance identified more than 50,000 cases of acute respiratory infection among survivors in Aceh Province, Indonesia.[61] Acute respiratory infections have likewise been common following several large hydrologic disasters in the United States.[11,33,35,36,62,63] Pertussis was diagnosed in an infant who was rescued from a rooftop in New Orleans after Hurricane Katrina.[11] In most instances, upper respiratory infections are viral in origin, while lower respiratory infections (pneumonia) are likely attributable to common bacterial (eg, *Streptococcus pneumoniae*) and viral pathogens. Management should follow standard clinical practices.

Immersion and near-drowning after a hydrologic event can lead to aspiration of contaminated floodwater, with subsequent inoculation of bacteria into the respiratory tract. Following the 2004 Indian Ocean tsunami, multiple cases of gram-negative and polymicrobial aspiration pneumonitis and pneumonia were reported among survivors.[21,26,64–66] Common gram-negative organisms isolated in sputum culture included *P aeruginosa*, *Klebsiella* species, *E coli*, and *Aeromonas* species. Among severely injured European tourists repatriated to their native countries following the tsunami, several multidrug-resistant gram-negative organisms were recovered from upper respiratory cultures, likely acquired from environmental and healthcare exposure.[21] Aspiration-related melioidosis, manifesting with multilobar pneumonia, pulmonary abscess, and sepsis, was also reported in Thailand and Indonesia among tsunami survivors.[64,67] Although *B pseudomallei* is endemic to southeast Asia and northern Australia, sporadic cases of melioidosis have been described in the Americas, with 1 case occurring after floodwater exposure in Puerto Rico.[68] Inhalation of aerosolized particles (eg, high-pressure washing of contaminated environments) may also predispose individuals to gram-negative and polymicrobial pneumonia during the postimpact phase after a hydrologic event.[6] In general, patients with pneumonia not responding to conventional antibiotic regimens for community-acquired pneumonia should undergo microbiological investigation for unusual or polymicrobial infections.

Pulmonary tuberculosis can present unique challenges to public health after a hydrologic disaster when populations are displaced. Following Hurricane Katrina, a homeless man who was evacuated from New Orleans to Philadelphia was identified on entry screening with suspicious symptoms, isolated, and diagnosed with tuberculosis.[11] Additional new tuberculosis cases were identified among evacuees to 3 other states.[69] All the while, intense public health efforts were underway to track 195 individuals with known tuberculosis throughout Alabama, Louisiana, and Mississippi to confirm continuation of their treatment.[11] Transmitted through airborne droplet nuclei, *Mycobacterium tuberculosis* can linger for hours in enclosed and poorly ventilated spaces, posing significant infection risks in crowded living conditions. Chronic cough (>3 weeks), fever, chills, night sweats, and recent weight loss in high-risk patients (eg, immunosuppression, drug use, incarceration, close household contact with another person with pulmonary tuberculosis, or birth in a tuberculosis-endemic region) should all raise concern for tuberculosis.

ZOONOTIC INFECTIONS

Zoonotic infections stem from pathogens that are transmitted from animals to people. Chief among these, leptospirosis is a significant concern after hydrologic events associated with flooding and population displacement. More than a million estimated cases of leptospirosis contribute upwards of 59,000 deaths annually, with the highest morbidity and mortality seen in resource-poor countries.[70] Leptospirosis is caused by spirochetes from the genus *Leptospira*, which are free-living in freshwater and moist soil, and widely distributed in temperate and tropical regions around the world. Animals, particularly rodents, can become infected and serve as reservoirs, shedding high concentrations of *Leptospira* in urine back into the environment. Subsequent human infection occurs when nonintact skin (eg, abrasions or lacerations) and mucous membranes (conjunctiva, nasopharynx) come in direct contact with contaminated water and other environmental sources of *Leptospira*. Leptospirosis is common in endemic regions in the setting of heavy rainfall, freshwater flooding, increases in rodent population due to poor sanitation, and situations that place rodents and people in close proximity with one another.[2] Several outbreaks have been reported after flooding related to typhoons and unusually heavy rainfall throughout southeast Asia, Australia, and South America.[71-77] A fourfold increase in leptospirosis cases was identified in Puerto Rico shortly after Hurricane Hortense in 1996.[78] Another rise in cases in Puerto Rico following Hurricane Maria in late 2017 remains under investigation.

After a 5 to 14 day incubation period, patients with leptospirosis develop a flu-like illness with fever, chills, malaise, myalgias, headache, cough, nausea, vomiting, and diarrhea. Conjunctival suffusion is often present. Most cases of leptospirosis are self-limited; however, a subset can be complicated by aseptic meningitis, jaundice, renal failure, pulmonary hemorrhage, or acute respiratory distress syndrome. Diagnosis of leptospirosis is often clinical as confirmatory laboratory testing may take considerable time, depending on availability. Serology (eg, microscopic agglutination test, enzyme-linked immunosorbent assay) and increasingly molecular diagnostics (eg, polymerase chain reaction assay) support definitive diagnosis; blood culture has low sensitivity and can take several weeks. Antibiotic therapy for mild cases should consist of oral doxycycline or amoxicillin; intravenous penicillin or ceftriaxone is used to treat severe disease. Those with severe disease may require hospital admission, renal replacement therapy, ventilatory support, or even extracorporeal membrane oxygenation (ECMO).[79] Chemoprophylaxis with doxycycline following severe floods in endemic countries after high-risk exposure and during outbreaks may be effective in reducing leptospirosis cases.[73,76,80]

Animal bites are a common traumatic injury following the displacement of human and animal populations. After Hurricane Ike in 2008, many bites resulted from contact with domesticated pets (primarily dogs and cats) known to victims, some complicated by soft tissue infection.[81] Delayed wound care and lack of antibiotic prophylaxis can increase the risk for infections related to oral flora of the biting animal or human skin flora, particularly with deep wounds. Canine and feline oral flora include *Pasteurella multocida*, *Capnocytophaga canimorsus*, *Staphylococcus*, *Streptococcus*, and anaerobes; *Bartonella henselae* is found primarily in cat saliva.[82] Antibiotic prophylaxis after a dog or cat bite with amoxicillin-clavulanate provides adequate coverage in many instances.[12] Mild infections can likewise be treated with amoxicillin-clavulanate if MRSA is not a concern; severe infections may be treated with ampicillin-sulbactam or other broad-spectrum antibiotic regimens with coverage of anaerobes and antibiotic-resistant organisms when appropriate. Management of infections related to unusual and uncommon types of animal bites should be based on anticipated oral flora, wound culture, and infectious disease consultation.[82]

Although rare in the United States and other countries with established animal vaccination programs, rabies remains endemic in many parts of the world, with infections largely attributed to animal bites, primarily involving dogs.[83] Prophylaxis following an animal bite or other high-risk contact (eg, bat exposure), including the administration of human rabies immune globulin (HRIG) and rabies vaccine, should be guided by local epidemiology, risk assessment, public health infrastructure for animal testing and monitoring, and availability of HRIG and vaccine in resource-limited settings.[84,85]

VECTOR-BORNE DISEASES

Infectious diseases transmitted by arthropod vectors, particularly mosquitos, are variably influenced by hydrologic disasters and their aftermath in endemic regions. Initial high winds and heavy flooding can reduce vector populations and disrupt existing breeding sites, decreasing the risk of infection during the impact phase. Standing water left behind may establish new vector breeding sites in the postimpact and recovery phase. Differing levels of exposure to disease-carrying vectors and active public health interventions to control vectors further shape the landscape of vector-borne disease after a hydrologic disaster.

Dengue virus (DENV) is an arthropod-borne virus (arbovirus) that is transmitted by the *Aedes aegypti* and *Aedes albopictus* mosquito. Common throughout the tropics, DENV is responsible for an estimated 390 million infections annually, of which a quarter manifest with clinically significant disease.[86] Heavy precipitation and other climatic changes have predicted increases in DENV infection in several endemic regions weeks to months later.[87–90] In Cuba, heavy rainfall from Hurricane Michelle may have further potentiated an ongoing DENV outbreak in 2001.[91] Severe flooding may have a similar additive effect in endemic resource-poor settings, as seen in 2010 during a severe DENV epidemic in Pakistan.[92] Dengue cases briefly exceeded epidemic threshold 2 months after Typhoon Haiyan struck the Philippines in late 2013; however, no large outbreak occurred due in large part to aggressive nationwide vector control activities in affected areas.[93] A similar response following flash flooding in Honiara, Solomon Islands, likely also prevented any large DENV outbreaks despite significant population displacement.[94]

Symptoms of DENV infection, including fever, headache, retro-orbital pain, arthralgias, myalgias, rash, and hemorrhagic manifestations (eg, epistaxis, gingival bleeding, petechia, ecchymosis, gastrointestinal bleeding, or vaginal bleeding), develop within 4 to 7 days after inoculation. Leukopenia, thrombocytopenia, and transaminitis are common. A fraction of patients may develop severe disease with plasma leakage, severe bleeding, hypotension, and multiorgan failure. Diagnosis of DENV infection is clinical. Laboratory confirmation is made by serologic or molecular testing (reverse transcriptase polymerase chain reaction, RT-PCR). Treatment is supportive, with aggressive fluid hydration and administration of acetaminophen for fever and pain control.[95] Aspirin, ibuprofen, and other nonsteroidal anti-inflammatory drugs are to be avoided given the risk of exacerbating bleeding. Management of severe DENV infection may require critical care interventions including blood transfusion, renal replacement therapy, and hemodynamic support with vasopressors.

Malaria is a protozoal infection that is transmitted by the *Anopheles* mosquito throughout most tropical regions. In 2013, an estimated 95 to 284 million cases occurred worldwide, resulting in anywhere from 703,000 to 1,032,000 deaths.[96] Of the 5 species known to cause human disease, *Plasmodium falciparum* accounts for most worldwide disease and associated mortality. Malaria outbreaks have been reported after heavy rainfall and severe flooding in southeast Asia and sub-Saharan Africa where disease is endemic and populations are highly vulnerable to infection.[97–100] In 1963, Haiti was the site of a malaria epidemic totaling some 75,000 cases following heavy rainfall and flooding from Hurricane Flora 2 months prior.[101]

The incubation period for malaria ranges anywhere from 7 to 30 days, depending on the infecting *Plasmodium* species. Initial symptoms are protean including fever, chills, rigors, diaphoresis, malaise, myalgias, arthralgias, headache, cough, nausea, vomiting, abdominal pain, and diarrhea. As the infection progresses, fever can become cyclic. With severe malaria, patients may develop significant anemia, altered mental status (including encephalopathy with cerebral malaria), renal failure, liver failure, coagulopathy, metabolic acidosis, acute respiratory distress syndrome, and septic shock. Diagnosis is classically made by identification and quantification of parasitemia in thick and thin blood smears with light microscopy. In resource-limited settings and endemic countries, rapid detection tests (RDTs) targeting specific antigens have emerged as a reliable means for diagnosing uncomplicated *P falciparum* malaria.[102] A positive RDT is highly specific for *P falciparum*, but a negative result cannot rule infection. It is recommended that all RDTs be confirmed with traditional blood smears. Antimalarial therapy is imperative and should be guided by prevailing regional malaria epidemiology and drug resistance patterns.[103,104] Young children, immunocompromised patients, those with severe malaria and/or high parasitemia, and other patients at high-risk for complications should be hospitalized for treatment and may require critical care.

HUMAN REMAINS AND INFECTIOUS DISEASES

Human remains and their potential to spread infectious diseases after a natural disaster have long been a concern among many. However, most initial deaths associated with a hydrologic disaster are caused by traumatic injuries or drowning and not infection. Human remains pose little risk to the general public in regions not endemic for certain infectious diseases (eg, *V cholerae*, *M tuberculosis*).[105–108] No known epidemics of infectious disease after recent natural disasters have been attributed to the presence of human remains.[108]

Without a living human host, most medically significant pathogens do not survive for a considerable time, particularly in the setting of desiccation. Although bloodborne pathogens (eg, human immunodeficiency virus, hepatitis C virus) can persist in human remains, infection generally requires body fluid exposure with nonintact skin or mucous membranes or a percutaneous injury (eg, needle, bone fragment).[105] In regions with endemic infectious diseases, human remains resulting from a hydrologic disaster are unlikely to transmit infection except in unique circumstances. For example, *V cholerae* is environmentally resilient and naturally exists in aquatic environments. Corpses harboring *V cholerae* could contaminate drinking water sources during an ongoing epidemic, contributing to spread of disease alongside more significant factors (eg, overcrowding, poor sanitation), but are not likely to be the primary trigger for an epidemic.[108] Remains of a person with pulmonary tuberculosis in which respirations have ceased are unlikely to disseminate *M tuberculosis,* although certain precautions should be taken to further reduce exposure (eg, covering the mouth of the body to prevent escape of air and ensuring adequate ventilation of the surrounding environment during handling of remains).[105] Avoiding death rituals that involve close unprotected family contact with corpses associated with pathogens known to be transmitted in this manner (eg, *V cholerae*, Ebola virus) is highly prudent, irrespective of a coinciding hydrologic disaster.[109,110] In general, the risk of infectious diseases from human remains is negligible compared with that of survivors of a disaster.

GUIDANCE FOR EMERGENCY RESPONDERS

Prevention of infectious diseases following a hydrologic disaster requires systems-based public health and emergency management strategies that address population displacement. Evacuation of survivors from contaminated environments and access to safe shelter, clean water and food, and basic health care services are integral components of a coordinated disaster response. Avoidance of overcrowding, promotion of personal hygiene, restoration of a functional sanitation infrastructure, and aggressive vector control in vulnerable regions help further mitigate the risk of communicable infectious diseases. Awareness of the spectrum of infectious disease possible after a hydrologic disaster informs early recognition, definitive diagnosis, and management, and helps prevent transmission to others, depending on the causative pathogen.

Emergency physicians, nurses, fire and emergency medical services professionals, and other first responders providing aid in a hydrologic disaster can reduce their risk of infectious disease through preparation, attention to preventive health, and use of appropriate personal protective equipment. Prior to a disaster, providers should ensure they are current with routinely recommended immunizations, including tetanus and influenza, in accordance with annual CDC guidance (www.cdc.gov/vaccines/schedules/hcp/adult.html). In addition, health care professionals should receive immunization against hepatitis B virus; those anticipating responses in countries with high or intermediate hepatitis A endemicity should also receive HAV immunization. Other immunizations related to responses outside the United States may be considered in consultation with an infectious disease or travel medicine specialist, or based on routinely updated recommendations for travelers, such as the CDC Yellow Book (www.cdc.gov/travel).

At the time of disaster, medical planning should include information gathering about ongoing infectious disease outbreaks as well as diseases endemic to the anticipated area of operations, particularly if deploying internationally. The CDC travelers' health Web site (including the Yellow Book) and International Society for Infectious Diseases' internet-based Program for Monitoring Emerging Diseases (ProMed; www.promedmail.org) are regularly updated resources that provide timely information for assessing infectious disease risks by geographic region. If mosquitos and other arthropods are likely to be a concern, appropriate clothing minimizing exposed skin and use of insect repellent can help reduce bites, particularly important in areas with known endemic vector-borne diseases. Likewise, chemoprophylaxis for certain endemic diseases (eg, malaria and leptospirosis) may be considered, particularly if high-risk exposures are anticipated (eg, sleeping outdoors and immersion in contaminated water).

Use of appropriate personal protective equipment while providing health care after a hydrologic disaster should follow standard precautions; transmission-based precautions (eg, airborne, droplet, and contact precautions) should be guided by clinical suspicion for certain pathogens, particularly when caring for a patient with respiratory complaints, uncontrolled diarrhea, or draining wounds. Hand hygiene underpins all infection prevention practices, perhaps even more so in disaster settings where resources are limited. For rescuers and those likely to be significantly exposed or immersed in floodwater, protective clothing and equipment minimizing skin and mucous membrane contact with contaminated water are advised whenever possible. Following such exposures, clothing, equipment, and responders should undergo decontamination (eg, soap and clean water) to remove residual microbial and chemical burden from floodwater. For those likely to navigate through or handle debris, appropriate head protection, eyewear, work gloves, and boots protect against traumatic injury in contaminated environments. Masks or respirators may be considered if there is potential for aerosolization of floodwater or other environmental particulates. Growing literature focusing on emergency responders and deployment health during past hydrologic disasters can help inform future preventive strategies.[111–113]

Access to safe, uncontaminated food and water is critical to preventing infectious diseases among disaster responders as much as it is to the affected populations they serve. Responders should remain vigilant for signs or symptoms of infection and seek medical care when indicated during and after participation in disaster aid, as some illnesses may not clinically manifest until after returning home.

SUMMARY

Infectious diseases have long been associated with hydrologic events and their aftermath, although outbreaks are uncommon in developed countries with intact emergency management and public health infrastructures. Most communicable infections surface among displaced populations in the setting of inadequate shelter, overcrowding, poor sanitation, and lack of access to clean food and water. Increased awareness and knowledge of the potential infectious disease risks after a hydrologic disaster optimize emergency care to survivors and safeguards the health of disaster responders.

REFERENCES

1. Lechat MF. The epidemiology of health effects of disasters. Epidemiol Rev 1990; 12:192–8.
2. Watson JT, Gayer M, Connolly MA. Epidemics after natural disasters. Emerg Infect Dis 2007;13:1–5.
3. Kouadio IK, Aljunid S, Kamigaki T, et al. Infectious diseases following natural disasters: prevention and control measures. Expert Rev Anti Infect Ther 2012;10: 95–104.
4. Ivers LC, Ryan ET. Infectious diseases of severe weather-related and flood-related natural disasters. Curr Opin Infect Dis 2006;19:408–14.
5. Cann KF, Thomas DR, Salmon RL, et al. Extreme water-related weather events and waterborne disease. Epidemiol Infect 2013;141:671–86.
6. Allworth A. Infectious disease considerations related to sudden flooding disasters for the emergency physician. Emerg Med Australas 2011;23:120–2.
7. Lee SH, Choi CP, Eun HC, et al. Skin problems after a tsunami. J Eur Acad Dermatol Venereol 2006;20:860–3.
8. Tempark T, Lueangarun S, Chatproedprai S, et al. Flood-related skin diseases: a literature review. Int J Dermatol 2013;52:1168–76.
9. Bandino JP, Hang A, Norton SA. The infectious and noninfectious dermatological consequences of flooding: a field manual for the responding provider. Am J Clin Dermatol 2015;16:399–424.
10. Dayrit JF, Bintanjoyo L, Andersen LK, et al. Impact of climate change on dermatological conditions related to flooding: update from the International Society of Dermatology Climate Change Committee. Int J Dermatol 2018; 57(8):901–10.

11. Centers for Disease Control and Prevention. Infectious disease and dermatologic conditions in evacuees and rescue workers after Hurricane Katrina–multiple states, August-September, 2005. MMWR Morb Mortal Wkly Rep 2005;54: 961–4.

12. Stevens DL, Bisno AL, Chambers HF, et al. Practice guidelines for the diagnosis and management of skin and soft tissue infections: 2014 update by the Infectious Diseases Society of America. Clin Infect Dis 2014;59:147–59.

13. Lim PL. Wound infections in tsunami survivors: a commentary. Ann Acad Med Singapore 2005;34:582–5.

14. Diaz JH, Lopez FA. Skin, soft tissue and systemic bacterial infections following aquatic injuries and exposures. Am J Med Sci 2015;349:269–75.

15. Strom MS, Paranjpye RN. Epidemiology and pathogenesis of Vibrio vulnificus. Microbes Infect 2000;2:177–88.

16. Centers for Disease Control and Prevention. *Vibrio* illnesses after Hurricane Katrina–multiple states, August-September 2005. MMWR Morb Mortal Wkly Rep 2005;54:928–31.

17. Liu JW, Lee IK, Tang HJ, et al. Prognostic factors and antibiotics in *Vibrio vulnificus* septicemia. Arch Intern Med 2006;166:2117–23.

18. Chao WN, Tsai CF, Chang HR, et al. Impact of timing of surgery on outcome of *Vibrio vulnificus*-related necrotizing fasciitis. Am J Surg 2013;206:32–9.

19. Hiransuthikul N, Tantisiriwat W, Lertutsahakul K, et al. Skin and soft-tissue infections among tsunami survivors in southern Thailand. Clin Infect Dis 2005;41: e93–6.

20. Presley SM, Rainwater TR, Austin GP, et al. Assessment of pathogens and toxicants in New Orleans, LA, following Hurricane Katrina. Environ Sci Technol 2006;40:468–74.

21. Maegele M, Gregor S, Steinhausen E, et al. The long-distance tertiary air transfer and care of tsunami victims: injury pattern and microbiological and psychological aspects. Crit Care Med 2005;33:1136–40.

22. Doung-ngern P, Vatanaprasan T, Chungpaibulpatana J, et al. Infections and treatment of wounds in survivors of the 2004 Tsunami in Thailand. Int Wound J 2009;6:347–54.

23. Lin PC, Lin HJ, Guo HR, et al. Epidemiological characteristics of lower extremity cellulitis after a typhoon flood. PLoS One 2013;8:e65655.

24. Nieminen T, Vaara M. *Burkholderia pseudomallei* infections in Finnish tourists injured by the December 2004 tsunami in Thailand. Euro Surveill 2005;10: E050303.4.

25. Svensson E, Welinder-Olsson C, Claesson BA, et al. Cutaneous melioidosis in a Swedish tourist after the tsunami in 2004. Scand J Infect Dis 2006;38:71–4.

26. Garzoni C, Emonet S, Legout L, et al. Atypical infections in tsunami survivors. Emerg Infect Dis 2005;11:1591–3.

27. Appelgren P, Farnebo F, Dotevall L, et al. Late-onset posttraumatic skin and soft-tissue infections caused by rapid-growing mycobacteria in tsunami survivors. Clin Infect Dis 2008;47:e11–6.

28. Long SW, Kachroo P, Musser JM, et al. Whole-genome sequencing of a human clinical isolate of emm28 *Streptococcus pyogenes* causing necrotizing fasciitis acquired contemporaneously with Hurricane Harvey. Genome Announc 2017;5 [pii:e01269-17].

29. Andresen D, Donaldson A, Choo L, et al. Multifocal cutaneous mucormycosis complicating polymicrobial wound infections in a tsunami survivor from Sri Lanka. Lancet 2005;365:876–8.

30. Snell BJ, Tavakoli K. Necrotizing fasciitis caused by *Apophysomyces elegans* complicating soft-tissue and pelvic injuries in a tsunami survivor from Thailand. Plast Reconstr Surg 2007;119:448–9.

31. Aceh Epidemiology Group. Outbreak of tetanus cases following the tsunami in Aceh Province, Indonesia. Glob Public Health 2006;1:173–7.

32. Liang JL, Tiwari T, Moro P, et al. Prevention of pertussis, tetanus, and diphtheria with vaccines in the United States: recommendations of the Advisory Committee on Immunization Practices (ACIP). MMWR Recomm Rep 2018;67:1–44.

33. Centers for Disease Control and Prevention. Tropical Storm Allison rapid needs assessment–Houston, Texas, June 2001. MMWR Morb Mortal Wkly Rep 2002; 51:365–9.

34. Wade TJ, Sandhu SK, Levy D, et al. Did a severe flood in the Midwest cause an increase in the incidence of gastrointestinal symptoms? Am J Epidemiol 2004; 159:398–405.

35. Centers for Disease Control and Prevention. Hurricane Ike rapid needs assessment - Houston, Texas, September 2008. MMWR Morb Mortal Wkly Rep 2009; 58:1066–71.

36. Noe RS, Schnall AH, Wolkin AF, et al. Disaster-related injuries and illnesses treated by American Red Cross disaster health services during Hurricanes Gustav and Ike. South Med J 2013;106:102–8.

37. Wade TJ, Lin CJ, Jagai JS, et al. Flooding and emergency room visits for gastrointestinal illness in Massachusetts: a case-crossover study. PLoS One 2014;9: e110474.

38. Ali M, Nelson AR, Lopez AL, et al. Updated global burden of cholera in endemic countries. PLoS Negl Trop Dis 2015;9:e0003832.

39. Qadri F, Khan AI, Faruque AS, et al. Enterotoxigenic *Escherichia coli* and *Vibrio cholerae* diarrhea, Bangladesh, 2004. Emerg Infect Dis 2005;11:1104–7.

40. Schwartz BS, Harris JB, Khan AI, et al. Diarrheal epidemics in Dhaka, Bangladesh, during three consecutive floods: 1988, 1998, and 2004. Am J Trop Med Hyg 2006;74:1067–73.

41. Harris AM, Chowdhury F, Begum YA, et al. Shifting prevalence of major diarrheal pathogens in patients seeking hospital care during floods in 1998, 2004, and 2007 in Dhaka, Bangladesh. Am J Trop Med Hyg 2008;79:708–14.

42. Centers for Disease Control and Prevention. Two cases of toxigenic *Vibrio cholerae* O1 infection after Hurricanes Katrina and Rita–Louisiana, October 2005. MMWR Morb Mortal Wkly Rep 2006;55:31–2.

43. Leibovici-Weissman Y, Neuberger A, Bitterman R, et al. Antimicrobial drugs for treating cholera. Cochrane Database Syst Rev 2014;(6):CD008625.

44. Shane AL, Mody RK, Crump JA, et al. 2017 Infectious Diseases Society of America clinical practice guidelines for the diagnosis and management of infectious diarrhea. Clin Infect Dis 2017;65:1963–73.

45. Vollaard AM, Ali S, van Asten HA, et al. Risk factors for typhoid and paratyphoid fever in Jakarta, Indonesia. JAMA 2004;291:2607–15.

46. Ni W, Ding G, Li Y, et al. Effects of the floods on dysentery in north central region of Henan Province, China from 2004 to 2009. J Infect 2014;69:430–9.

47. Lin CJ, Wade TJ, Hilborn ED. Flooding and *Clostridium difficile* infection: a case-crossover analysis. Int J Environ Res Public Health 2015;12:6948–64.

48. Atmar RL, Opekun AR, Gilger MA, et al. Determination of the 50% human infectious dose for Norwalk virus. J Infect Dis 2014;209:1016–22.

49. Centers for Disease Control and Prevention. Norovirus outbreak among evacuees from Hurricane Katrina–Houston, Texas, September 2005. MMWR Morb Mortal Wkly Rep 2005;54:1016–8.

50. Yee EL, Palacio H, Atmar RL, et al. Widespread outbreak of norovirus gastroenteritis among evacuees of Hurricane Katrina residing in a large "megashelter" in Houston, Texas: lessons learned for prevention. Clin Infect Dis 2007;44:1032–9.

51. Ridpath AD, Bregman B, Jones L, et al. Challenges to implementing communicable disease surveillance in New York City evacuation shelters after Hurricane Sandy, November 2012. Public Health Rep 2015;130:48–53.

52. Sugunan AP, Roy S, Murhekar MV, et al. Outbreak of rotaviral diarrhoea in a relief camp for tsunami victims at Car Nicobar Island, India. J Public Health (Oxf) 2007;29:449–50.

53. Jones FK, Ko AI, Becha C, et al. Increased rotavirus prevalence in diarrheal outbreak precipitated by localized flooding, Solomon Islands, 2014. Emerg Infect Dis 2016;22:875–9.

54. Stanaway JD, Flaxman AD, Naghavi M, et al. The global burden of viral hepatitis from 1990 to 2013: findings from the Global Burden of Disease Study 2013. Lancet 2016;388:1081–8.

55. McCarthy MC, He J, Hyams KC, et al. Acute hepatitis E infection during the 1988 floods in Khartoum, Sudan. Trans R Soc Trop Med Hyg 1994;88:177.

56. Pal S, Juyal D, Sharma M, et al. An outbreak of hepatitis A virus among children in a flood rescue camp: a post-disaster catastrophe. Indian J Med Microbiol 2016;34:233–6.

57. Gao L, Zhang Y, Ding G, et al. Identifying flood-related infectious diseases in Anhui Province, China: a spatial and temporal analysis. Am J Trop Med Hyg 2016;94:741–9.

58. Mamun Al M, Rahman S, Khan M, et al. HEV infection as an aetiologic factor for acute hepatitis: experience from a tertiary hospital in Bangladesh. J Health Popul Nutr 2009;27:14–9.

59. Bellos A, Mulholland K, O'Brien KL, et al. The burden of acute respiratory infections in crisis-affected populations: a systematic review. Confl Health 2010;4:3.

60. Campanella N. Infectious diseases and natural disasters: the effects of Hurricane Mitch over Villanueva municipal area, Nicaragua. Public Health Rev 1999;27:311–9.

61. World Health Organization. Epidemic-prone disease surveillance and response after the tsunami in Aceh Province, Indonesia. Wkly Epidemiol Rec 2005;80:160–4.

62. Centers for Disease Control and Prevention. Surveillance in hurricane evacuation centers–Louisiana, September-October 2005. MMWR Morb Mortal Wkly Rep 2006;55:32–5.

63. Centers for Disease Control and Prevention. Injury and illness surveillance in hospitals and acute-care facilities after Hurricanes Katrina And Rita–New Orleans area, Louisiana, September 25-October 15, 2005. MMWR Morb Mortal Wkly Rep 2006;55:35–8.

64. Athan E, Allworth AM, Engler C, et al. Melioidosis in tsunami survivors. Emerg Infect Dis 2005;11:1638–9.

65. Kateruttanakul P, Paovilai W, Kongsaengdao S, et al. Respiratory complication of tsunami victims in Phuket and Phang-Nga. J Med Assoc Thai 2005;88:754–8.

66. Yorsaengrat W, Chungpaibulpatana J, Tunki B, et al. Respiratory complication of tsunami diaster victims in Vachira Phuket Hospital. J Med Assoc Thai 2006;89:518–21.

67. Chierakul W, Winothai W, Wattanawaitunechai C, et al. Melioidosis in 6 tsunami survivors in southern Thailand. Clin Infect Dis 2005;41:982–90.

68. Christenson B, Fuxench Z, Morales JA, et al. Severe community-acquired pneumonia and sepsis caused by *Burkholderia pseudomallei* associated with flooding in Puerto Rico. Bol Asoc Med P R 2003;95:17–20.

69. Centers for Disease Control and Prevention. Tuberculosis control activities after Hurricane Katrina–New Orleans, Louisiana, 2005. MMWR Morb Mortal Wkly Rep 2006;55:332–5.

70. Costa F, Hagan JE, Calcagno J, et al. Global morbidity and mortality of leptospirosis: a systematic review. PLoS Negl Trop Dis 2015;9:e0003898.

71. Kawaguchi L, Sengkeopraseuth B, Tsuyuoka R, et al. Seroprevalence of leptospirosis and risk factor analysis in flood-prone rural areas in Lao PDR. Am J Trop Med Hyg 2008;78:957–61.

72. Su HP, Chan TC, Chang CC. Typhoon-related leptospirosis and melioidosis, Taiwan, 2009. Emerg Infect Dis 2011;17:1322–4.

73. Dechet AM, Parsons M, Rambaran M, et al. Leptospirosis outbreak following severe flooding: a rapid assessment and mass prophylaxis campaign; Guyana, January-February 2005. PLoS One 2012;7:e39672.

74. Amilasan AS, Ujiie M, Suzuki M, et al. Outbreak of leptospirosis after flood, the Philippines, 2009. Emerg Infect Dis 2012;18:91–4.

75. Smith JK, Young MM, Wilson KL, et al. Leptospirosis following a major flood in Central Queensland, Australia. Epidemiol Infect 2013;141:585–90.

76. Chusri S, McNeil EB, Hortiwakul T, et al. Single dosage of doxycycline for prophylaxis against leptospiral infection and leptospirosis during urban flooding in southern Thailand: a non-randomized controlled trial. J Infect Chemother 2014;20:709–15.

77. Mohd Radi MF, Hashim JH, Jaafar MH, et al. Leptospirosis outbreak after the 2014 major flooding event in Kelantan, Malaysia: a spatial-temporal analysis. Am J Trop Med Hyg 2018;98:1281–95.

78. Sanders EJ, Rigau-Perez JG, Smits HL, et al. Increase of leptospirosis in dengue-negative patients after a hurricane in Puerto Rico in 1996 [correction of 1966]. Am J Trop Med Hyg 1999;61:399–404.

79. Delmas B, Jabot J, Chanareille P, et al. Leptospirosis in ICU: a retrospective study of 134 consecutive admissions. Crit Care Med 2018;46:93–9.

80. Schneider MC, Velasco-Hernandez J, Min KD, et al. The use of chemoprophylaxis after floods to reduce the occurrence and impact of leptospirosis outbreaks. Int J Environ Res Public Health 2017;14.

81. Warner GS. Increased incidence of domestic animal bites following a disaster due to natural hazards. Prehosp Disaster Med 2010;25:188–90.

82. Abrahamian FM, Goldstein EJ. Microbiology of animal bite wound infections. Clin Microbiol Rev 2011;24:231–46.

83. Hampson K, Coudeville L, Lembo T, et al. Estimating the global burden of endemic canine rabies. PLoS Negl Trop Dis 2015;9:e0003709.

84. Manning SE, Rupprecht CE, Fishbein D, et al. Human rabies prevention–United States, 2008: recommendations of the Advisory Committee on Immunization Practices. MMWR Recomm Rep 2008;57:1–28.

85. Rupprecht CE, Briggs D, Brown CM, et al. Use of a reduced (4-dose) vaccine schedule for postexposure prophylaxis to prevent human rabies: recommendations of the Advisory Committee on Immunization Practices. MMWR Recomm Rep 2010;59:1–9.

86. Bhatt S, Gething PW, Brady OJ, et al. The global distribution and burden of dengue. Nature 2013;496:504–7.

87. Hashizume M, Dewan AM, Sunahara T, et al. Hydroclimatological variability and dengue transmission in Dhaka, Bangladesh: a time-series study. BMC Infect Dis 2012;12:98.

88. Sang S, Gu S, Bi P, et al. Predicting unprecedented dengue outbreak using imported cases and climatic factors in Guangzhou, 2014. PLoS Negl Trop Dis 2015;9:e0003808.

89. Chuang TW, Chaves LF, Chen PJ. Effects of local and regional climatic fluctuations on dengue outbreaks in southern Taiwan. PLoS One 2017;12:e0178698.

90. Sirisena P, Noordeen F, Kurukulasuriya H, et al. Effect of climatic factors and population density on the distribution of dengue in Sri Lanka: a GIS based evaluation for prediction of outbreaks. PLoS One 2017;12:e0166806.

91. Hsieh YH, de Arazoza H, Lounes R. Temporal trends and regional variability of 2001-2002 multiwave DENV-3 epidemic in Havana City: did Hurricane Michelle contribute to its severity? Trop Med Int Health 2013;18:830–8.

92. Hassan U, Loya A, Mehmood MT, et al. Dengue fever outbreak in Lahore. J Coll Physicians Surg Pak 2013;23:231–3.

93. Aumentado C, Cerro BR, Olobia L, et al. The prevention and control of dengue after Typhoon Haiyan. Western Pac Surveill Response J 2015;6(Suppl 1):60–5.

94. Shortus M, Musto J, Bugoro H, et al. Vector-control response in a post-flood disaster setting, Honiara, Solomon Islands, 2014. Western Pac Surveill Response J 2016;7:38–43.

95. World Health Organization. Dengue: guidelines for diagnosis, treatment, prevention and control. New edition. Geneva (Switzerland): World Health Organization; 2009.

96. Murray CJ, Ortblad KF, Guinovart C, et al. Global, regional, and national incidence and mortality for HIV, tuberculosis, and malaria during 1990-2013: a systematic analysis for the Global Burden of Disease Study 2013. Lancet 2014;384: 1005–70.

97. Brown V, Abdir Issak M, Rossi M, et al. Epidemic of malaria in north-eastern Kenya. Lancet 1998;352:1356–7.

98. Kondo H, Seo N, Yasuda T, et al. Post-flood–infectious diseases in Mozambique. Prehosp Disaster Med 2002;17:126–33.

99. Memon MS, Solangi S, Lakho S, et al. Morbidity and mortality of malaria during monsoon flood of 2011: South East Asia experience. Iran J Public Health 2014; 43:28–34.

100. Boyce R, Reyes R, Matte M, et al. Severe flooding and malaria transmission in the western Ugandan highlands: implications for disease control in an era of global climate change. J Infect Dis 2016;214:1403–10.

101. Mason J, Cavalie P. Malaria epidemic in Haiti following a hurricane. Am J Trop Med Hyg 1965;14:533–9.

102. Abba K, Deeks JJ, Olliaro P, et al. Rapid diagnostic tests for diagnosing uncomplicated P. falciparum malaria in endemic countries. Cochrane Database Syst Rev 2011;(7):CD008122.

103. Centers for Disease Control and Prevention. Guidelines for treatment of malaria in the United States. Atlanta (GA): Centers for Disease Control and Prevention; 2013.

104. World Health Organization. Guidelines for the treatment of malaria. 3rd edition. Geneva (Switzerland): World Health Organization; 2015.

105. Morgan O. Infectious disease risks from dead bodies following natural disasters. Rev Panam Salud Publica 2004;15:307–12.
106. de Ville de Goyet C. Epidemics caused by dead bodies: a disaster myth that does not want to die. Rev Panam Salud Publica 2004;15:297–9.
107. Kirkis EJ. A myth too tough to die: the dead of disasters cause epidemics of disease. Am J Infect Control 2006;34:331–4.
108. Pan American Health Organization. Management of dead bodies after disasters: a field manual for first responders. 2nd edition. Washington (DC): Pan American Health Organization; 2016.
109. Sack RB, Siddique AK. Corpses and the spread of cholera. Lancet 1998;352: 1570.
110. Dietz PM, Jambai A, Paweska JT, et al. Epidemiology and risk factors for Ebola virus disease in Sierra Leone-23 May 2014 to 31 January 2015. Clin Infect Dis 2015;61:1648–54.
111. O'Leary DR, Rigau-Perez JG, Hayes EB, et al. Assessment of dengue risk in relief workers in Puerto Rico after Hurricane Georges, 1998. Am J Trop Med Hyg 2002;66:35–9.
112. Tak S, Bernard BP, Driscoll RJ, et al. Floodwater exposure and the related health symptoms among firefighters in New Orleans, Louisiana 2005. Am J Ind Med 2007;50:377–82.
113. Rusiecki JA, Thomas DL, Chen L, et al. Disaster-related exposures and health effects among US Coast Guard responders to hurricanes Katrina and Rita: a cross-sectional study. J Occup Environ Med 2014;56:820–33.

Antimicrobial Stewardship in the Emergency Department

Michael Pulia, MD, MS[a],*, Robert Redwood, MD, MPH[b,1],
Larissa May, MD, MSPH[c]

KEYWORDS

- Antibiotics • Antimicrobial stewardship • Emergency department
- Quality improvement • Infectious diseases

KEY POINTS

- The emergency department is a critical setting for antimicrobial stewardship efforts given the frequency of infectious disease encounters and its major role in hospital admissions and acute care outpatient encounters.
- Institutional support, especially for a physician champion, is critical for the success of any emergency department–based antimicrobial stewardship intervention.
- The biomarker procalcitonin and influenza assays are effective means to differentiate viral from bacteria causes of respiratory tract infections and thereby safely reduce unnecessary antibiotic prescribing.
- Emergency department stewardship efforts for urinary tract infections should focus on avoiding routine screening urinalyses for patients without urinary complaints and reducing treatment of asymptomatic bacteriuria.
- Clinical cure rates for uncomplicated abscesses are marginally improved with antibiotics following incision and drainage. The decision to prescribe antibiotics should involve shared decision making, which includes discussion of the risk/benefit ratio.

Disclosure Statement: M. Pulia: Cempra (advisory board), Cepheid (grant funding, honoraria), Roche Diagnostics (grant funding), Thermo Fisher Scientific (advisory board, consulting). R. Redwood: No disclosures. L. May: Cepheid (grant funding, honoraria), Roche Diagnostics (grant funding, advisory board), BioFire (consulting).
Dr M. Pulia's effort on this article was supported in part by grant funding from the Agency for Healthcare Research and Quality (K08HS024342).
[a] BerbeeWalsh Department of Emergency Medicine, University of Wisconsin-Madison School of Medicine and Public Health, 800 University Bay Drive, Suite 300, Madison, WI 53705, USA;
[b] Department of Family Medicine and Community Health, University of Wisconsin Madison School of Medicine and Public Health, 1100 Delaplaine Ct, Madison, WI 53715; [c] Department of Emergency Medicine, University of California Davis, 4150 V Street, Suite 2100, Sacramento, CA 95817, USA
[1] Present address: 2817 New Pinery Road, Portage, WI 53901.
* Coresponding author. 800 University Bay Drive, Suite 310, Madison, WI 53705.
E-mail address: mspulia@medicine.wisc.edu

Emerg Med Clin N Am 36 (2018) 853–872
https://doi.org/10.1016/j.emc.2018.06.012
0733-8627/18/© 2018 Elsevier Inc. All rights reserved.
emed.theclinics.com

INTRODUCTION

Antimicrobials are unique among all classes of therapeutics in that they decrease in effectiveness over time and in direct relation to the frequency of use.[1] Pathogen resistance develops in response to selective pressure associated with all antibiotic prescribing but is accelerated by inappropriate use. Antimicrobials are critically important medications that affect not only the patient receiving them but also the surrounding community. A substantial increase in global rates of infections related to resistant pathogens, in combination with limited new antimicrobial agents in development, has raised concerns of an impending "postantibiotic era" with potential catastrophic consequences for human health.[2]

To address this public health crisis, tremendous efforts have begun to curb the widespread inappropriate use of antimicrobials in human health and agriculture.[3–5] Antimicrobial stewardship refers to efforts aimed at optimizing the use of anti-infective medications. There is a substantial body of literature supporting the ability of hospital antimicrobial stewardship programs to reduce costs while also exerting a positive impact on clinical outcomes.[6] The emergency department (ED) has traditionally been underrepresented as a focus for antimicrobial stewardship efforts. However, policy changes, such as the Joint Commission's antibiotic stewardship accreditation standard (enacted January 1, 2017) and inclusion of stewardship quality metrics in the Centers for Medicare & Medicaid Services Physician Quality Reporting System,[7,8] will increasingly require ED providers to engage in these efforts.[9] This review serves as a primer on antimicrobial stewardship tailored for emergency care providers. To achieve this, we present antimicrobial stewardship from a public health and individual patient safety perspective, review the key domains of stewardship, identify the ED as a critical setting for stewardship efforts, summarize commonly implemented stewardship interventions, and provide stewardship strategies for the most common bacterial infections encountered in the ED.

Public Health Impact of Antimicrobial Misuse

Antimicrobial resistance is a phenomenon in which antimicrobials apply selective pressure on pathogens that, in turn, develop defense mechanisms against that antimicrobial agent's mode of action.[10] Antimicrobial resistance has been occurring since the advent of the first antimicrobial agents; however, the speed and severity of this naturally occurring phenomenon is accelerated by the misuse of antimicrobials.[11] One recent example of this was the increase in macrolide prescribing throughout the 1990s (+388% in ambulatory care).[12,13] Streptococcus pneumoniae isolates resistance to macrolides rose dramatically during and after this time period, going from 10% in 1994 to 35% in 1995 and to 50% in 2009.[14]

From 2000 to 2010, antimicrobial use increased by 36% globally and the trend shows no signs of slowing.[15] Moreover, the United States uses a disproportionate amount of antimicrobials per capita, ranking third in the world for total antimicrobial consumption.[15] Antimicrobial resistance is widely regarded as a global epidemic and the conservative estimate for worldwide deaths directly attributable to antimicrobial resistance is 700,000 per year. That figure, however, is projected to swell to 10 million by the year 2050 if current trends continue.[11] Unchecked, the cumulative loss of economic output from antimicrobial resistance by 2050 would amount to 20 to 35 trillion US dollars or roughly double the current US gross domestic product.[11]

Patient Safety Aspects of Antimicrobial Prescribing

Inappropriate and excessive use of antimicrobials remains a major public health threat; however, messaging to health care professionals and the public has frequently overlooked individual patient safety concerns. Recent literature suggests that clinicians who demonstrated increased awareness of potential harm from antibiotics during the clinical decision-making process prescribed fewer antibiotics.[16] The risk of antibiotic-associated adverse events varies by class and the overall incidence may be 20%.[17,18] These adverse events can range from minor side effects (eg, diarrhea) to life threatening (eg, anaphylaxis). Antibiotics are the second most common cause of ED visits for adverse drug events with approximately 1 in 1000 prescriptions resulting in an ED visit.[18,19] Although penicillins and cephalosporins account for the highest volume of adverse drug events encountered in the ED, sulfonamides and clindamycin have the highest rates of adverse events per prescription.[18] Of increasing concern is the rising rate of *Clostridium difficile* infection (CDI) and resistant bacteria causing health care–associated infections. Antibiotics are the primary risk factor for development of CDI, estimated at nearly half a million cases and 15,000 attributable deaths each year.[20] Furthermore, an estimated 2 million illnesses and 23,000 deaths annually occur from resistant bacteria in the United States alone.[21]

The Five Ds of Antimicrobial Stewardship

The application of antimicrobial stewardship to human health care has focused on curbing inappropriate use. There are four "Ds" required for optimal antimicrobial prescribing: drug, dose, duration, de-escalation.[22] Ideally, the prescriber selects the right drug (eg, most narrow spectrum), at the right dose (eg, adjusted for patient renal function), for the right duration (eg, shortest to successfully treat infection), and considers de-escalation whenever possible (eg, narrow spectrum based on culture results). A fifth "D" of stewardship, which is perhaps most critical in the context of emergency care, is diagnosis. Prescribing of antibiotics for inappropriate diagnoses (ie, nonresponsive conditions) is prevalent in the ED for all common infection types. This includes upper respiratory tract infections (eg, bronchitis, sinusitis), urinary tract infections (UTI; eg, asymptomatic bacteriuria [ASB]), and skin and soft tissue infections (eg, pseudocellulitis).[23–28]

The Emergency Department: A Critical Setting for Antimicrobial Stewardship

The ED is increasingly the central hub of the US health care system. Annual ED visits continue to climb each year and according to National Hospital Ambulatory Medical Care Survey data annual US ED visits totaled 136.9 million or 43 per 100 persons in 2015.[29] The ED straddles the inpatient and outpatient environment, serving as the primary gateway of entry into the hospital (>80% of all of admissions) and a primary location for acute care encounters (>25%).[30,31] In fact, a recently published analysis of the US health care system concluded that roughly 50% of all medical care occurs in the ED.[32]

Infection is one of the most common reasons that patients seek acute, unscheduled care. The Centers for Disease Control and Prevention (CDC) estimate that 11% (16 million) of annual US ED diagnoses were related to infection.[33] Worsening infection also accounts for 11% of short-term readmissions following ED discharge among Medicare recipients.[34]

Reflecting the infection-related visit rates, antimicrobials are one of the most commonly prescribed drug classes in the ED. The CDC estimates that in 2015 US EDs generated more than 28 million antibiotic prescriptions.[29] Although national data specific to overall ED antibiotic prescribing appropriateness are lacking, a recent single center study in a Veterans Affairs hospital ED identified that 39% of all antimicrobial use was inappropriate.[35] This result is consistent with estimated inappropriate antibiotic use in the inpatient and outpatient clinic settings.[26,36,37]

Cost Impact of Stewardship Interventions

Although not specifically established for the ED setting, inpatient antimicrobial stewardship programs have had substantial cost savings for health systems. A 2016 meta-analysis identified that most stewardship intervention studies demonstrate significant cost savings, through reduced length of stay and drug costs, when included as an outcome.[38] Additionally, a 2017 meta-analysis reported significant reductions in colonization and infection with multidrug-resistance organisms (37%–51%) and CDI (32%).[39] These benefits are enhanced when paired with infection-control programs and CDI rates may be most directly affected by those stewardship programs that restrict use of certain antibiotics.[39,40] Reductions in difficult-to-treat health care–associated infections caused by resistant bacteria and CDIs would yield substantial cost savings for US hospitals given the associated increased lengths of stay and substantial penalties applied by Centers for Medicare & Medicaid Services related to these conditions.[41–43]

ANTIMICROBIAL STEWARDSHIP INTERVENTIONS FOR THE EMERGENCY DEPARTMENT

Antimicrobial stewardship interventions can generally be characterized into two broad categories: system-level and provider-level. An alternative method of categorizing stewardship interventions uses the classification of "horizontal" to indicate broad, system-level interventions aimed at reducing inappropriate antibiotic prescribing overall (eg, formulary restrictions), whereas "vertical" refers to interventions targeting specific antibiotics or infection types.[44] Naturally, there is some overlap between these classifications because antimicrobial stewardship interventions often involve multiple components and system-level care change processes often simultaneously influence behavior at the provider level. In 2016, a joint guideline on implementing antimicrobial stewardship programs was published by the Infectious Diseases Society of America and the Society for Healthcare Epidemiology of America.[45] This document includes evidence-based recommendations for the most commonly used stewardship interventions and is an excellent resource for those looking to initiate ED stewardship programs.[46]

OVERVIEW OF SYSTEMS-LEVEL INTERVENTIONS

Physician and pharmacist leadership is an essential first step when operationalizing an ED antimicrobial stewardship program. Antimicrobial stewardship efforts should be multidisciplinary, collaborative, patient-centered, and fully supported by hospital administrators. An ED physician champion can serve as liaison between the stewardship program leadership and front-line clinicians to facilitate intervention implementation and provision of bidirectional feedback. Successful antimicrobial stewardship in the ED is multifaceted; however, system-level interventions fit broadly into four categories: (1) culture follow-up programs, (2) formulary restrictions, (3) pharmacist initiatives, and (4) antibiograms.

Emergency Department Culture Follow-up Programs

In the ED setting, all patients diagnosed with an acute infection are discharged home without available culture and susceptibility results. As such, structured culture follow-up programs are one of the first process improvements that should be considered to improve antimicrobial stewardship in the ED. The basic concept of a structured culture follow-up program is that all clinical cultures are to be reviewed by ED staff with attention to any discrepancies between the empirically prescribed antimicrobial therapy and the reported culture and sensitivity. If a patient is receiving inappropriate or suboptimal antimicrobial therapy, the ED staff (typically a nurse or pharmacist) consults with the emergency physician and adjusts the regimen. If appropriate, a new prescription is called to the patient's outpatient pharmacy and the patient is contacted and counseled about the culture results and new antimicrobial prescription. Direct contact with the patient is key to effective stewardship, because staff may need to counsel patients about regimen compliance and answer any patient questions. As dedicated ED pharmacists become more commonplace, research suggests that the pharmacist-physician dyad outperforms the nurse-physician in this role.[47] One study found that having ED pharmacists take over the culture follow-up program saved 50 hours of cumulative emergency physician clinician time per month and decreased infection-related readmissions by 12% with no change in reported adverse drug events.[48]

Emergency Department Formulary Restrictions

Because the initial encounter for many episodes of care occurs in the ED, antimicrobial decisions made by emergency care providers often impact subsequent inpatient and outpatient therapy choices. As such, limiting the ED use of certain broad-spectrum antibiotics is one strategy to ensure that the efficacy of these agents is preserved over time.[49] A common method for implementing formulary restrictions is to establish a defined ED formulary that excludes specific antibiotics.[50] Another formulary restriction method is to establish ED criteria for use of certain antimicrobials. In this case, the ED prescriber must give their rationale for the selection of a particular antimicrobial. Typically, this is accomplished via computer-physician order entry, where the prescriber must select the criteria for use from a prepopulated menu.[51] The decision to restrict an antimicrobial or antimicrobial class is typically based on local resistance patterns and cost considerations when there is a less expensive but equally effective alternative antibiotic. Unintended consequences, such as delays in administration of broad-spectrum therapy in sepsis, should be considered in any formulary restriction policy.

Emergency Department Pharmacist

The presence of a dedicated ED pharmacist is often considered a key component of a collaborative, multidisciplinary ED practice, rather than a stand-alone, measurable intervention.[52] Nevertheless, multiple studies have demonstrated that ED pharmacists can exert a specific positive impact on antimicrobial stewardship through various roles, including: assisting in the appropriate selection and dosing of empiric antibiotics, enforcing formulary restrictions, adjusting regimens based on organ function/illness severity, structured follow-up on positive cultures, providing education on antimicrobial stewardship, and performing quality improvement projects related to antimicrobial stewardship.[47,48,53–62]

Emergency Department Antibiograms

An ED antibiogram is "a periodic summary of antimicrobial susceptibilities of local bacterial isolates [from the ED], submitted to the hospital's clinical microbiology laboratory."[63] It is typically updated annually and used by clinicians and pharmacists to assess ED susceptibility rates, as an aid in selecting empiric antimicrobial therapy, and in monitoring ED resistance trends over time. In practice, many low-volume facilities do not have an ED-specific antibiogram because the minimal number of isolates required to report resistance for a particular organism are not available. Solutions to this problem include constructing a biannual antibiogram or pooling data with other local EDs to construct a regional ED antibiogram. Common challenges that occur when first reporting a dedicated ED antibiogram include difficulty separating ED data from hospital-wide data, difficulty separating screening data from diagnostic data, and difficulty ensuring that the data from admitted patients are not counted twice.

Antibiograms should be used to guide ED-specific recommendations for empiric treatment of all common bacterial infections.

Overview of Behavioral Interventions

The ED has unique challenges to implementing quality improvement interventions because of frequent interruptions, high-volume care, the need for rapid decisions with limited information, variation in staff over different shifts, and concerns related to patient satisfaction.[64–66] Furthermore, even though emergency care providers may appreciate the public health implications of growing antimicrobial resistance, changing practice is difficult for a multitude of reasons. To ensure each patient gets the right antibiotic at the right dose and for the right duration, or avoid an antibiotic when not indicated, effective interventions to change prescribing behavior are critically needed.

Traditional educational approaches are not effective at producing long-lasting changes in clinical practice. Although education-only interventional studies have been published, it is more common to see education included as part of a steward intervention bundle.[67,68] These typically encompass provision of education on best practice guidelines and provision of associated clinical decision support systems. For example, clinical decision support systems have been demonstrated to improve ED antibiotic decision making for community-acquired pneumonia and uncomplicated UTIs.[69–71]

Beyond simple education-based interventions, evidence from behavioral economics and the psychology decision-making literature suggests that audit and feedback, academic detailing (ie, one-on-one education), behavioral nudges, and peer comparisons can improve prescribing outcomes.[72–74] Because emergency care providers often rely on heuristics given constraints of time and limited information, behavioral interventions that take into account workflow and decision-making processes have the potential to significantly impact change by targeting specific barriers and facilitators. For example, multifaceted stewardship interventions have been demonstrated to improve ED antibiotic prescribing for pneumonia,[75–78] UTIs,[79,80] skin and soft tissue infections,[81] and sepsis.[82]

Audit and feedback

Randomized controlled trials (RCT) of audit and feedback conducted in primary care practices demonstrate that feedback can significantly improve appropriate antibiotic prescribing.[72,83] One large RCT conducted in this setting used a peer comparison feedback intervention that took advantage of social motivation and found that being labeled a top performer or not top performer was an effective means to reduce inappropriate antibiotic prescribing for respiratory tract infections.[72] However, several studies have demonstrated a reversal of stewardship gains after discontinuation of audit and feedback, suggesting the need for ongoing efforts to achieve sustainability.[84,85]

Public commitments

Simple interventions that rely on social motivation and accountability to patients and peers, such as posters placed in examination rooms and letters with a commitment to avoid potentially harmful antibiotic use, has resulted in 20% absolute reduction in prescribing.[73] Given the higher acuity and rapid pace of ED care relative to clinic settings (ie, illness or time restrictions preventing patients from reading posters) and absence of treatment areas associated with individual physicians, the effectiveness of physician pledges in this setting is unknown. Emergency care providers may be more likely to be judicious about antibiotic avoidance when they have committed publicly to avoiding patient harm and related materials can be used for patient education.

OVERVIEW OF DIAGNOSTIC INTERVENTIONS

Diagnostic stewardship interventions are divided into three categories: (1) cultures, (2) organism identification assays, and (3) biomarkers. Although traditional cultures are not available to impact prescribing at the point of care, they are a critical component to enhance the downstream tailoring of antibiotic therapy for post-ED care in the inpatient and outpatient setting. Infection-specific cultures (eg, sputum, urine, wound) may assist in the tailoring or discontinuation of antibiotic therapy but are not routinely advised for uncomplicated UTIs, skin and soft tissue infections, or pneumonia. Additionally, although blood cultures are a core component of sepsis care, routine blood cultures should not be obtained for uncomplicated pneumonias, UTIs (including pyelonephritis), or skin and soft tissue infections because of low clinical utility and the risk of contamination resulting in false positives and unnecessary antibiotic prescribing.[86–89]

With the emergence of molecular assays that can rapidly identify organisms, such as methicillin-resistant *Staphylococcus aureus* (MRSA), there has been increased interest in using these in the ED for stewardship applications. These compliment more traditional organism identification assays, such as group A β-hemolytic *Streptococcus* for pharyngitis and influenza. Finally, procalcitonin (PCT) is a biomarker approved in 2017 by the Food and Drug Administration to assist with antibiotic prescribing decisions for respiratory tract infections.[90] PCT joins C-reactive protein, which is the other biomarker that has been tested as an antibiotic stewardship intervention.[91] Each of these interventions is covered next in more detail in their respective condition specific stewardship section.

CONDITION-SPECIFIC STEWARDSHIP APPROACHES
Respiratory Tract Infections

Antibiotic prescriptions for nonbacterial respiratory tract infections (eg, bronchitis, sinusitis, otitis media, nonspecific URI) represent the most frequent source of unnecessary antibiotic prescribing in ambulatory care settings.[26] Although simply avoiding antibiotic prescribing for nonindicated conditions would make a significant impact on stewardship, there are clinical scenarios that involve diagnostic uncertainty, which can also drive overuse. For example, patients with viral respiratory infections (eg, influenza) may have radiographic infiltrates on chest radiograph, which traditionally would prompt a diagnosis of pneumonia and prescription of antibiotics. One potential solution to this dilemma are influenza assays, which have been demonstrated in a series of studies to reduce the number of patients presenting to the ED with respiratory tract infection symptoms who receive antibiotic therapy.[92–95] More broadly, recently commercialized multiplex rapid viral panels have been proposed as a potential solution to improve antibiotic prescribing for respiratory conditions.[45,96,97] However, several clinical studies, one of which included discharged ED patients, suggest that the broader viral panel results did not significantly change antibiotic prescribing outside of those involving a positive influenza result.[98,99] It remains to be seen whether incorporating rapid multiplex viral panel results as part of an ED antimicrobial stewardship program could improve their impact.[45]

PCT is a biomarker upregulated by the presence of bacterial infection and attenuated by viral infections.[100] A 2017 Cochrane review that included data from 32 RCTs concluded that PCT-guided antibiotic therapy in the acute care setting is effective in reducing antibiotic prescribing without any adverse effect on patient safety or outcomes.[101] Based on the available data, PCT was approved by the Food and Drug Administration in 2017 to assist with antibiotic decision making in patients with lower respiratory tract infections (eg, pneumonia).[90] The impact of PCT on US ED antibiotic prescribing is unknown because it has not been widely adopted. Epidemiologic data indicate that a bacterial pathogen was identified in less than 15% of patients admitted with pneumonia as diagnosed by the presence of an infiltrate on chest radiograph.[102] This fact suggests a large potential role for PCT in helping to identify pneumonias that are not bacterial in origin.

In cases where the provider has decided to treat suspected pneumonia with antibiotics, stewardship should focus on the selection of optimal empiric therapy. Although recommended for community-acquired pneumonia in the 2007 guideline, increasing national rates of macrolide resistance among S pneumonia isolates means there is a diminishing role for macrolide monotherapy in the treatment of community-acquired pneumonia.[103,104] Selection of β-lactam plus doxycycline or azithromycin versus a respiratory fluoroquinolone should be based on patient factors (eg, comorbidities, potential for medication interactions) and local resistance patterns. Another important area for improved stewardship is to eliminate the use of reflex broad-spectrum antibiotic prescribing for patients meeting the traditional definition of health care–associated pneumonia (HCAP): recent admission, residing in a long-term care settings, chemotherapy, or hemodialysis.[105] Because of its poor discriminatory ability for patients at risk for pneumonia caused by resistant organisms referred to as PES (Pseudomonas aeruginosa, Enterobacteriaceae extended-spectrum β-lactamase-positive, and MRSA),[106] HCAP is no longer considered an appropriate basis for initiation of broad-spectrum antibiotics in ED patients being admitted with pneumonia.[107,108] A recently published prediction score, drug resistance in pneumonia, demonstrated improved diagnostic performance characteristics as compared with HCAP but has not yet been widely validated.[109] Initial studies suggest drug resistance in pneumonia (DRIP) can reduce broad-spectrum antibiotic prescribing without adverse clinical outcomes but further research is needed before widespread implementation.[110–114]

Urinary Tract Infections and Asymptomatic Bacteriuria

UTIs are one of the most common discharge diagnoses made in the ED and the CDC reports that treatment of UTIs in US hospitals could be improved in nearly 40% of cases.[36] To optimize ED stewardship for UTIs efforts should focus on improved diagnostic processes (eg, when to order a urinalysis [UA] and how to correctly interpret it), reduced overtreatment of ASB, and selection of appropriate empiric antibiotics.

Because of the persistence of myths around the diagnosis of UTI, optimizing the ordering of UAs and urine cultures can have a profound impact on antibiotic prescribing.[115] In ideal circumstances, the UA should only be used as a diagnostic test for UTI in the setting of clinical symptoms and suspicion for infection. Because it can identify the presence of bacteria in asymptomatic patients, a UA should not be routinely sent as a screening test for UTI.[116] Provider-level examples of inappropriate UA ordering include confirming a verbal nursing order for a UA on a patient with no urinary symptoms because the patient is confused, because the sample "looks dirty," or simply because "the patient had to pee, so I collected a sample doc…should I send it?"[117] Perhaps even more commonplace are the system-level examples of inappropriate

UA ordering. One common example is UAs sent on asymptomatic patients because the order is included on a default order set (eg, abdominal pain, psychiatric clearance, trauma). In either scenario, ordering a UA for a patient with a low pretest probability for UTI puts the ED clinician in a position where the positive predictive value of the UA is greatly diminished and the likelihood of the patient receiving unnecessary antibiotics is greatly increased.

The potential for misdiagnosis and overtreatment is compounded when urine cultures are ordered inappropriately, because the urine culture results are typically reviewed days later, often by a staff member who is not personally familiar with the patient's signs and symptoms. The two most basic stewardship interventions to reduce ordering of inappropriate urine cultures are to avoid the use of reflex urine cultures and to remove urine cultures from most order sets. Emergency care providers can also combat the ordering of inappropriate urine cultures by implementing two key practice changes. First, they can recognize patient populations that are high-risk for ASB (indwelling Foley catheter, long-term care) and avoid sending a UA or urine culture if the patient is not having symptoms. Second, they can add clarity to the situation and improve downstream care by documenting a diagnosis of "asymptomatic bacteriuria" if a UA (whether ordered intentionally or unintentionally) shows bacteria for an asymptomatic patient.

The key to understanding why a significant portion of antimicrobials given for UTI are unnecessary hinges on one's appreciation of what ASB is and what patient populations are at-risk for having ASB. ASB is defined as "isolation of bacteria in an appropriately collected urine sample from an individual without signs or symptoms referable to a urinary infection."[118] Transient ASB is common in healthy reproductive-age women (2%–5% prevalence) and even more common during pregnancy (2%–11% prevalence).[119] These patients may test "positive" 1 day and then have an unremarkable UA the next day after voiding. If the patient is tested during a period of transient ASB, they are at risk for being prescribed unnecessary antimicrobials.

In certain specialty populations, patients' bladders are colonized with nonpathogenic bacteria, meaning that they test "positive" at any time. In the long-term care population, the prevalence of ASB varies widely (5%–50%) because the presence of ASB typically corresponds to the patient's level of functional impairment. For example, up to 50% of patients with spinal cord injury or paralysis exhibit ASB. Most notably, the prevalence of ASB in patients with indwelling catheters is nearly 100%, meaning that *any* UA sent in this patient population looks "positive" if the ED clinician does not have a high index of suspicion for ASB.[118]

Emergency care providers commonly treat ASB, because this practice was standard of care for decades. The logical fallacy is that ASB progresses to pyelonephritis. This pathophysiology was observed in pregnant patients when the urine culture was first developed and the assumption was that the same was true for all patients. This false assumption led to the general treatment of ASB in all patient populations. In fact, according to national infectious disease guidelines, treating ASB is only acceptable in three niche clinical scenarios: (1) preurologic procedure, (2) immediately post-renal transplant, and (3) *once* in early pregnancy (only if present on two separate urine cultures).[116]

Another common but controversial example of treating ASB that merits its own discussion is whether or not to order a UA on older adults presenting with altered mental status or functional decline with no urinary symptoms, fever, or clinical instability. The current literature suggests that UTI is not a common cause of altered mental status in the elderly and that the premature incorrect diagnosis of UTI can lead to anchoring bias and prevent the clinician from uncovering the true (often multifactorial) cause of the altered mental status (eg, dehydration, hypoxia, polypharmacy, sundowning, sensory impairment).[120,121] Schulz and colleagues[115] summarize a reasonable approach to this challenging patient population, asserting that older adults "with acute mental status changes accompanied by bacteriuria and pyuria, without clinical instability or other signs or symptoms of UTI, can reasonably be observed for resolution of confusion for 24 to 48 hours without antibiotics, while searching for other causes of confusion."

Another opportunity for stewardship in UTI care involves the selection of appropriate empiric therapy. Ciprofloxacin, once the mainstay of outpatient UTI and pyelonephritis treatment, is rapidly losing its efficacy against *Escherichia coli* with resistance rates averaging 35% in the United Sates.[122] Therefore it should no longer be considered a universal first-line agent for UTI and empiric therapy should be based on local resistance patterns (ie, ED antibiogram). For most patients with an uncomplicated UTI and normal renal function, we recommend nitrofurantoin or trimethoprim and sulfamethoxazole (TMP-SMX) if local *E coli* resistance rates are less than 20%.

Catheter-Associated Urinary Tract Infections

Catheter-associated UTIs are a significant source of hospital-acquired infection and thus represent a core component of ED infection prevention and antimicrobial stewardship. One national study estimated that 65% of urinary catheters placed in the ED potentially could have been avoided.[123] At the provider-level, clinicians should be aware that urinary catheters should not be placed for incontinence, ease of nursing care, or urine output measuring.[124] All catheters placed in the ED should have a plan for removal in place at the time of initial placement, so that clinical inertia does not result in a catheter being in place longer than is medically necessary. If an ED has a nurse-initiated protocol for catheter placement, the HOUDINI acronym outlines appropriate reasons for placement of a urinary catheter: *H*ematuria, gross; *O*bstruction, urinary; *U*rologic surgery; *D*ecubitus ulcer—open sacral or perineal wound in incontinent patient; *I*nput and output critical for patient management or hemodynamic instability; *N*o code/comfort care/hospice care; *I*mmobility caused by physical constraints.[125]

Skin and Soft Tissue Infections

Antimicrobial stewardship considerations in the management of skin and soft tissue infections vary depending on the type of infection. The avoidance of antibiotics following incision and drainage (I&D) of uncomplicated abscesses has been a mainstay of ED antimicrobial stewardship since it was included as part of the American College of Emergency Physician's initial Choosing Wisely recommendations in 2013.[126] This guidance was based on a series of RCTs that failed to demonstrate clinical benefit for systemic antibiotics following I&D.[127]

However, two recently published large RCTs did demonstrate a statistically significant reduction in treatment failure and development of recurrent abscesses with TMP-SMX and clindamycin following I&D.[128,129] These results have prompted some to conclude that antibiotics should become standard of care following I&D of uncomplicated abscesses.[130] Given the societal ramifications of potential increased bacterial resistance related to routine antibiotic prescribing for the hundreds of thousands of patients with uncomplicated abscesses treated in the United States alone each year, a critical analysis of these trial results is necessary.

First, it is important to recognize that the narrow margin of benefit observed for antibiotics in these trials is associated with high numbers needed to treat ranging from 7 to 14.[128,129] Even if applying the results from Daum and colleagues,[129] highest demonstrated margin of benefit observed using a composite definition of treatment failure, which included development of future abscesses, approximately 70% of patients do not require antibiotics to successfully resolve their abscess. Additionally, there were no cases of sepsis or infection-related mortality observed among the more than 2000 trial participants, suggesting that withholding antibiotics for uncomplicated abscesses would not compromise patient safety.[128,129]

Moving forward, emergency care providers should attempt to balance the marginal treatment benefit from post-I&D antibiotics with patient safety and public health considerations. One potential solution is to engage in shared decision making, which includes discussions about the numbers needed to treat for this condition and safety risks related to antibiotics. To assist with risk stratification, results from a subgroup analysis of the Talan and colleagues[131] RCT suggest that patients with a history of MRSA or fever are more likely to benefit from antibiotic therapy. Delayed antibiotic prescribing, which substantially reduces the number of antibiotic prescriptions filled without increasing complication rates in patients with suspected respiratory tract infections, is another potential strategy.[132] When providers make a decision to prescribe, the common practice of double coverage for group A ß-hemolytic streptococcus and MRSA (eg, cephalexin plus TMP-SMX) should be avoided given clinical cure rates more than 80% are achieved with TMP-SMX alone.[27,133,134] In terms of dosing, clinical cure rates were similar with lower doses of TMP-SMX (160/800 mg twice daily) as compared with double doses (320/1600 mg twice daily).[128,129] Given increased resistance of S aureus isolates to clindamycin in the United States, use of this antibiotic in the treatment of abscesses should be guided by local antibiograms.[135]

Another potential solution to enhance antimicrobial stewardship in the management of uncomplicated abscesses is the use of rapid molecular MRSA assays.[136] One RCT demonstrated that these assays effectively assist emergency care providers in tailoring antibiotic therapy toward the causative bacteria in abscesses, whereas a retrospective study did not show significant improvements because of low uptake of the results by clinicians.[137,138] The tailoring of therapy is important because antibiotics commonly used to cover MRSA (TMP-SMX and clindamycin) are associated with more than twice the risk of adverse reaction compared with antibiotics with activity against methicillin-sensitive S aureus (eg, cephalexin).[18] The rapid detection of MRSA could also be helpful in risk stratification because patients with MRSA-related abscesses were also more likely to benefit from antibiotics in the Talan et al. RCT subgroup analysis.[131]

In the case of cellulitis, the primary areas of focus for stewardship should be improving diagnostic accuracy and appropriate antibiotic selection. A recent study published in the dermatology literature concluded that a significant portion (~30%) of ED cellulitis admissions may actually represent noninfectious dermatologic conditions termed pseudocellulitis.[23] Although this was a retrospective single-center study, the author correctly suggest emergency care providers should be vigilant for cellulitis mimics, such as "venous stasis dermatitis, lymphedema, deep venous thrombosis, gout, and contact dermatitis."[23] Diagnostic accuracy in the ED is improved through simple strategies, such as passive leg raise to observe abatement of erythema as a sign of nonbacterial cause and first considering alternative edema-causing conditions before making the unlikely diagnosis of bilateral lower extremity cellulitis.[139] The double coverage approach for uncomplicated cellulitis has been evaluated in two RCTs, neither of which observed a reduction in treatment failure with the addition of TMP-SMX to a ß-hemolytic streptococcus-active antibiotic (eg, cephalexin).[140,141] Uncomplicated, nonpurulent cellulitis should therefore only be treated after careful consideration of potential mimics and be managed with a single antibiotic active against group A ß-hemolytic Streptococcus.

Sexually Transmitted Infections

Sexually transmitted infections (STI) are the most common notifiable diseases seen in ED settings. There was a nearly 40% increase in the number of STI visits to EDs for the time period 2011 to 2013 compared with 2008 to 2010, versus a 2% increase for all diagnoses.[142] A total of 17% of all STI patients are seen in hospital based EDs, with patients presenting to EDs being more likely to be younger, nonwhite, and to have public insurance.[143]

Clinical judgment is often inadequate for diagnosis of STIs, leading to standard practice that involves use of empiric therapy to prevent public health transmission. Given growing evidence of resistant gonorrhea,[144] overuse of antibiotics to treat STDs is an imperative topic to address. A RCT of rapid STI testing with real-time result reporting during the ED visit coupled with specimen self-collection found only 12.9% of patients with symptoms consistent with STI tested positive for chlamydia or gonorrhea. Compared with control subjects (batched nucleic acid amplification testing), patients in the rapid molecular diagnostic group were significantly less likely to receive unnecessary empiric antibiotic treatment, less likely to report missed antibiotic doses, and more likely to be notified of their results. There were no significant differences in charges or health care use measures.[145] These results were mirrored in a recently published quasi-experimental study that also demonstrated the feasibility of rapid STI testing in the ED and observed an associated increase in appropriate antibiotic use.[146]

SUMMARY

Given the increasing role of the ED in the US health care system and magnitude of antibiotic use that occurs in this setting, antimicrobial stewardship programs are an important area of focus to improve clinical outcomes, optimize patient safety, and protect antibiotics as a critical public health resource. Opportunities to enhance antimicrobial stewardship are abundant in the ED. Each of the most common infection types (respiratory tract, urinary tract, skin and soft tissue) have aspects of antibiotic prescribing that could be significantly enhanced and we suggest these are starting points for those looking to initiate ED-based stewardship quality improvement interventions. The most effective stewardship interventions involve a bundle approach, building on the strengths of multiple systems and provider-level approaches to achieve sustainable improvements in appropriate antibiotic prescribing.

REFERENCES

1. McGowan JE Jr. Antimicrobial resistance in hospital organisms and its relation to antibiotic use. Rev Infect Dis 1983;5(6):1033–48.
2. WHO. Global action plan on antimicrobial resistance. WHO. Available at: http://apps.who.int/iris/bitstream/10665/193736/1/9789241509763_eng.pdf?ua=1. Accessed March 2, 2018.
3. Collignon PC, Conly JM, Andremont A, et al. World Health Organization ranking of antimicrobials according to their importance in human medicine: a critical step for developing risk management strategies to control antimicrobial resistance from food animal production. Clin Infect Dis 2016;63(8):1087–93.
4. National Strategy to Combat Antibiotic Resistance. Available at: https://www.cdc.gov/drugresistance/federal-engagement-in-ar/national-strategy/index.html. Accessed March 2, 2018.
5. The FAO action plan on antimicrobial resistance: 2016-2020. United Nations. Available at: http://www.fao.org/3/a-i5996e.pdf. Accessed March 2, 2018.

6. Plachouras D, Hopkins S. Antimicrobial stewardship: we know it works; time to make sure it is in place everywhere. Cochrane Database Syst Rev 2017;2: ED000119.
7. ACEP PQRS quality details: 2016 regulatory highlights. Available at: https://www.acep.org/Legislation-and-Advocacy/Federal-Issues/Quality-Issues/2016-Regulatory-Highlights/. Accessed April 7, 2016.
8. Medicare C for, Baltimore MS 7500 SB, USA M. 2016 Physician Quality Reporting System Measures List. 2018. Available at: https://www.cms.gov/apps/ama/license.asp?file=/PQRS/downloads/PQRS_2016_Measure_List_01072016.xlsx. Accessed March 26, 2018.
9. Joint Commission on Hospital Accreditation. APPROVED: new antimicrobial stewardship standard. Jt Comm Perspect 2016;36(7):1, 3–4, 8.
10. Murray BE, Moellering RC. Patterns and mechanisms of antibiotic resistance. Med Clin North Am 1978;62(5):899–923.
11. O'Neil J. Antimicrobial resistance: tackling a crisis for the health and wealth of nations. 2014. Available at: https://amr-review.org/sites/default/files/AMR%20Review%20Paper%20-%20Tackling%20a%20crisis%20for%20the%20health%20and%20wealth%20of%20nations_1.pdf. Accessed February 27, 2018.
12. Neuman MI, Ting SA, Meydani A, et al. National study of antibiotic use in emergency department visits for pneumonia, 1993 through 2008. Acad Emerg Med 2012;19(5):562–8.
13. McCaig LF, Besser RE, Hughes JM. Antimicrobial-drug prescription in ambulatory care settings, United States, 1992–2000. Emerg Infect Dis 2003;9(4):432–7.
14. Jenkins SG, Farrell DJ. Increase in pneumococcus macrolide resistance, United States. Emerg Infect Dis 2009;15(8):1260–4.
15. Van Boeckel TP, Gandra S, Ashok A, et al. Global antibiotic consumption 2000 to 2010: an analysis of national pharmaceutical sales data. Lancet Infect Dis 2014; 14(8):742–50.
16. Klein EY, Martinez EM, May L, et al. Categorical risk perception drives variability in antibiotic prescribing in the emergency department: a mixed methods observational study. J Gen Intern Med 2017;32(10):1083–9.
17. Tamma PD, Avdic E, Li DX, et al. Association of adverse events with antibiotic use in hospitalized patients. JAMA Intern Med 2017;177(9):1308–15.
18. Shehab N, Patel PR, Srinivasan A, et al. Emergency department visits for antibiotic-associated adverse events. Clin Infect Dis 2008;47(6):735–43.
19. Shehab N, Lovegrove MC, Geller AI, et al. US emergency department visits for outpatient adverse drug events, 2013-2014. JAMA 2016;316(20):2115–25.
20. Lessa FC, Mu Y, Bamberg WM, et al. Burden of *Clostridium difficile* infection in the United States. N Engl J Med 2015;372(9):825–34.
21. U.S. Department of Health and Human Services Centers for Disease Control and Prevention. Antibiotic resistance threats in the United States, 2013. 2013. Available at: https://www.cdc.gov/drugresistance/threat-report-2013/pdf/ar-threats-2013-508.pdf#page=5. Accessed February 23, 2018.
22. Joseph J, Rodvold KA. The role of carbapenems in the treatment of severe nosocomial respiratory tract infections. Expert Opin Pharmacother 2008;9(4): 561–75.
23. Weng QY, Raff AB, Cohen JM, et al. Costs and consequences associated with misdiagnosed lower extremity cellulitis. JAMA Dermatol 2017;153(2):141–6.
24. Watson JR, Sánchez PJ, Spencer JD, et al. Urinary tract infection and antimicrobial stewardship in the emergency department. Pediatr Emerg Care 2018;34(2): 93–5.

25. Elshimy G, Mariano V, Joy CM, et al. Are urinalyses used inappropriately in the diagnosis of urinary tract infections? Open Forum Infect Dis 2017;4(suppl_1): S350.
26. Fleming-Dutra KE, Hersh AL, Shapiro DJ, et al. Prevalence of inappropriate antibiotic prescriptions among US ambulatory care visits, 2010-2011. JAMA 2016; 315(17):1864–73.
27. Pallin DJ, Camargo CA, Schuur JD. Skin infections and antibiotic stewardship: analysis of emergency department prescribing practices, 2007-2010. West J Emerg Med 2014;15(3):282–9.
28. Gonzales R, Camargo CA, MacKenzie T, et al. Antibiotic treatment of acute respiratory infections in acute care settings. Acad Emerg Med 2006;13(3):288–94.
29. 2015 NHAMCS emergency department summary tables. 2018. Available at: https:// www.cdc.gov/nchs/data/nhamcs/web_tables/2015_ed_web_tables.pdf. Accessed March 25, 2018.
30. Gonzalez Morganti K, Bauhoff S, Blanchard JC, et al. The evolving roles of emergency departments in the United States. 2013. Available at: https://www.rand. org/content/dam/rand/pubs/research_reports/RR200/RR280/RAND_RR280.pdf. Accessed March 16, 2018.
31. Kocher KE, Dimick JB, Nallamothu BK. Changes in the source of unscheduled hospitalizations in the United States. Med Care 2013;51(8):689–98.
32. Marcozzi D, Carr B, Liferidge A, et al. Trends in the contribution of emergency departments to the provision of hospital-associated health care in the USA. Int J Health Serv 2018;48(2):267–88.
33. U.S. Department of Health and Human Services Centers for Disease Control and Prevention. National Hospital Ambulatory Medical Care Survey: 2014 Emergency Department Summary Tables. 2014. Available at: https://www.cdc.gov/ nchs/data/nhamcs/web_tables/2014_ed_web_tables.pdf. Accessed February 27, 2018.
34. Gabayan GZ, Sun BC, Asch SM, et al. Qualitative factors in patients who die shortly after emergency department discharge. Acad Emerg Med 2013;20(8): 778–85.
35. Timbrook TT, Caffrey AR, Ovalle A, et al. Assessments of opportunities to improve antibiotic prescribing in an emergency department: a period prevalence survey. Infect Dis Ther 2017;6(4):497–505.
36. Fridkin S, Baggs J, Fagan R, et al. Vital signs: improving antibiotic use among hospitalized patients. MMWR Morb Mortal Wkly Rep 2014;63(9):194–200.
37. Durkin MJ, Jafarzadeh SR, Hsueh K, et al. Outpatient antibiotic prescription trends in the United States: a national cohort study. Infect Control Hosp Epidemiol 2018;1–6. https://doi.org/10.1017/ice.2018.26.
38. Schuts EC, Hulscher MEJL, Mouton JW, et al. Current evidence on hospital antimicrobial stewardship objectives: a systematic review and meta-analysis. Lancet Infect Dis 2016;16(7):847–56.
39. Baur D, Gladstone BP, Burkert F, et al. Effect of antibiotic stewardship on the incidence of infection and colonisation with antibiotic-resistant bacteria and Clostridium difficile infection: a systematic review and meta-analysis. Lancet Infect Dis 2017;17(9):990–1001.
40. Feazel LM, Malhotra A, Perencevich EN, et al. Effect of antibiotic stewardship programmes on Clostridium difficile incidence: a systematic review and meta-analysis. J Antimicrob Chemother 2014;69(7):1748–54.
41. CMS Hospital-acquired condition reduction program fiscal year 2018 fact sheet. Available at: https://www.cms.gov/Medicare/Medicare-Fee-for-Service-Payment/

AcuteInpatientPPS/Downloads/FY2018-HAC-Reduction-Program-Fact-Sheet.pdf. Accessed March 16, 2018.

42. Mitchell BG, Gardner A. Prolongation of length of stay and *Clostridium difficile* infection: a review of the methods used to examine length of stay due to health-care associated infections. Antimicrob Resist Infect Control 2012;1(1):14.

43. Roberts RR, Hota B, Ahmad I, et al. Hospital and societal costs of antimicrobial-resistant infections in a Chicago teaching hospital: implications for antibiotic stewardship. Clin Infect Dis 2009;49(8):1175–84.

44. Patel PK. Applying the horizontal and vertical paradigm to antimicrobial stewardship. Infect Control Hosp Epidemiol 2017;38(5):532–3.

45. Barlam TF, Cosgrove SE, Abbo LM, et al. Executive summary: implementing an antibiotic stewardship program: guidelines by the Infectious Diseases Society of America and the Society for Healthcare Epidemiology of America. Clin Infect Dis 2016;62(10):1197–202.

46. Barlam TF, Cosgrove SE, Abbo LM, et al. Implementing an antibiotic stewardship program: guidelines by the Infectious Diseases Society of America and the Society for Healthcare Epidemiology of America. Clin Infect Dis 2016;62(10):e51–77.

47. Davis LC, Covey RB, Weston JS, et al. Pharmacist-driven antimicrobial optimization in the emergency department. Am J Health Syst Pharm 2016;73(5 Suppl 1):S49–56.

48. Randolph TC, Parker A, Meyer L, et al. Effect of a pharmacist-managed culture review process on antimicrobial therapy in an emergency department. Am J Health Syst Pharm 2011;68(10):916–9.

49. Knox KL, Holmes AH. Regulation of antimicrobial prescribing practices: a strategy for controlling nosocomial antimicrobial resistance. Int J Infect Dis 2002;6: S8–13.

50. Fagan M, Lindbæk M, Reiso H, et al. A simple intervention to reduce inappropriate ciprofloxacin prescribing in the emergency department. Scand J Infect Dis 2014;46(7):481–5.

51. Reed EE, Stevenson KB, West JE, et al. Impact of formulary restriction with prior authorization by an antimicrobial stewardship program. Virulence 2013;4(2): 158–62.

52. ASHP statement on pharmacy services to the emergency department. American Society of Health-System Pharmacists. Available at: http://www.ashp.org/ s_ashp/docs/files/BP07/New_ED.pdf. Accessed March 27, 2015.

53. Trinh TD, Klinker KP. Antimicrobial stewardship in the emergency department. Infect Dis Ther 2015;4(Suppl 1):39–50.

54. Fairbanks RJ, Hays DP, Webster DF, et al. Clinical pharmacy services in an emergency department. Am J Health Syst Pharm 2004;61(9):934–7.

55. Baker SN, Acquisto NM, Ashley ED, et al. Pharmacist-managed antimicrobial stewardship program for patients discharged from the emergency department. J Pharm Pract 2012;25(2):190–4.

56. Acquisto NM, Baker SN. Antimicrobial stewardship in the emergency department. J Pharm Pract 2011;24(2):196–202.

57. DeFrates SR, Weant KA, Seamon JP, et al. Emergency pharmacist impact on health care-associated pneumonia empiric therapy. J Pharm Pract 2013;26(2): 125–30.

58. Weant KA, Baker SN. Emergency medicine pharmacists and sepsis management. J Pharm Pract 2013;26(4):401–5.

59. DeWitt KM, Weiss SJ, Rankin S, et al. Impact of an emergency medicine pharmacist on antibiotic dosing adjustment. Am J Emerg Med 2016;34(6):980–4.

60. Lingenfelter E, Drapkin Z, Fritz K, et al. ED pharmacist monitoring of provider antibiotic selection aids appropriate treatment for outpatient UTI. Am J Emerg Med 2016;34(8):1600–3.
61. Bailey AM, Stephan M, Weant KA, et al. Dosing of appropriate antibiotics and time to administration of first doses in the pediatric emergency department. J Pediatr Pharmacol Ther 2015;20(4):309–15.
62. Hunt A, Nakajima S, Hall Zimmerman L, et al. Impact of prospective verification of intravenous antibiotics in an ED. Am J Emerg Med 2016;34(12):2392–6.
63. Joshi S. Hospital antibiogram: a necessity. Indian J Med Microbiol 2010;28(4): 277–80.
64. Chisholm CD, Collison EK, Nelson DR, et al. Emergency department workplace interruptions are emergency physicians "interrupt-driven" and "multitasking"? Acad Emerg Med 2000;7(11):1239–43.
65. IFEM Framework for Quality and Safety in the Emergency Department. Available at: https://www.ifem.cc/wp-content/uploads/2016/03/Framework-for-Quality-and-Safety-in-the-Emergency-Department-2012.doc.pdf. Accessed June 15, 2018.
66. Chisholm CD, Weaver CS, Whenmouth L, et al. A task analysis of emergency physician activities in academic and community settings. Ann Emerg Med 2011;58(2):117–22.
67. Klein LE, Charache P, Johannes RS. Effect of physician tutorials on prescribing patterns of graduate physicians. J Med Educ 1981;56(6):504–11.
68. Metlay JP, Camargo CA, MacKenzie T, et al. Cluster-randomized trial to improve antibiotic use for adults with acute respiratory infections treated in emergency departments. Ann Emerg Med 2007;50(3):221–30.
69. Buising KL, Thursky KA, Black JF, et al. Improving antibiotic prescribing for adults with community acquired pneumonia: does a computerised decision support system achieve more than academic detailing alone? A time series analysis. BMC Med Inform Decis Mak 2008;8(1):35.
70. Demonchy E, Dufour J-C, Gaudart J, et al. Impact of a computerized decision support system on compliance with guidelines on antibiotics prescribed for urinary tract infections in emergency departments: a multicentre prospective before-and-after controlled interventional study. J Antimicrob Chemother 2014; 69(10):2857–63.
71. Dean NC, Jones BE, Jones JP, et al. Impact of an electronic clinical decision support tool for emergency department patients with pneumonia. Ann Emerg Med 2015;66(5):511–20.
72. Meeker D, Linder JA, Fox CR, et al. Effect of behavioral interventions on inappropriate antibiotic prescribing among primary care practices: a randomized clinical trial. JAMA 2016;315(6):562–70.
73. Meeker D, Knight TK, Friedberg MW, et al. Nudging guideline-concordant antibiotic prescribing: a randomized clinical trial. JAMA Intern Med 2014;174(3): 425–31.
74. Spellberg B. Antibiotic judo: working gently with prescriber psychology to overcome inappropriate use. JAMA Intern Med 2014;174(3):432–3.
75. Marrie TJ, Lau CY, Wheeler SL, et al. A controlled trial of a critical pathway for treatment of community-acquired pneumonia. JAMA 2000;283(6):749–55.
76. Ambroggio L, Thomson J, Murtagh Kurowski E, et al. Quality improvement methods increase appropriate antibiotic prescribing for childhood pneumonia. Pediatrics 2013;131(5):e1623–31.
77. Ostrowsky B, Sharma S, DeFino M, et al. Antimicrobial stewardship and automated pharmacy technology improve antibiotic appropriateness for

community-acquired pneumonia. Infect Control Hosp Epidemiol 2013;34(6): 566–72.

78. Julian-Jimenez A, Palomo de los Reyes MJ, Parejo Miguez R, et al. Improved management of community-acquired pneumonia in the emergency department. Arch Bronconeumol 2013;49(6):230–40.

79. Hecker MT, Fox CJ, Son AH, et al. Effect of a stewardship intervention on adherence to uncomplicated cystitis and pyelonephritis guidelines in an emergency department setting. PLoS One 2014;9(2):e87899.

80. Percival KM, Valenti KM, Schmittling SE, et al. Impact of an antimicrobial stewardship intervention on urinary tract infection treatment in the ED. Am J Emerg Med 2015;33(9):1129–33.

81. Trajano R, Ondak S, Tancredi D, et al. Emergency department specific antimicrobial stewardship intervention reduces antibiotic duration and selection for discharged adult and pediatric patients with skin and soft-tissue infections. Open Forum Infect Dis 2017;4(Suppl 1):S274.

82. Francis M, Rich T, Williamson T, et al. Effect of an emergency department sepsis protocol on time to antibiotics in severe sepsis. CJEM 2010;12(4):303–10.

83. Gerber JS, Prasad PA, Fiks AG, et al. Effect of an outpatient antimicrobial stewardship intervention on broad-spectrum antibiotic prescribing by primary care pediatricians: a randomized trial. JAMA 2013;309(22):2345–52.

84. Linder JA, Meeker D, Fox CR, et al. Effects of behavioral interventions on inappropriate antibiotic prescribing in primary care 12 months after stopping interventions. JAMA 2017;318(14):1391–2.

85. Gerber JS, Prasad PA, Fiks AG, et al. Durability of benefits of an outpatient antimicrobial stewardship intervention after discontinuation of audit and feedback. JAMA 2014;312(23):2569–70.

86. Makam AN, Auerbach AD, Steinman MA. Blood culture use in the emergency department in patients hospitalized for community-acquired pneumonia. JAMA Intern Med 2014;174(5):803–6.

87. Mills AM, Chen EH. Are blood cultures necessary in adults with cellulitis? Ann Emerg Med 2005;45(5):548–9.

88. Velasco M, Martínez JA, Moreno-Martínez A, et al. Blood cultures for women with uncomplicated acute pyelonephritis: are they necessary? Clin Infect Dis 2003; 37(8):1127–30.

89. Dellinger RP, Levy MM, Rhodes A, et al. Surviving sepsis campaign: international guidelines for management of severe sepsis and septic shock: 2012. Crit Care Med 2013;41(2):580–637.

90. Voelker R. Test aids antibiotic decisions. JAMA 2017;317(13):1308.

91. Gonzales R, Aagaard EM, Camargo CA Jr, et al. C-reactive protein testing does not decrease antibiotic use for acute cough illness when compared to a clinical algorithm. J Emerg Med 2011;41(1):1–7.

92. Blaschke AJ, Shapiro DJ, Pavia AT, et al. A national study of the impact of rapid influenza testing on clinical care in the emergency department. J Pediatric Infect Dis Soc 2014;3(2):112–8.

93. Noyola DE, Demmler GJ. Effect of rapid diagnosis on management of influenza A infections. Pediatr Infect Dis J 2000;19(4):303–7.

94. Esposito S, Marchisio P, Morelli P, et al. Effect of a rapid influenza diagnosis. Arch Dis Child 2003;88(6):525–6.

95. Bonner AB, Monroe KW, Talley LI, et al. Impact of the rapid diagnosis of influenza on physician decision-making and patient management in the pediatric

emergency department: results of a randomized, prospective, controlled trial. Pediatrics 2003;112(2):363–7.

96. Rogers BB, Shankar P, Jerris RC, et al. Impact of a rapid respiratory panel test on patient outcomes. Arch Pathol Lab Med 2015;139(5):636–41.

97. Huang H-S, Tsai C-L, Chang J, et al. Multiplex PCR system for the rapid diagnosis of respiratory virus infection: systematic review and meta-analysis. Clin Microbiol Infect 2017. https://doi.org/10.1016/j.cmi.2017.11.018.

98. Green DA, Hitoaliaj L, Kotansky B, et al. Clinical utility of on-demand multiplex respiratory pathogen testing among adult outpatients. J Clin Microbiol 2016; 54(12):2950–5.

99. Semret M, Schiller I, Jardin BA, et al. Multiplex respiratory virus testing for antimicrobial stewardship: a prospective assessment of antimicrobial use and clinical outcomes among hospitalized adults. J Infect Dis 2017;216(8):936–44.

100. Assicot M, Bohuon C, Gendrel D, et al. High serum procalcitonin concentrations in patients with sepsis and infection. Lancet 1993;341(8844):515–8.

101. Schuetz P, Wirz Y, Sager R, et al. Procalcitonin to initiate or discontinue antibiotics in acute respiratory tract infections. Cochrane Database Syst Rev 2017;(10):CD007498.

102. Jain S, Self WH, Wunderink RG, et al. Community-acquired pneumonia requiring hospitalization among U.S. adults. N Engl J Med 2015;373(5):415–27.

103. Niederman MS. Macrolide-resistant pneumococcus in community-acquired pneumonia. Is there still a role for macrolide therapy? Am J Respir Crit Care Med 2015;191(11):1216–7.

104. ResistanceMap. Available at: https://resistancemap.cddep.org/. Accessed October 27, 2017.

105. Abrahamian FM, DeBlieux PM, Emerman CL, et al. Health care-associated pneumonia: identification and initial management in the ED. Am J Emerg Med 2008;26(6):1–11.

106. Prina E, Ranzani OT, Polverino E, et al. Risk factors associated with potentially antibiotic-resistant pathogens in community-acquired pneumonia. Ann Am Thorac Soc 2015;12(2):153–60.

107. Chalmers JD, Rother C, Salih W, et al. Healthcare-associated pneumonia does not accurately identify potentially resistant pathogens: a systematic review and meta-analysis. Clin Infect Dis 2014;58(3):330–9.

108. Dean NC, Webb BJ. Health care–associated pneumonia is mostly dead. Long live the acronym PES? Ann Am Thorac Soc 2015;12(2):239–40.

109. Webb BJ, Dascomb K, Stenehjem E, et al. Derivation and multicenter validation of the drug resistance in pneumonia clinical prediction score. Antimicrob Agents Chemother 2016;60(5):2652–63.

110. Self WH, Wunderink RG, Williams DJ, et al. Comparison of clinical prediction models for resistant bacteria in community-onset pneumonia. Acad Emerg Med 2015;22(6):730–40.

111. Webb BJ, Dascomb K, Stenehjem E, et al. Predicting risk of drug-resistant organisms in pneumonia: moving beyond the HCAP model. Respir Med 2015; 109(1):1–10.

112. Webb BJ, Stenehjem E, Dascomb K, et al. Reply to Babbel et al., "Application of the DRIP score at a Veterans Affairs Hospital". Antimicrob Agents Chemother 2018;62(3). https://doi.org/10.1128/AAC.02337-17.

113. Babbel D, Sutton J, Rose R, et al. Application of the DRIP score at a Veterans Affairs hospital. Antimicrob Agents Chemother 2018;62(3). https://doi.org/10.1128/AAC.02277-17.

114. Farkas A, Sassine J, Mathew JP, et al. Outcomes associated with the use of a revised risk assessment strategy to predict antibiotic resistance in community-onset pneumonia: a stewardship perspective. J Antimicrob Chemother 2018. https://doi.org/10.1093/jac/dky202.

115. Schulz L, Hoffman RJ, Pothof J, et al. Top ten myths regarding the diagnosis and treatment of urinary tract infections. J Emerg Med 2016;51(1):25–30.

116. Nicolle LE. Asymptomatic bacteriuria: when to screen and when to treat. Infect Dis Clin North Am 2003;17(2):367–94.

117. Redwood R, Knobloch MJ, Pellegrini DC, et al. Reducing unnecessary culturing: a systems approach to evaluating urine culture ordering and collection practices among nurses in two acute care settings. Antimicrob Resist Infect Control 2018;7:4.

118. Nicolle LE, Bradley S, Colgan R, et al. Infectious Diseases Society of America guidelines for the diagnosis and treatment of asymptomatic bacteriuria in adults. Clin Infect Dis 2005;40(5):643–54.

119. Hooton TM, Scholes D, Stapleton AE, et al. A prospective study of asymptomatic bacteriuria in sexually active young women. N Engl J Med 2000;343(14): 992–7.

120. Tambyah PA, Maki DG. Catheter-associated urinary tract infection is rarely symptomatic: a prospective study of 1,497 catheterized patients. Arch Intern Med 2000;160(5):678–82.

121. Beveridge LA, Davey PG, Phillips G, et al. Optimal management of urinary tract infections in older people. Clin Interv Aging 2011;6:173–80.

122. Fasugba O, Gardner A, Mitchell BG, et al. Ciprofloxacin resistance in community- and hospital-acquired Escherichia coli urinary tract infections: a systematic review and meta-analysis of observational studies. BMC Infect Dis 2015;15:545.

123. Schuur JD, Chambers JG, Hou PC. Urinary catheter use and appropriateness in U.S. emergency departments, 1995-2010. Acad Emerg Med 2014;21(3):292–300.

124. Carter EJ, Pallin DJ, Mandel L, et al. Emergency department catheter-associated urinary tract infection prevention: multisite qualitative study of perceived risks and implemented strategies. Infect Control Hosp Epidemiol 2016;37(02):156–62.

125. Adams D, Bucior H, Day G, et al. HOUDINI: make that urinary catheter disappear – nurse-led protocol. J Infect Prev 2012;13(2):44–6.

126. ACEP Joins Choosing Wisely Campaign. ACEP Now. Available at: http://www.acepnow.com/article/acep-joins-choosing-wisely-campaign/. Accessed December 19, 2017.

127. Singer AJ, Thode HC Jr. Systemic antibiotics after incision and drainage of simple abscesses: a meta-analysis. Emerg Med J 2014;31(7):576–8.

128. Talan DA, Mower WR, Krishnadasan A, et al. Trimethoprim-sulfamethoxazole versus placebo for uncomplicated skin abscess. N Engl J Med 2016;374(9): 823–32.

129. Daum RS, Miller LG, Immergluck L, et al. A placebo-controlled trial of antibiotics for smaller skin abscesses. N Engl J Med 2017;376(26):2545–55.

130. Vermandere M, Aertgeerts B, Agoritsas T, et al. Antibiotics after incision and drainage for uncomplicated skin abscesses: a clinical practice guideline. BMJ 2018;360:k243.

131. Talan DA, Moran GJ, Krishnadasan A, et al. Subgroup analysis of antibiotic treatment for skin abscesses. Ann Emerg Med 2018;71(1):21–30.

132. Spurling GK, Del Mar CB, Dooley L, et al. Delayed antibiotic prescriptions for respiratory infections. Cochrane Database Syst Rev 2017;(9):CD004417.

133. Schmitz G, Goodwin T, Singer A, et al. The treatment of cutaneous abscesses: comparison of emergency medicine providers' practice patterns. West J Emerg Med 2013;14(1):23–8.

134. May L, Harter K, Yadav K, et al. Practice patterns and management strategies for purulent skin and soft-tissue infections in an urban academic ED. Am J Emerg Med 2012;30(2):302–10.

135. Sutter DE, Milburn E, Chukwuma U, et al. Changing susceptibility of *Staphylococcus aureus* in a US Pediatric Population. Pediatrics 2016;137(4). https://doi.org/10.1542/peds.2015-3099.

136. Pulia M, Calderone M, Hansen B, et al. Feasibility of rapid polymerase chain reaction for detection of methicillin-resistant *Staphylococcus aureus* colonization among emergency department patients with abscesses. Open Access Emerg Med 2013;5:17–22.

137. May LS, Rothman RE, Miller LG, et al. A randomized clinical trial comparing use of rapid molecular testing for *Staphylococcus aureus* for patients with cutaneous abscesses in the emergency department with standard of care. Infect Control Hosp Epidemiol 2015;36(12):1423–30.

138. Terp S, Krishnadasan A, Bowen W, et al. Introduction of rapid methicillin-resistant *Staphylococcus aureus* polymerase chain reaction testing and antibiotic selection among hospitalized patients with purulent skin infections. Clin Infect Dis 2014;58(8):e129–32.

139. McCreary EK, Heim ME, Schulz LT, et al. Top 10 myths regarding the diagnosis and treatment of cellulitis. J Emerg Med 2017;53(4):485–92.

140. Moran GJ, Krishnadasan A, Mower WR, et al. Effect of cephalexin plus trimethoprim-sulfamethoxazole vs cephalexin alone on clinical cure of uncomplicated cellulitis. JAMA 2017;317(20):2088–96.

141. Pallin DJ, Binder WD, Allen MB, et al. Comparative effectiveness of cephalexin plus trimethoprim-sulfamethoxazole versus cephalexin alone for treatment of uncomplicated cellulitis: a randomized controlled trial. Clin Infect Dis 2013;56(12):1754–62.

142. Pearson WS, Peterman TA, Gift TL. An increase in sexually transmitted infections seen in US emergency departments. Prev Med 2017;100:143–4.

143. Ware CE, Ajabnoor Y, Mullins PM, et al. A retrospective cross-sectional study of patients treated in US EDs and ambulatory care clinics with sexually transmitted infections from 2001 to 2010. Am J Emerg Med 2016;34(9):1808–11.

144. Kirkcaldy RD, Harvey A, Papp JR, et al. *Neisseria gonorrhoeae* antimicrobial susceptibility surveillance: the gonococcal isolate surveillance project, 27 sites, United States, 2014. MMWR Surveill Summ 2016;65(7):1–19.

145. May L, Ware CE, Jordan JA, et al. A randomized controlled trial comparing the treatment of patients tested for chlamydia and gonorrhea after a rapid polymerase chain reaction test versus standard of care testing. Sex Transm Dis 2016;43(5):290–5.

146. Rivard KR, Dumkow LE, Draper HM, et al. Impact of rapid diagnostic testing for chlamydia and gonorrhea on appropriate antimicrobial utilization in the emergency department. Diagn Microbiol Infect Dis 2017;87(2):175–9.

Infection Prevention for the Emergency Department
Out of Reach or Standard of Care?

Stephen Y. Liang, MD, MPHS[a,b,]*, Madison Riethman, MPH, CPH[c],
Josephine Fox, MPH, RN, CIC[d]

KEYWORDS

- Infection prevention • Hand hygiene • Environmental cleaning
- Central line–associated bloodstream infection
- Catheter-associated urinary tract infection • Ventilator-associated pneumonia
- Emergency department

KEY POINTS

- The emergency department (ED) presents unique challenges to infection control and prevention.
- Hand hygiene is a fundamental strategy for preventing the transmission of infectious disease in health care settings.
- Transmission-based precautions, environmental cleaning, and appropriate reprocessing of reusable medical devices provide added layers of protection to counter the spread of infectious disease.
- Health care–associated infections (eg, catheter-associated urinary tract infection, ventilator-associated pneumonia, central line–associated bloodstream infection) are often preventable but require systems-based strategies.
- Future research and innovation are needed to optimize infection prevention practices in the ED.

Disclosure Statement: S.Y. Liang reports no conflicts of interest in this work. S.Y. Liang is the recipient of a KM1 Comparative Effectiveness Research Career Development Award (KM1CA156708-01) and received support through the Clinical and Translational Science Award (CTSA) program (UL1RR024992) of the National Center for Advancing Translational Sciences as well as the Barnes-Jewish Patient Safety & Quality Career Development Program, which is funded by the Foundation for Barnes-Jewish Hospital.
[a] Division of Emergency Medicine, Washington University School of Medicine, 4523 Clayton Avenue, Campus Box 8072, St Louis, MO 63110, USA; [b] Division of Infectious Diseases, Washington University School of Medicine, 4523 Clayton Avenue, Campus Box 8051, St Louis, MO 63110, USA; [c] Communicable Disease, Clark County Public Health, Center for Community Health, 1601 East Fourth Plain Boulevard, Building 17, PO Box 9825, Vancouver, WA 98666, USA; [d] Infection Prevention, Barnes-Jewish Hospital, Mailstop 90-75-593, 4590 Children's Place, St Louis, MO 63108, USA
* Corresponding author. 4523 Clayton Avenue, Campus Box 8051, St Louis, MO 63110.
E-mail address: syliang@wustl.edu

Emerg Med Clin N Am 36 (2018) 873–887
https://doi.org/10.1016/j.emc.2018.06.013
0733-8627/18/© 2018 Elsevier Inc. All rights reserved.

Emergency departments (EDs) are the vanguard of modern health care systems, serving as a primary point of access to timely and life-saving medical care for the acutely ill or injured. In 2014, more than 137.8 million patient visits were made to US EDs, at a rate of 432 per 1000 population.[1] More than half of the 34.5 million inpatient admissions that occur annually in the United States originate in an ED. During mass casualty events, natural disasters, and public health emergencies, EDs play an integral part in local and regional response, absorbing rapid surges of patients requiring emergent medical attention. On a day-to-day basis, EDs function as a safety net for diverse and often vulnerable populations that might not otherwise receive routine health care. Infectious diseases factor prominently among the reasons patients seek care in the ED. Emergency clinicians must be well versed not only in the diagnosis and management but also in the control and prevention of infectious diseases.

Infection control and prevention have traditionally focused on inpatient health care settings with the objectives of reducing transmission of communicable infectious diseases and averting health care–associated infections. As a hybrid environment bridging ambulatory and hospital care, the ED presents unique challenges to this work.[2,3] By virtue of a concentrated geographic footprint, ED patients and healthcare professionals (HCP) routinely come in close contact with one another in busy waiting rooms as well as treatment areas. Undifferentiated clinical presentations of infectious disease delay recognition, patient isolation, and HCP use of appropriate personal protective equipment (PPE), increasing the potential for transmission of disease. Variable patient acuity, frequent HCP-patient interactions, and simultaneous care of multiple patients create obstacles to infection prevention practices, particularly when invasive procedures are necessary. Finite inpatient beds and isolation rooms lead to the boarding of patients with infectious illness in the ED. Overcrowding, be it from high patient volume or delays in hospital admission, can lead to the evaluation and treatment of patients in nontraditional environs such as a hallway or other overflow sites. Finally, rapid room turnovers frequently strain environmental cleaning services, allowing the persistence of infectious microorganisms on health care surfaces.

Infection prevention has garnered greater recognition as an essential component of high-quality emergency care.[2,3] In this review, the authors introduce the emergency clinician to the growing body of literature focused on hand hygiene, transmission-based precautions, environmental cleaning, high-level disinfection and sterilization of reusable medical devices, and the prevention of health care–associated infections in the ED.

HAND HYGIENE

Hand hygiene is a fundamental principle of infection prevention. Health care provider hands have the capacity to transmit pathogens from one patient to another.[4–6] Microorganisms present on patient skin, from either infection or colonization, or shed into the health care environment can contaminate the hands of an HCP through direct patient contact or interaction with their environment (eg, bed rails, bed linen, bedside furniture, or patient care equipment). When these microorganisms are able to persist on skin and hand hygiene is lacking or inadequate, HCP hands can transmit them to another patient through direct contact or interaction with their environment. In the absence of visible soiling, routine hand hygiene using an alcohol-based hand rub is an effective and time-efficient means for reducing the cross-transmission of pathogenic microorganisms in health care settings.[4] Hand washing with soap and water is advised when HCP hands are grossly soiled or when caring for patients with suspected *Clostridium difficile* or norovirus infection, because alcohol-based products lack efficacy and mechanical friction associated with hand washing aids in the removal of these pathogens. Although most emergency clinicians are accustomed to performing hand hygiene upon room entry and exit (ie, "foam in, foam out") and before any procedure, the Centers for Disease Control and Prevention (CDC) and the World Health Organization (WHO) recommend hand hygiene before and/or after key actions, best codified within the latter's "My Five Moments for Hand Hygiene"[4,6] (**Fig. 1**).

Adherence to hand hygiene in the ED has historically been low, particularly among physicians.[7–9] Hand hygiene rates among emergency clinicians span anywhere from less than 10% to more than 90%,[10–22] with adherence assessed by trained observers in most of the existing literature. Perceived barriers to hand hygiene in the ED include urgent clinical situations requiring lifesaving intervention, insufficient time, and ambiguity about when to perform hand hygiene.[22] Glove use has also been associated with poor hand hygiene in emergency and trauma settings.[13,15,20] Although gloves provide an essential barrier to blood and other potentially infectious body substances as part of standard precautions,[23,24] their use does not obviate hand hygiene, because hand contamination can still occur during glove removal or through microscopic tears in the gloves themselves.

In a study examining more than 5865 hand hygiene opportunities in an urban academic ED, patient location in a hallway was the strongest predictor for poor HCP hand hygiene (relative risk = 88.9%, 95% confidence interval [CI] 85.9%–92.1%).[13] Similarly, a study of 1673 hand hygiene opportunities in another urban academic ED also found that hand hygiene adherence was lower in hallway care areas compared with semiprivate care areas (odds ratio [OR] = 0.73, 95% CI 0.55–0.97).[19] Adherence was even more significantly impacted when the ED was at its highest level of overcrowding, quantified using the National Emergency Department Overcrowding Scale (OR = 0.39, 95% CI 0.28–0.55).[19] In a Canadian study, time to physician assessment greater than 1.5 hours, a measure of ED

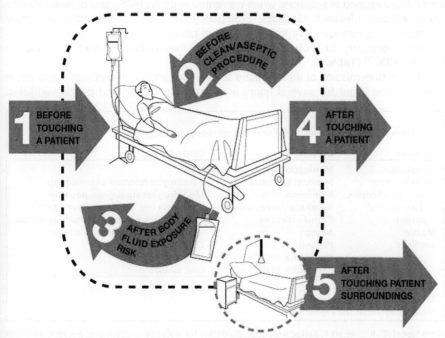

Fig. 1. WHO's "My five moments for hand hygiene." (*Data from* http://www.who.int/infection-prevention/tools/hand-hygiene/en/. Accessed May 29, 2018.)

workload and overcrowding, was also associated with decreased hand hygiene adherence (OR = 0.67, 95% CI, 0.51–0.89).[16] Emergency clinicians should understand how these unique aspects of ED care influence hand hygiene behavior and increase the risk for transmission of infection during vulnerable periods.

Educational interventions to improve ED hand hygiene have included distribution of written policies and other instructional materials, in-person teaching followed by observation with direct feedback, use of fluorescent markers to demonstrate cross-transmission of microorganisms through contact, and posting visual reminders in patient care areas.[9,15,25] Other efforts have focused on improving access to hand hygiene products in the ED, including the use of wearable hand sanitizer dispensers.[26–28] Workflow standardization and optimization can help reduce the number of hand hygiene opportunities and increase adherence during necessary moments.[15] Multimodal interventions combining HCP education, a culture of safety, recruitment of ED clinician champions, improved access to hand hygiene products, and routine auditing with feedback have led to significant albeit modest improvements in adherence in at least 2 quasi-experimental ED-based studies.[18,29,30] More research is needed in ED settings to identify simple and sustainable strategies to promote and maximize hand hygiene adherence.

TRANSMISSION-BASED PRECAUTIONS

Transmission-based precautions target microorganisms spread through airborne droplet nuclei, large particle droplets, or direct contact using a combination of PPE and patient isolation. In most instances, the decision to initiate transmission-based precautions in the ED will hinge on the patient's presenting clinical syndrome and a differential diagnosis of infectious diseases that may be responsible. Failure to initiate transmission-based precautions when warranted exposes HCPs and patients alike to communicable infectious diseases. Emergency clinicians should understand how common microorganisms are transmitted from person-to-person as well as the precautions necessary to protect themselves and their patients based on guidance from the CDC[31] (**Table 1**).

Airborne transmission of an infectious disease occurs via droplet nuclei (≤ 5 μm in size) that can linger for several hours at a time in enclosed and poorly ventilated

Table 1
Transmission-based precautions for selected microorganisms

Airborne	Droplet	Contact
Tuberculosis	Meningococcus	MRSA
Varicella zoster virus (chickenpox, disseminated zoster)	Seasonal influenza	Vancomycin-resistant *Enterococcus*
	Rhinovirus	Multidrug-resistant gram-negative
	Respiratory syncytial virus	bacteria (eg, carbapenem-resistant
	German measles	*Enterobacteriaceae*, extended-spectrum
Measles	Mumps	β-lactamase producing bacteria)
Smallpox	Pertussis	*C difficile*
	Diphtheria	Norovirus
	Pneumonic plague	Lice, scabies
Highly pathogenic influenza		
Severe acute respiratory syndrome		
Middle East respiratory syndrome		

From Siegel JD, Rhinehart E, Jackson M, et al. Guideline for isolation precautions: preventing transmission of infectious agents in healthcare settings. 2007. Available at: https://www.cdc.gov/infectioncontrol/guidelines/isolation/index.html. Accessed May 29, 2018.

spaces. Tuberculosis, measles, and varicella (including disseminated zoster) are classic airborne diseases that pose a risk to emergency clinicians. Several emerging pathogens, including smallpox, highly pathogenic influenza, severe acute respiratory syndrome coronavirus (SARS-CoV), and the Middle East respiratory syndrome coronavirus (MERS-CoV), are readily transmitted in this manner as well. Airborne precautions mandate HCP use of an N95 or powered air-purifying respirator during patient care and prompt placement of the infected patient within a single-occupancy airborne infection isolation room (capable of generating negative room pressure and ≥12 air exchanges per hour).[31] EDs are decidedly vulnerable and highly likely to be involved in the initial care of a patient infected with an airborne pathogen. Use of screening tools and clinical decision-making instruments can aid recognition of airborne infections based on symptoms, risk factors, and objective clinical findings[32–34] and may in turn help expedite initiation of airborne precautions in the ED. Education and access to appropriately fitting PPE are necessary if adherence to these precautions is to be improved.[35] Finally, limited availability of isolation rooms remains a significant barrier for many EDs, particularly when caring for multiple patients requiring airborne precautions.[36,37] The added time required to completely exchange the air in an isolation room after a patient has left imposes further burden on its availability for the next patient.

Droplet transmission occurs via large particles (>5 μm in size) that travel short distances and generally do not loiter in the air for long periods. Seasonal influenza, meningococcal meningitis, and a wide range of other respiratory viral and bacterial infections fall under the umbrella of droplet transmission. Droplet precautions consist of HCP use of a surgical mask whenever working within a 3-foot radius of the infected patient.[31] Isolation is implemented either through physical separation (>3 feet) from other patients and use of a privacy curtain, or placement of the infected patient within a single-occupancy room. Access to PPE, particularly during peak respiratory virus season, and diminished awareness of when to use them can hinder adherence to droplet precautions in the ED.[38] Education and reminders to HCPs, including through the electronic medical record, can improve adherence.[39] Promoting respiratory hygiene through patient education on cough etiquette, hand hygiene, masking and separation of patients with respiratory complaints in the ED waiting room at the time of triage, and optimization of HCP adherence to droplet precautions may also help reduce transmission of respiratory pathogens, but requires significant patient engagement.[40,41]

Microorganisms transmitted through direct contact include health care–associated pathogens, such as methicillin-resistant *Staphylococcus aureus* (MRSA), vancomycin-resistant *Enterococcus*, multidrug-resistant gram-negative bacteria, and *C difficile* as well as viruses associated with respiratory (eg, highly pathogenic influenza, SARS-CoV, MERS-CoV) and gastrointestinal infections (eg, norovirus). Contact precautions entail the use of protective gown and gloves to prevent HCP acquisition of these microorganisms on their hands, skin, or attire and preferably patient isolation within a single-occupancy room.[31] In the absence of a prior history of colonization or infection with a health care–associated pathogen, empiric contact precautions are generally recommended for patients with uncontained wound drainage or diarrhea with stool incontinence. However, significant variations in contact precaution policy exist among EDs.[42] Although several studies have demonstrated transmission of health care–associated pathogens to protective gown and gloves during routine patient care in hospital settings,[43–45] little is known about their risk of transmission within the ED to HCPs or other patients. As the evidence surrounding contact precautions and health care–associated pathogens continues to evolve, modified ED policies more focused on clinical conditions likely to contaminate the health care environment or deemed highly contagious may help facilitate implementation and improve adherence to contact precautions in the ED.[46,47]

ENVIRONMENTAL CLEANING

The ED health care environment itself may serve as a reservoir for microorganisms. Although the ED microbiome has not been well characterized, limited prevalence studies have recovered MRSA from up to 7% of environmental surfaces sampled in 2 urban academic EDs.[48,49] In the absence of hand hygiene, HCP hands that come in direct contact with contaminated environmental surfaces in patient care areas can transfer microorganisms to other patients.[50,51] Evidence also suggests that patients may acquire health care–associated pathogens when hospitalized in a room previously occupied by a patient infected or colonized with that pathogen.[52,53] Effective environmental cleaning therefore plays an essential part in preventing health care–associated infections.

The Healthcare Infection Control Practices Advisory Committee divides environmental surfaces into 2 categories: medical equipment surfaces and housekeeping surfaces (eg, floors, walls, tabletops).[54] Housekeeping surfaces are further separated into "high-touch" surfaces (eg, door handles, bedrails, light switches) and those with minimal hand contact (eg, floors, ceilings).[54] The frequency with which cleaning is necessary for each of these surfaces is determined by the potential for direct patient contact, the degree and frequency of hand contact, and the risk of contamination with body substances or environmental sources of microorganisms (eg, soil, dust, water).[54]

Research has demonstrated that environmental service (EVS) workers frequently fail to decontaminate "high-touch" surfaces, including those in the ED.[55,56] At the authors' facility, overall compliance with environmental cleaning of "high-touch" surfaces in ED treatment rooms was 32% when audited using a fluorescent marker to simulate contamination during routine quality improvement surveys (unpublished data, FOX, 2016). Surfaces with the highest rate of cleaning included the bed mattress (97%) and stretcher rail (72%). Surfaces with the lowest rate of cleaning included the procedure light handle (3%) and wall-mounted thermometer (0%). It is vital that ED, EVS, and infection prevention leaders work together to identify "high-touch" surfaces in treatment areas and prioritize their regular cleaning.[54] Emergency clinicians may perceive the time to correctly clean "high-touch" and other environmental surfaces as a barrier to providing prompt live-saving patient care. Pressure to turn over a treatment room or space expediently may lead to incomplete environmental surface disinfection. ED staff may be unaware of which cleaning and disinfection products are approved and compatible with medical equipment surfaces in the ED or the contact times necessary for these products to work effectively. Likewise, ED staff may be unfamiliar with which surfaces they are responsible for cleaning (eg, sensitive medical equipment) and which surfaces fall under the purview of EVS (eg, stretcher rails, countertops, door handles) at their facility, leading to confusion and poor compliance. In an ED in Brazil, coordinated efforts to educate nursing about environmental cleaning, standardize cleaning procedures and supplies, and conduct compliance audits with feedback increased compliance, but proved difficult to sustain over time.[55] Further studies addressing the dissemination and implementation of environmental cleaning best practices in EDs are greatly needed.

HIGH-LEVEL DISINFECTION AND STERILIZATION OF REUSABLE MEDICAL DEVICES

The Spaulding classification system guides reprocessing decisions for reusable medical devices.[57] Critical devices (eg, surgical instruments) enter sterile tissues or the vasculature and require sterilization. Semicritical devices contact intact mucous membranes or nonintact skin (eg, endoscopes) and necessitate either high-level disinfection or sterilization. High-level disinfection is defined as the complete elimination of microorganisms in or on a device, except for a small number of spores, using a chemical disinfectant (eg, glutaraldehyde, hydrogen peroxide). Noncritical devices (eg, stethoscopes, blood pressure cuffs) that only come in contact with intact skin may undergo low-level disinfection using an Environmental Protection Agency–registered product.

Although the standards and detailed methods by which different levels of reprocessing are achieved are beyond the scope of this review, it is important for emergency clinicians to recognize that several reusable medical devices common to ED clinical practice are considered semicritical, including reusable laryngoscopes, bronchoscopes, and endocavitary ultrasound probes. In one study, bacteria were isolated from 18.2% of laryngoscope blades and 28.2% of laryngoscope handles with knurled surfaces stored in emergency crash carts even before their use.[58] Human papillomavirus has been isolated from transvaginal ultrasound probes using polymerase chain reaction after patient contact, even with use of a probe cover and low-level disinfection.[59] Incorrect reprocessing of these reusable devices after ED use can result in unintentional transmission of pathogens between patients with the potential for subsequent infection.[60]

Most hospitals perform cleaning, disinfection, and sterilization of reusable medical devices in a central processing department to ensure standardization and quality control.[57] However, precleaning of the device at the point of use in the ED is crucial to ensure the completeness of reprocessing. Precleaning reduces the likelihood that patient body fluids and gross debris will adhere to and dry on the device, rendering cleaning and disinfection processes inadequate.[60] Some medical devices, such as endocavitary ultrasound probes, can safely undergo high-level disinfection in the ED using US Food and Drug Administration–approved technologies.[61] It is vital that ED leadership partner with infection prevention to assess reprocessing needs for reusable medical devices, ensure that reprocessing steps assigned to ED staff are performed correctly, and provide rigorous training on reprocessing to ED staff on a recurring basis.[57] Routine audits should be conducted to ensure competency with and adherence to cleaning, disinfection, sterilization, and proper device storage and transport procedures, followed by feedback to leadership.[57]

Considered noncritical devices, external ultrasound probes are widely used in many EDs for a variety of point-of-care diagnostic and therapeutic purposes. Bacterial contamination of ED ultrasound probes is common and can include clinically significant pathogens such as MRSA, particularly after contact with patients with skin and soft tissue infections.[62–65] Low-level disinfection is effective in eliminating bacterial growth. Although many academic EDs mandated probe disinfection after each patient use, standardized protocols emphasizing required contact times for various products were frequently lacking in one study.[66] Infection prevention strategies targeting ED point-of-care ultrasound remain an area in need of further investigation and innovation.[67] Several studies have also demonstrated significant bacterial contamination of stethoscopes, blood pressure cuffs, pulse oximeters, and other devices commonly used in the ED.[68–72] Although bacterial growth on noncritical reusable medical devices has yet to be linked to infection, their routine disinfection promotes cleanliness and professionalism.

DEVICE-ASSOCIATED INFECTIONS
Catheter-Associated Urinary Tract Infection

Although insertion of an indwelling urinary catheter (UC) is often necessary in emergency care, these devices also represent one of the largest preventable causes of health care–associated infection. Urinary tract infections contribute more than 12%

of all health care–associated infections, most of which are attributable to UCs.[73] UCs provide a direct avenue for bacteria to access and infect the bladder. Guidelines from the CDC and the Society for Healthcare Epidemiology of America (SHEA) recommend limiting use of UCs to the management of acute urinary retention and bladder outlet obstruction, accurate measurement of urine output in critically ill patients, clinical situations requiring prolonged immobilization (eg, pelvic fracture, spine trauma), and selected surgical procedures.[74,75] However, UCs are often inserted for inappropriate indications that may increase a patient's risk for a potentially preventable catheter-associated urinary tract infection (CAUTI).

In a study of the National Hospital Ambulatory Medical Survey, UCs were inserted at an annual rate of 2.2 to 3.3 per 100 adult ED visits between 1995 and 2010.[76] Among those admitted to the hospital with UCs inserted in the ED, 64.9% (95% CI 56.9%–72.9%) were considered potentially avoidable. In a teaching hospital in central Italy, 12.5% of all catheterized inpatients diagnosed with a CAUTI had their UC initially inserted in the ED.[77] In one US hospital, 8.7% of patients aged 65 years or older who received a UC in the ED developed a CAUTI.[78] Although CAUTI rates of ED-inserted UCs are not widely known, avoidance of unnecessary UC insertins across health care settings, including the ED, is an important and well-recognized CAUTI prevention strategy.[75]

Several barriers to appropriate UC utilization exist in the ED. Scenario-based assessments found wide variations in practice pattern and what HCPs thought constituted an appropriate clinical scenario for UC use.[79] Focus groups involving ED nurses identified lack of clarity and ownership in determining appropriateness of UC insertion, difficulty negotiating with families when a UC was not indicated, inadequate nurse education and evaluation of competency with UC insertion, and suboptimal collaboration and communication with hospital administration as barriers to safe and appropriate UC use in the ED.[80] In a qualitative study of 6 US EDs considered early adopters of CAUTI prevention strategies, inappropriate reasons for UC insertion, limited physician involvement in UC insertion decisions, patterns of UC overuse, and poor insertion technique were all considered ED-specific risk factors for CAUTI.[81] In a study of UC procedures performed in an academic ED, at least one major breach in aseptic technique (eg, breach or contamination of the sterile field, contamination of the UC during preparation or insertion) was observed in more than half of all insertion attempts, underscoring the need for improved education and auditing of UC insertion practices with HCP feedback.[82]

Emergency clinician engagement in identifying and addressing barriers to appropriate UC utilization can lead to significant reductions in ED UC insertions and is therefore essential to any CAUTI prevention strategy.[83] Multifaceted approaches combining ED HCP education, guidelines, and decision-making tools emphasizing clearly defined criteria for appropriate UC use supported by physician and nurse champions have been shown to be effective in curbing unnecessary ED UC use.[84–86] In a quality improvement initiative spanning 18 US EDs, implementation of a multifaceted intervention led to an overall reduction in UC insertions of more than 30%, with the greatest reductions seen at hospitals with a baseline UC use of ≥5%.[84]

Central-Line Associated Bloodstream Infection

Central venous catheters are often inserted as part of the resuscitation of a critically ill patient or when peripheral venous access is not available. Colonization of a catheter by microorganisms present on the patient's skin or the hands of a HCP at the time of insertion can lead to a central line–associated bloodstream infection (CLABSI). Using administrative and billing data, the CLABSI rate of ED-inserted catheters in an urban academic medical center was found to be 1.93 per 1000 catheter-days (95% CI 0.50–3.36), comparable to that of the intensive care unit (ICU).[87] In a prospective observational study at another urban academic medical center, the ED rate was 2.0 per 1000 catheter-days (95% CI 1.0–3.8), concurrent to an institutional ICU rate of 2.3 per 1000 catheter-days (95% CI 1.9–2.7).[88]

Tremendous strides have been made in reducing CLABSI rates through the implementation of insertion and maintenance bundles. Guidelines from multiple organizations support a systems-based approach comprising education, procedure checklists, a standardized catheter cart or kit, hand hygiene, use of maximal sterile barrier precautions (sterile surgical gown, sterile gloves, mask, cap, and large sterile drape), avoidance of femoral catheter insertion given its high rate of infection, chlorhexidine-alcohol skin antisepsis, and use of ultrasound guidance for internal jugular catheter insertion.[89,90] Successful implementation of CLABSI prevention bundles in EDs requires staff engagement, clinician champion recruitment, clear delineation of staff responsibilities, workflow redesign, observer empowerment to ensure compliance, and feedback to HCPs on bundle compliance and CLABSI rates associated with ED-inserted catheters.[91]

Ventilator-Associated Pneumonia

Emergency airway management in the critically ill patient frequently calls for endotracheal intubation and the use of mechanical ventilation. Ventilator-associated pneumonia (VAP) arises when bacteria present within environmental reservoirs (eg, a contaminated respiratory circuit) or the patient's oropharynx or gastrointestinal tract gain entry to the lungs through microaspiration, with subsequent infection. VAP is defined as the diagnosis of a new pneumonia after $\geq$48 hours of mechanical ventilation, not present at the time of intubation. At least half of all cases of VAP are thought to be preventable.[92] Endotracheal intubation in the ED and prolonged ED stay have been associated with higher VAP rates when compared with the ICU.[93–98]

SHEA guidelines outline several basic VAP prevention strategies supported by good evidence and that pose little risk of harm to the patient, including elevating the head of the bed to 30° to 45°, minimizing sedation whenever possible, subglottic suctioning, and changing visibly soiled or malfunctioning ventilator circuits.[99] Avoidance of intubation with the use of noninvasive positive pressure ventilation in clinically appropriate situations may also be considered. In one academic ED, a VAP prevention bundle comprising several of these interventions along with other common and more labor-intensive ICU practices (eg, oral care, sedation titration, and vacations) led to a significant reduction in VAP rates, even after accounting for complexities in establishing true rates.[100] Nursing engagement is integral to the successful implementation of these bundles.[100,101]

SUMMARY

Infection prevention is part of our basic responsibility to patients as clinicians to *first, do no harm*. Although EDs pose unique operational and environmental challenges not often encountered in traditional inpatient or ambulatory settings, a growing body of evidence demonstrates that effective and sustainable infection prevention in emergency care settings is achievable, although not without cost or commitment, or need for future research and innovation.[2,3,102] Hand hygiene remains the bedrock of preventing the spread of infectious diseases. Transmission-based precautions, environmental cleaning, and appropriate reprocessing of reusable medical devices each provide additional levels of protection to patients and HCPs alike. Health care–associated infections are preventable in many instances but require systems-based approaches.

As frontline HCPs' on the leading edge of health care, emergency clinicians can and already play an invaluable role in infection prevention.

REFERENCES

1. Moore BJSC, Owens PL. Trends in emergency department visits, 2006-2014. HCUP statistical brief #227. Rockville (MD): Agency for Healthcare Research and Quality; 2017.
2. Carter EJ, Pouch SM, Larson EL. Common infection control practices in the emergency department: a literature review. Am J Infect Control 2014;42:957–62.
3. Liang SY, Theodoro DL, Schuur JD, et al. Infection prevention in the emergency department. Ann Emerg Med 2014;64:299–313.
4. Boyce JM, Pittet D, Healthcare Infection Control Practices Advisory Committee, et al. Guideline for Hand Hygiene in Health-Care Settings. Recommendations of the Healthcare Infection Control Practices Advisory Committee and the HIC-PAC/SHEA/APIC/IDSA Hand Hygiene Task Force. Society for Healthcare Epidemiology of America/Association for Professionals in Infection Control/Infectious Diseases Society of America. MMWR Recomm Rep 2002;51:1–45 [quiz: CE1–4].
5. Pittet D, Allegranzi B, Sax H, et al. Evidence-based model for hand transmission during patient care and the role of improved practices. Lancet Infect Dis 2006;6: 641–52.
6. World Health Organization. WHO guidelines on hand hygiene in health care. Geneva (Switzerland): World Health Organization; 2009.
7. Rumgay S, Macdonald S, Robertson CE. Hand-washing patterns and infection control in the accident and emergency department. Arch Emerg Med 1984;1: 157–9.
8. Meengs MR, Giles BK, Chisholm CD, et al. Hand washing frequency in an emergency department. Ann Emerg Med 1994;23:1307–12.
9. Dorsey ST, Cydulka RK, Emerman CL. Is handwashing teachable?: failure to improve handwashing behavior in an urban emergency department. Acad Emerg Med 1996;3:360–5.
10. Al-Damouk M, Pudney E, Bleetman A. Hand hygiene and aseptic technique in the emergency department. J Hosp Infect 2004;56:137–41.
11. Pittet D, Simon A, Hugonnet S, et al. Hand hygiene among physicians: performance, beliefs, and perceptions. Ann Intern Med 2004;141:1–8.
12. Saint S, Bartoloni A, Virgili G, et al. Marked variability in adherence to hand hygiene: a 5-unit observational study in Tuscany. Am J Infect Control 2009;37: 306–10.
13. Venkatesh AK, Pallin DJ, Kayden S, et al. Predictors of hand hygiene in the emergency department. Infect Control Hosp Epidemiol 2011;32:1120–3.
14. Sánchez-Payá J, Hernández-García I, Camargo Ángeles R, et al. Hand hygiene in the emergency department: degree of compliance, predictors and change over time. Emergencias 2012;24:107–12.
15. Scheithauer S, Kamerseder V, Petersen P, et al. Improving hand hygiene compliance in the emergency department: getting to the point. BMC Infect Dis 2013; 13:367.
16. Muller MP, Carter E, Siddiqui N, et al. Hand hygiene compliance in an emergency department: the effect of crowding. Acad Emerg Med 2015;22:1218–21.
17. Yanagizawa-Drott L, Kurland L, Schuur JD. Infection prevention practices in Swedish emergency departments: results from a cross-sectional survey. Eur J Emerg Med 2015;22:338–42.

18. Arntz PR, Hopman J, Nillesen M, et al. Effectiveness of a multimodal hand hygiene improvement strategy in the emergency department. Am J Infect Control 2016;44:1203–7.
19. Carter EJ, Wyer P, Giglio J, et al. Environmental factors and their association with emergency department hand hygiene compliance: an observational study. BMJ Qual Saf 2016;25:372–8.
20. Haac B, Rock C, Harris AD, et al. Hand hygiene compliance in the setting of trauma resuscitation. Injury 2017;48:165–70.
21. Zottele C, Magnago T, Dullius A, et al. Hand hygiene compliance of healthcare professionals in an emergency department. Rev Esc Enferm USP 2017;51: e03242.
22. Jeanes A, Coen PG, Drey NS, et al. The development of hand hygiene compliance imperatives in an emergency department. Am J Infect Control 2018;46: 441–7.
23. Centers for Disease Control and Prevention. Recommendations for prevention of HIV transmission in health-care settings. MMWR Morb Mortal Wkly Rep 1987; 36(Suppl 2):1S–18S.
24. Centers for Disease Control and Prevention. Guidelines for prevention of transmission of human immunodeficiency virus and hepatitis B virus to health-care and public-safety workers. MMWR Morb Mortal Wkly Rep 1989;38(Suppl 6): 1–37.
25. Wiles LL, Roberts C, Schmidt K. Keep it clean: a visual approach to reinforce hand hygiene compliance in the emergency department. J Emerg Nurs 2015; 41:119–24.
26. Larson EL, Albrecht S, O'Keefe M. Hand hygiene behavior in a pediatric emergency department and a pediatric intensive care unit: comparison of use of 2 dispenser systems. Am J Crit Care 2005;14:304–11 [quiz: 12].
27. Haas JP, Larson EL. Impact of wearable alcohol gel dispensers on hand hygiene in an emergency department. Acad Emerg Med 2008;15:393–6.
28. Stackelroth J, Sinnott M, Shaban RZ. Hesitation and error: does product placement in an emergency department influence hand hygiene performance? Am J Infect Control 2015;43:913–6.
29. Saint S, Conti A, Bartoloni A, et al. Improving healthcare worker hand hygiene adherence before patient contact: a before-and-after five-unit multimodal intervention in Tuscany. Qual Saf Health Care 2009;18:429–33.
30. di Martino P, Ban KM, Bartoloni A, et al. Assessing the sustainability of hand hygiene adherence prior to patient contact in the emergency department: a 1-year postintervention evaluation. Am J Infect Control 2011;39:14–8.
31. Siegel JD, Rhinehart E, Jackson M, et al, Health Care Infection Control Practices Advisory Committee. 2007 guideline for isolation precautions: preventing transmission of infectious agents in health care settings. Am J Infect Control 2007;35: S65–164.
32. Solari L, Acuna-Villaorduna C, Soto A, et al. A clinical prediction rule for pulmonary tuberculosis in emergency departments. Int J Tuberc Lung Dis 2008;12: 619–24.
33. Moran GJ, Barrett TW, Mower WR, et al. Decision instrument for the isolation of pneumonia patients with suspected pulmonary tuberculosis admitted through US emergency departments. Ann Emerg Med 2009;53:625–32.
34. Koenig KL, Alassaf W, Burns MJ. Identify-isolate-inform: a tool for initial detection and management of measles patients in the emergency department. West J Emerg Med 2015;16:212–9.

35. Asimos AW, Kaufman JS, Lee CH, et al. Tuberculosis exposure risk in emergency medicine residents. Acad Emerg Med 1999;6:1044–9.
36. Fusco FM, Schilling S, De Iaco G, et al. Infection control management of patients with suspected highly infectious diseases in emergency departments: data from a survey in 41 facilities in 14 European countries. BMC Infect Dis 2012;12:27.
37. Garner K, Wheeler JG, Yamauchi T. Airborne pathogen isolation capability in emergency departments of US children's hospitals. Am J Infect Control 2016; 44:1747–9.
38. Martel J, Bui-Xuan EF, Carreau AM, et al. Respiratory hygiene in emergency departments: compliance, beliefs, and perceptions. Am J Infect Control 2013;41: 14–8.
39. May L, Lung D, Harter K. An intervention to improve compliance with transmission precautions for influenza in the emergency department: successes and challenges. J Emerg Med 2012;42:79–85.
40. Rothman RE, Irvin CB, Moran GJ, et al. Respiratory hygiene in the emergency department. Ann Emerg Med 2006;48:570–82.
41. Longtin Y, Akakpo C, Rutschmann OT, et al. Evaluation of patients' mask use after the implementation of cough etiquette in the emergency department. Infect Control Hosp Epidemiol 2009;30:904–8.
42. Pallin DJ, Camargo CA Jr, Yokoe DS, et al. Variability of contact precaution policies in US emergency departments. Infect Control Hosp Epidemiol 2014;35:310–2.
43. Snyder GM, Thom KA, Furuno JP, et al. Detection of methicillin-resistant Staphylococcus aureus and vancomycin-resistant enterococci on the gowns and gloves of healthcare workers. Infect Control Hosp Epidemiol 2008;29:583–9.
44. Hayden MK, Blom DW, Lyle EA, et al. Risk of hand or glove contamination after contact with patients colonized with vancomycin-resistant enterococcus or the colonized patients' environment. Infect Control Hosp Epidemiol 2008;29:149–54.
45. Morgan DJ, Liang SY, Smith CL, et al. Frequent multidrug-resistant Acinetobacter baumannii contamination of gloves, gowns, and hands of healthcare workers. Infect Control Hosp Epidemiol 2010;31:716–21.
46. Kotkowski K, Ellison RT 3rd, Barysauskas C, et al. Association of hospital contact precaution policies with emergency department admission time. J Hosp Infect 2017;96:244–9.
47. Skyum F, Andersen V, Chen M, et al. Infectious gastroenteritis and the need for strict contact precaution procedures in adults presenting to the emergency department: a Danish register-based study. J Hosp Infect 2018;98:391–7.
48. Otter JA, Passaretti CL, French GL, et al. Low frequency of environmental contamination with methicillin-resistant Staphylococcus aureus in an inner city emergency department and a human immunodeficiency virus outpatient clinic. Am J Infect Control 2011;39:151–3.
49. Kei J, Richards JR. The prevalence of methicillin-resistant staphylococcus aureus on inanimate objects in an urban emergency department. J Emerg Med 2011;41:124–7.
50. Weber DJ, Rutala WA, Miller MB, et al. Role of hospital surfaces in the transmission of emerging health care-associated pathogens: norovirus, Clostridium difficile, and Acinetobacter species. Am J Infect Control 2010;38:S25–33.
51. Otter JA, Yezli S, Salkeld JA, et al. Evidence that contaminated surfaces contribute to the transmission of hospital pathogens and an overview of strategies to address contaminated surfaces in hospital settings. Am J Infect Control 2013;41:S6–11.

52. Cohen B, Liu J, Cohen AR, et al. Association between healthcare-associated infection and exposure to hospital roommates and previous bed occupants with the same organism. Infect Control Hosp Epidemiol 2018;39:541–6.

53. Cohen B, Cohen CC, Loyland B, et al. Transmission of health care-associated infections from roommates and prior room occupants: a systematic review. Clin Epidemiol 2017;9:297–310.

54. Sehulster LM, Chinn RYW, Arduino MJ, et al. Guidelines for environmental infection control in health-care facilities. Recommendations from Centers for Disease Control and Prevention and the Healthcare Infection Control Practices Advisory Committee (HICPAC). MMWR Recomm Rep 2003;52(RR-10):1–42.

55. Frota OP, Ferreira AM, Koch R, et al. Surface cleaning effectiveness in a walk-in emergency care unit: influence of a multifaceted intervention. Am J Infect Control 2016;44:1572–7.

56. Carling PC, Parry MF, Von Beheren SM, Healthcare Environmental Hygiene Study Group. Identifying opportunities to enhance environmental cleaning in 23 acute care hospitals. Infect Control Hosp Epidemiol 2008;29:1–7.

57. Rutala WA, Weber DJ, Healthcare Infection Control Practices Advisory Committee (HICPAC). Guideline for disinfection and sterilization in healthcare facilities, 2008. Available from: https://www.cdc.gov/infectioncontrol/pdf/guidelines/disinfection-guidelines.pdf. Accessed May 29, 2018.

58. Choi JH, Cho YS, Lee JW, et al. Bacterial contamination and disinfection status of laryngoscopes stored in emergency crash carts. J Prev Med Public Health 2017;50:158–64.

59. Ma ST, Yeung AC, Chan PK, et al. Transvaginal ultrasound probe contamination by the human papillomavirus in the emergency department. Emerg Med J 2013. https://doi.org/10.1136/emermed-2012-201407.

60. Rutala WA, Weber DJ. Disinfection, sterilization, and antisepsis: an overview. Am J Infect Control 2016;44:e1–6.

61. Abramowicz JS, Evans DH, Fowlkes JB, et al, WFUMB Safety Committee. Guidelines for cleaning transvaginal ultrasound transducers between patients. Ultrasound Med Biol 2017;43:1076–9.

62. Frazee BW, Fahimi J, Lambert L, et al. Emergency department ultrasonographic probe contamination and experimental model of probe disinfection. Ann Emerg Med 2011;58:56–63.

63. Rodriguez G, Quan D. Bacterial growth on ED ultrasound machines. Am J Emerg Med 2011;29:816–7.

64. Sanz GE, Theoret J, Liao MM, et al. Bacterial contamination and cleanliness of emergency department ultrasound probes. CJEM 2011;13:384–9.

65. Keys M, Sim BZ, Thom O, et al. Efforts to attenuate the spread of infection (EASI): a prospective, observational multicentre survey of ultrasound equipment in Australian emergency departments and intensive care units. Crit Care Resusc 2015;17:43–6.

66. Hoyer R, Adhikari S, Amini R. Ultrasound transducer disinfection in emergency medicine practice. Antimicrob Resist Infect Control 2016;5:12.

67. Shokoohi H, Armstrong P, Tansek R. Emergency department ultrasound probe infection control: challenges and solutions. Open Access Emerg Med 2015;7:1–9.

68. Jones JS, Hoerle D, Riekse R. Stethoscopes: a potential vector of infection? Ann Emerg Med 1995;26:296–9.

69. Nunez S, Moreno A, Green K, et al. The stethoscope in the emergency department: a vector of infection? Epidemiol Infect 2000;124:233–7.

70. Davis C. Blood pressure cuffs and pulse oximeter sensors: a potential source of cross-contamination. Australas Emerg Nurs J 2009;12:104–9.

71. Tang PH, Worster A, Srigley JA, et al. Examination of staphylococcal stethoscope contamination in the emergency department (pilot) study (EXSSCITED pilot study). CJEM 2011;13:239–44.

72. Fafliora E, Bampalis VG, Lazarou N, et al. Bacterial contamination of medical devices in a Greek emergency department: impact of physicians' cleaning habits. Am J Infect Control 2014;42:807–9.

73. Magill SS, Edwards JR, Bamberg W, et al. Multistate point-prevalence survey of health care-associated infections. N Engl J Med 2014;370:1198–208.

74. Gould CV, Umscheid CA, Agarwal RK, et al, Healthcare Infection Control Practices Advisory Committee. Guideline for prevention of catheter-associated urinary tract infections 2009. Infect Control Hosp Epidemiol 2010;31:319–26.

75. Lo E, Nicolle LE, Coffin SE, et al. Strategies to prevent catheter-associated urinary tract infections in acute care hospitals: 2014 update. Infect Control Hosp Epidemiol 2014;35:464–79.

76. Schuur JD, Chambers JG, Hou PC. Urinary catheter use and appropriateness in U.S. emergency departments, 1995-2010. Acad Emerg Med 2014;21:292–300.

77. Barbadoro P, Labricciosa FM, Recanatini C, et al. Catheter-associated urinary tract infection: role of the setting of catheter insertion. Am J Infect Control 2015;43:707–10.

78. Hazelett SE, Tsai M, Gareri M, et al. The association between indwelling urinary catheter use in the elderly and urinary tract infection in acute care. BMC Geriatr 2006;6:15.

79. Viswanathan K, Rosen T, Mulcare MR, et al. Emergency department placement and management of indwelling urinary catheters in older adults: knowledge, attitudes, and practice. J Emerg Nurs 2015;41:414–22.

80. Mizerek E, Wolf L. To foley or not to foley: emergency nurses' perceptions of clinical decision making in the use of urinary catheters in the emergency department. J Emerg Nurs 2015;41:329–34.

81. Carter EJ, Pallin DJ, Mandel L, et al. Emergency department catheter-associated urinary tract infection prevention: multisite qualitative study of perceived risks and implemented strategies. Infect Control Hosp Epidemiol 2016;37:156–62.

82. Manojlovich M, Saint S, Meddings J, et al. Indwelling urinary catheter insertion practices in the emergency department: an observational study. Infect Control Hosp Epidemiol 2016;37:117–9.

83. Scott RA, Oman KS, Makic MB, et al. Reducing indwelling urinary catheter use in the emergency department: a successful quality-improvement initiative. J Emerg Nurs 2014;40:237–44 [quiz: 93].

84. Fakih MG, Heavens M, Grotemeyer J, et al. Avoiding potential harm by improving appropriateness of urinary catheter use in 18 emergency departments. Ann Emerg Med 2014;63:761–8.e1.

85. Mulcare MR, Rosen T, Clark S, et al. A novel clinical protocol for placement and management of indwelling urinary catheters in older adults in the emergency department. Acad Emerg Med 2015;22:1056–66.

86. Saint S, Gaies E, Fowler KE, et al. Introducing a catheter-associated urinary tract infection (CAUTI) prevention guide to patient safety (GPS). Am J Infect Control 2014;42:548–50.

87. LeMaster CH, Schuur JD, Pandya D, et al. Infection and natural history of emergency department-placed central venous catheters. Ann Emerg Med 2010;56:492–7.

88. Theodoro D, Olsen MA, Warren DK, et al. Emergency department central line-associated bloodstream infections (CLABSI) incidence in the era of prevention practices. Acad Emerg Med 2015;22:1048–55.

89. O'Grady NP, Alexander M, Burns LA, et al. Guidelines for the prevention of intravascular catheter-related infections. Clin Infect Dis 2011;52:e162–93.

90. Marschall J, Mermel LA, Fakih M, et al. Strategies to prevent central line-associated bloodstream infections in acute care hospitals: 2014 update. Infect Control Hosp Epidemiol 2014;35:753–71.

91. Lemaster CH, Hoffart N, Chafe T, et al. Implementing the central venous catheter infection prevention bundle in the emergency department: experiences among early adopters. Ann Emerg Med 2014. https://doi.org/10.1016/j.annemergmed.2013.09.006.

92. Umscheid CA, Mitchell MD, Doshi JA, et al. Estimating the proportion of healthcare-associated infections that are reasonably preventable and the related mortality and costs. Infect Control Hosp Epidemiol 2011;32:101–14.

93. Eckert MJ, Davis KA, Reed RL 2nd, et al. Urgent airways after trauma: who gets pneumonia? J Trauma 2004;57:750–5.

94. Eckert MJ, Davis KA, Reed RL 2nd, et al. Ventilator-associated pneumonia, like real estate: location really matters. J Trauma 2006;60:104–10 [discussion: 10].

95. Eckert MJ, Wade TE, Davis KA, et al. Ventilator-associated pneumonia after combined burn and trauma is caused by associated injuries and not the burn wound. J Burn Care Res 2006;27:457–62.

96. Carr BG, Kaye AJ, Wiebe DJ, et al. Emergency department length of stay: a major risk factor for pneumonia in intubated blunt trauma patients. J Trauma 2007;63:9–12.

97. Evans HL, Warner K, Bulger EM, et al. Pre-hospital intubation factors and pneumonia in trauma patients. Surg Infect (Larchmt) 2011;12:339–44.

98. Decelle L, Thys F, Zech F, et al. Ventilation-associated pneumonia after intubation in the prehospital or the emergency unit. Eur J Emerg Med 2013;20:61–3.

99. Klompas M, Branson R, Eichenwald EC, et al. Strategies to prevent ventilator-associated pneumonia in acute care hospitals: 2014 update. Infect Control Hosp Epidemiol 2014;35:915–36.

100. DeLuca LA Jr, Walsh P, Davidson DD Jr, et al. Impact and feasibility of an emergency department-based ventilator-associated pneumonia bundle for patients intubated in an academic emergency department. Am J Infect Control 2017;45:151–7.

101. Sinuff T, Muscedere J, Cook DJ, et al. Implementation of clinical practice guidelines for ventilator-associated pneumonia: a multicenter prospective study. Crit Care Med 2013;41:15–23.

102. Zimmerman PA, Mason M, Elder E. A healthy degree of suspicion: a discussion of the implementation of transmission based precautions in the emergency department. Australas Emerg Nurs J 2016;19:149–52.

UNITED STATES POSTAL SERVICE ® Statement of Ownership, Management, and Circulation (All Periodicals Publications Except Requester Publications)

1. Publication Title	2. Publication Number	3. Filing Date
EMERGENCY MEDICINE CLINICS OF NORTH AMERICA	000 – 714	9/18/2018

4. Issue Frequency	5. Number of Issues Published Annually	6. Annual Subscription Price
FEB, MAY, AUG, NOV	4	$336.00

7. Complete Mailing Address of Known Office of Publication (Not printer) (Street, city, county, state, and ZIP+4®)

ELSEVIER INC.
230 Park Avenue, Suite 800
New York, NY 10169

Contact Person
STEPHEN R. BUSHING

Telephone (Include area code)
215-239-3688

8. Complete Mailing Address of Headquarters or General Business Office of Publisher (Not printer)

ELSEVIER INC.
230 Park Avenue, Suite 800
New York, NY 10169

9. Full Names and Complete Mailing Addresses of Publisher, Editor, and Managing Editor (Do not leave blank)

Publisher (Name and complete mailing address)

TAYLOR E. BALL, ELSEVIER INC.
1600 JOHN F KENNEDY BLVD. SUITE 1800
PHILADELPHIA, PA 19103-2899

Editor (Name and complete mailing address)

PATRICK MANLEY, ELSEVIER INC.
1600 JOHN F KENNEDY BLVD. SUITE 1800
PHILADELPHIA, PA 19103-2899

Managing Editor (Name and complete mailing address)

PATRICK MANLEY, ELSEVIER INC.
1600 JOHN F KENNEDY BLVD. SUITE 1800
PHILADELPHIA, PA 19103-2899

10. Owner (Do not leave blank. If the publication is owned by a corporation, give the name and address of the corporation immediately followed by the names and addresses of all stockholders owning or holding 1 percent or more of the total amount of stock. If not owned by a corporation, give the names and addresses of the individual owners. If owned by a partnership or other unincorporated firm, give its name and address as well as those of each individual owner. If the publication is published by a nonprofit organization, give its name and address.)

Full Name	Complete Mailing Address
WHOLLY OWNED SUBSIDIARY OF REED/ELSEVIER, US HOLDINGS	1600 JOHN F KENNEDY BLVD. SUITE 1800 PHILADELPHIA, PA 19103-2899

11. Known Bondholders, Mortgagees, and Other Security Holders Owning or Holding 1 Percent or More of Total Amount of Bonds, Mortgages, or Other Securities. If none, check box   ☐ None

Full Name	Complete Mailing Address
N/A	

12. Tax Status (For completion by nonprofit organizations authorized to mail at nonprofit rates) (Check one)
The purpose, function, and nonprofit status of this organization and the exempt status for federal income tax purposes:
☒ Has Not Changed During Preceding 12 Months
☐ Has Changed During Preceding 12 Months (Publisher must submit explanation of change with this statement)

PS Form 3526, July 2014 [Page 1 of 4 (see instructions page 4)] PSN 7530-01-000-9631   PRIVACY NOTICE: See our privacy policy on www.usps.com.

---

13. Publication Title			14. Issue Date for Circulation Data Below
EMERGENCY MEDICINE CLINICS OF NORTH AMERICA			MAY 2018

15. Extent and Nature of Circulation			Average No. Copies Each Issue During Preceding 12 Months	No. Copies of Single Issue Published Nearest to Filing Date
a. Total Number of Copies (Net press run)			180	345
b. Paid Circulation (By Mail and Outside the Mail)	(1)	Mailed Outside-County Paid Subscriptions Stated on PS Form 3541 (Include paid distribution above nominal rate, advertiser's proof copies, and exchange copies)	106	194
	(2)	Mailed In-County Paid Subscriptions Stated on PS Form 3541 (Include paid distribution above nominal rate, advertiser's proof copies, and exchange copies)	0	0
	(3)	Paid Distribution Outside the Mails Including Sales Through Dealers and Carriers, Street Vendors, Counter Sales, and Other Paid Distribution Outside USPS®	35	66
	(4)	Paid Distribution by Other Classes of Mail Through the USPS (e.g., First-Class Mail®)	0	0
c. Total Paid Distribution (Sum of 15b (1), (2), (3), and (4))			141	260
d. Free or Nominal Rate Distribution (By Mail and Outside the Mail)	(1)	Free or Nominal Rate Outside-County Copies included on PS Form 3541	30	68
	(2)	Free or Nominal Rate In-County Copies Included on PS Form 3541	0	0
	(3)	Free or Nominal Rate Copies Mailed at Other Classes Through the USPS (e.g., First-Class Mail)	0	0
	(4)	Free or Nominal Rate Distribution Outside the Mail (Carriers or other means)	30	68
e. Total Free or Nominal Rate Distribution (Sum of 15d (1), (2), (3) and (4))			30	68
f. Total Distribution (Sum of 15c and 15e)			171	328
g. Copies not Distributed (See Instructions to Publishers #4 (page #3))			9	17
h. Total (Sum of 15f and g)			180	345
i. Percent Paid (15c divided by 15f times 100)			82.46%	79.27%

* If you are claiming electronic copies, go to line 16 on page 3. If you are not claiming electronic copies, skip to line 17 on page 3.

16. Electronic Copy Circulation	Average No. Copies Each Issue During Preceding 12 Months	No. Copies of Single Issue Published Nearest to Filing Date
a. Paid Electronic Copies	0	0
b. Total Paid Print Copies (Line 15c) + Paid Electronic Copies (Line 16a)	141	260
c. Total Print Distribution (Line 15f) + Paid Electronic Copies (Line 16a)	171	328
d. Percent Paid (Both Print & Electronic Copies) (16b divided by 16c × 100)	82.46%	79.27%

☒ I certify that 50% of all my distributed copies (electronic and print) are paid above a nominal price.

17. Publication of Statement of Ownership
☒ If the publication is a general publication, publication of this statement is required. Will be printed
in the NOVEMBER 2018 issue of this publication.   ☐ Publication not required.

18. Signature and Title of Editor, Publisher, Business Manager, or Owner		Date
STEPHEN R. BUSHING – INVENTORY DISTRIBUTION CONTROL MANAGER		9/18/2018

I certify that all information furnished on this form is true and complete. I understand that anyone who furnishes false or misleading information on this form or who omits material or information requested on the form may be subject to criminal sanctions (including fines and imprisonment) and/or civil sanctions (including civil penalties).

PS Form 3526, July 2014 (Page 2 of 4)   PRIVACY NOTICE: See our privacy policy on www.usps.com.

Printed and bound by CPI Group (UK) Ltd, Croydon, CR0 4YY

08/05/2025

01864737-0001